Shoulder Arthroplasty

Louis U. Bigliani, MD

Frank E. Stinchfield Professor and Chairman, Department of Orthopaedic Surgery, Columbia University Medical Center, New York, New York, USA

Evan L. Flatow, MD

Lasker Professor of Orthopaedic Surgery, Chief of Shoulder Surgery, Department of Orthopaedic Surgery, Mount Sinai Medical Center, Mount Sinai School of Medicine, New York, New York, USA

Editors

Shoulder Arthroplasty

With 191 Illustrations, 30 in Full Color

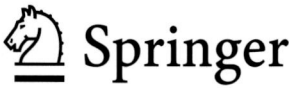 Springer

Louis U. Bigliani, MD
Frank E. Stinchfield Professor
    and
Chairman
Department of Orthopaedic Surgery
Columbia University Medical Center
New York, NY 10032
USA

Evan L. Flatow, MD
Lasker Professor of
    Orthopaedic Surgery
Chief of Shoulder Surgery
Department of Orthopaedic Surgery
Mount Sinai Medical Center
Mount Sinai School of Medicine
New York, NY 10029
USA

ISBN 0-387-22336-3   Printed on acid-free paper.

Printed in China   (BS/EVB)

9 8 7 6 5 4 3 2 1   SPIN 10938416

springeronline.com

To our families
for all of their support and understanding

Preface

The indications and use of shoulder arthroplasty have dramatically increased over the last decade, and this trend will continue in the future. The average age of our population is increasing, yet there is a strong desire to remain active and viable. The majority of people will not accept limitation of a joint function that compromises their life styles if a reasonable surgical solution is available.

Our knowledge of disease processes has broadened and improved our understanding about how best to manage these problems clinically. Technology and innovation have provided us with options that were not possible before. However, a successful shoulder arthroplasty depends not only on knowledge and modern technology but also on sound clinical judgment, accurate surgical technique, and appropriate postoperative rehabilitation.

This book provides a comprehensive approach to dealing with the most common indications for shoulder arthroplasty. In addition, it provides insight into some of the more complex problems. Detailed information concerning preoperative evaluation, approaches, technology, surgical technique, and postoperative therapy will allow the surgeon to make decisions that will help his patient remain active.

We thank the contributing authors for their work and commitment to this project. We appreciate the time they took from their practices and more importantly their families to complete this volume and provide an extraordinary text.

Louis U. Bigliani, MD
Evan L. Flatow, MD

Contents

Contents

Contributors

Christopher S. Ahmad, MD
Assistant Professor, Department of Orthopaedic Surgery, Columbia University Medical Center, New York, NY 10032, USA

Steven Aviles, MD
Third-Year Resident, Center for Shoulder, Elbow and Sports Medicine, Columbia University Medical Center, New York, NY 10032, USA

John Basti, PT
Lecturer, Department of Orthopaedics, Columbia University, New York, NY 10032, USA

Louis U. Bigliani, MD
Frank E. Stinchfield Professor and Chairman, Department of Orthopaedic Surgery, Columbia University Medical Center, New York, NY 10032, USA

Theodore A. Blaine, MD
Assistant Professor, Department of Orthopaedic Surgery; Associate Director, The Shoulder Service, New York Orthopaedic Hospital, Columbia University Medical Center, New York, NY 10032, USA

Evan L. Flatow, MD
Lasker Professor of Orthopaedic Surgery, Chief of Shoulder Surgery, Department of Orthopaedic Surgery, Mount Sinai Medical Center, Mount Sinai School of Medicine, New York, NY 10029, USA

Ian G. Kelly, BSc, MB, ChB, MD, FRCS(Edin), FRCPS(Glas)
Consultant Orthopaedic Surgeon, Honorary Clinical Senior Lecturer, University of Glasgow; Royal Infirmary, Glasgow G4 0SF, Scotland

Edward W. Lee, MD
Clinical Shoulder Fellow, Department of Orthopaedic Surgery, Mount Sinai School of Medicine, New York, NY 10029, USA

William N. Levine, MD
Assistant Professor, Department of Orthopaedic Surgery, Columbia University Medical Center, New York, NY 10032, USA

Angus D. MacLean, MB, ChB, AFRCS(Edin), MRCS(Glas)
Specialist Registrar, Orthopaedic Surgery, Royal Infirmary, Glasgow G4 0SF, Scotland

Gregory P. Nicholson, MD
Assistant Professor, Department of Orthopaedic Surgery, Rush University Medical Center; Midwest Orthopaedics at Rush, Chicago, IL 60612, USA

Kevin J. Setter, MD
Postdoctoral Clinical Fellow, Department of Orthopaedic Surgery, Columbia University Medical Center, New York, NY 10032, USA

Ilya Voloshin, MD
Fellow, The Shoulder Service, New York Orthopaedic Hospital, Columbia-Presbyterian Medical Center, New York, NY 10032, USA

Chapter 1

Surgical Approaches and Preoperative Evaluation

Kevin J. Setter, Ilya Voloshin, and Theodore A. Blaine

The majority of patients with shoulder arthritis present with pain and limited range of motion. Generally, they have failed a course of rest, NSAIDs, and physical therapy. For patients who are about to undergo total shoulder arthroplasty (TSA), certain facts need to be obtained from the history and physical examination that help with preoperative planning, as well as with intraoperative and postoperative decision making. Preoperative planning is essential when considering TSA. Preoperative templating can help with proper component sizing and positioning. Diligent preoperative assessment of the glenoid is critical to determine whether a glenoid could be placed or if any special considerations are necessary for proper placement. Proper technique during the approach during TSA aids in exposure, proper positioning of components, and appropriate soft tissue balancing.

Etiology

The most common pathologic condition leading to TSA is osteoarthritis of the glenohumeral joint. It accounts for more than 60% of all total shoulder arthroplasties performed [1]. Patients with osteoarthritis generally present with restricted range of motion that may limit vocational, recreational, or daily activities. Patients usually present over the age of 50. Although arthritis is a degenerative process, the inflammatory component of the disease often responds to nonsteroidal anti-inflammatory medication. Common radiographic finding associated with osteoarthritis include marginal osteophytes, subchondral sclerosis, subchondral cysts, and joint space narrowing. Full-thickness rotator cuff tears in this subgroup of patients are rare, occurring in only 5% to 10% [2–4].

Rheumatoid arthritis (RA) and other inflammatory conditions account for approximately 30% of all TSA [1]. Rheumatoid arthritis is characterized by symmetric and often medial wear, periarticular erosions, and osteopenia. The osteopenia may be secondary to the inflam-

1

matory disease itself or to medications associated with the disease. Most often these patients have been seen by an orthopedic surgeon for other issues related to their disease; the shoulder is rarely the first or only joint affected. Since the inflammatory process affects soft tissue as well as bone, the incidence of full rotator cuff tears in patients undergoing TSA for RA is significantly higher, occurring in up to 50%, with the average being approximately 25% [2–7].

Avascular necrosis account for approximately 3% of patients treated with TSA. The most common causes include corticosteroid use, alcohol abuse, sickle cell anemia, and idiopathic causes. One study has shown a 71% rate of progression of the disease to severe and disabling pain [8]. More than half of the patients who required surgical treatment for pain control required TSA. Cruess modified the Ficat staging system for osteonecrosis of the hip to apply to the shoulder [9–11]: stage I, no radiographic evidence of disease except by MRI; stage II, radiographic evidence of humeral head involvement, but no collapse; stage III, subchondral bone collapse or fracture (crescent sign); stage IV, humeral head collapse, no glenoid involvement; and stage V, humeral head and glenoid involvement. Shoulder arthroplasty is indicated for advanced stages of disease (stages III, IV, V) with successful results in the majority of patients [12]. In a relatively recent series in which shoulder arthroplasty was performed in 37 patients with advanced avascular necrosis, 89% of patients had satisfactory outcomes [13].

Capsulorraphy arthritis results from excessive anterior tightening of the soft tissues causing altered contact area and stresses on the glenoid [14]. Bigliani et al. have shown that anterior tightening increases contact stresses posteriorly on the glenoid [15]. This increased posterior stress can lead to erosion of the posterior glenoid and fixed subluxation of the humeral head. Preoperative evaluation includes axillary lateral radiographs or CT scan to assess the glenoid anatomy. In additional, it should be anticipated that extensive anterior soft tissue releases will be necessary at the time of surgery.

In 1983, Neer et al. described rotator cuff arthropathy (CTA) as arthritis associated with a massive rotator cuff tear and superior migration of the humeral head [16]. This superior migration leads to erosion of the undersurface of the acromion and blunting of the greater tuberosity. While successful results may be achieved with humeral head replacement and rotator cuff repair in these patients, early glenoid loosening may occur when TSA is performed for cuff tear arthropathy. We therefore consider CTA a contraindication for placement of a glenoid. The role of the *reverse* prosthesis (in which the glenoid becomes the fulcrum or *glenosphere* and the humerus becomes the socket) remains to be determined.

Indications and Contraindications

Studies have demonstrated the superior result of TSA over hemiarthroplasty in patients with glenohumeral arthritis [17–21]. Glenoid replacement should be performed when feasible and when contraindications (see following discussion) are not present. Three requirements are necessary for glenoid implantation [22, 23]:

1. Adequate bone stock: The glenoid vault must be of sufficient size to accept the prosthesis. Cemented glenoid fixation relies on both quality and quantity of cancellous bone available in the vault. It is also imperative to have concentric surfaces between the backside of the glenoid prosthesis and the remaining subchondral prepared glenoid surface. This decreases forces on the cement mantle and theoretically decreases the risk of glenoid loosening.

2. Functioning rotator cuff: Rates of glenoid loosening and component failure have been alarmingly high for patients with CTA treated with TSA [24–28]. At the present time, the best treatment for these patients is hemiarthroplasty. The role of the reverse ball and socket prosthesis can make on the treatment of CTA remains to be seen. Initially used in Europe and Canada, the reverse ball and socket prosthesis has been recently approved by the FDA in the United States.

3. Adequate soft tissue envelope: When placing a glenoid component in a patient with a severely contracted soft tissue envelope (capsule and rotator cuff), effective *overstuffing* of the joint may ensure. This would result in poor postoperative motion and stress on the subscapularis repair.

Contraindications to TSA with glenoid replacement include (1) Charcot arthropathy or neuropathic shoulder, (2) previous infection of the shoulder, (3) patients younger than 50 years of age, and (4) patients with neurological disorders.

Potential complications in young patients include aseptic loosening of the glenoid, which may result in significant glenoid bone loss. One potential solution for this problem may be the implantation of in growth metallic glenoid components. Tantalum (Implex, Allendale, NJ) has more favorable biomechanical properties that the metal used previously and an increased porosity. Short-term results have been encouraging; however, long term results have yet to be determined.

History

Examination of the patient with arthritis of the shoulder begins with a complete history. As with any other joint arthroplasty, patient age is important in determining timing of TSA. Hand dominance, as well as symptomatology of the contralateral shoulder, is also important to be determined. The patient's vocational and recreational activities should be determined. What desired activities is the pathology preventing the patient from accomplishing? What are the postoperative expectations and are they reasonable? These are important issues to discuss with the patient preoperatively. The onset and quality of the pain should also be determined. Arthritic pain generally is indolent and progressive in nature. An acute onset of increased pain, especially if associated with minor trauma may be indicative of other pathology such as a rotator cuff tear.

It is also crucial to document any form of previous treatment. Has the patient undergone a trial of rest or physical therapy? Not only the effectiveness of the therapy is determined, but also the duration and specifics of the program. A history of injections and whether or not they were effective is important. History of pain relief with an intraarticular injection is pathognomic for intraarticular pathology. Conversely, pain relief with subacromial and/or an acromioclavicular joint injection may indicate concurrent pathology that may need to be addressed at the time of TSA.

The functional limitations, both vocational and recreational, of the pain should also be ascertained. Any systemic symptoms indicative of an inflammatory arthropathy or infection should be elicited. Previous use of steroids or alcohol should be determined as they may indicate avascular necrosis. Previous fracture or surgery may indicate post-traumatic or capsulorrhaphy arthritis.

Physical Examination

Physical examination of the patient under consideration for a TSA should begin with examination of the neck. Palpation as well as range of motion of the cervical spine should be assessed and documented. Axial neck pain, radiculopathy, or any myelopathy should be noted. When indicated, an axial compression test should be performed to elicit any neurologic compression. Any signs of radicular or myelopathic pathology should be further investigated with either an EMG or MRI. Patients with rheumatoid arthritis frequently have cervical pathology, which may pose significant perioperative risk and therefore the cervical spine should always be evaluated in these patients. Aside from difficulties with intubation, patients with RA may have sufficient C1/2 instability, basilar invagination or lower c-spine instability, to warrant surgical treatment of the cervical spine before TSA in considered.

Next, a thorough inspection of the patient is made with the patient disrobed to the waist. Any scars may indicate previous surgery such as an instability repair. The patient should be inspected for any asymmetry or muscular atrophy from both anterior and posterior. Any atrophy of the supra or infraspinatus fossae should alert the examiner to the possibility of a significant rotator cuff pathology or neurologic injury. Deltoid atrophy could signal disuse or an axillary nerve lesion. Atrophy of the trapezius, drooping of the shoulder or asymmetric rotation of the scapulae should introduce the possibility of a long thoracic or accessory nerve palsy. If these are suspected, an EMG is recommended.

Range of motion (ROM), both active and passive, is then examined. Forward elevation, external rotation (both with the arm at the side and with the arm abducted 90 degrees), internal rotation and cross body adduction are recorded. The ROM of both the affected side and the contralateral side should be assessed and compared. Often it is easier to assess the patient's ROM with the patient in the supine position rather than upright. With active range of motion it is important to view the patient posteriorly. Symmetric and synchronous motion of the scapulothoracic articulation should be noted. Scapulothoracic dyskinesis or winging of the scapula may indicate a neurologic problem about the shoulder girdle and warrants a further work up. It is also important to assess the patient for associated pathology including AC joint and subacromial pathology, as these may need to be addressed at the time of TSA. Pain at the AC joint with palpation, forced cross body adduction or with the active compression test, indicates acromioclavicular pathology. Impingement signs include the Neer, Hawkin's and drop arm test. Bicep signs, such as Speed's and Yergenson's, must also be explored. The strength of the rotator cuff is assessed, and lag signs, including both external and internal rotation lag signs, are documented. Positive findings indicate a significant rotator cuff deficit. It is important to evaluate the integrity and competence of the subscapularis tendon with the belly-press and lift-off tests. The load and shift test is used to determine anteroposterior laxity. The sulcus sign is checked for inferior instability. The apprehension, relocation and anterior release tests can be used to investigate subtle instability. Generally, patients with arthritis are stiff and these tests are difficult to perform.

Diagnostic Tests

Radiographic Evaluation

Patients undergoing planning for a TSA should have a complete shoulder series that includes five views. This includes a true AP of the shoulder with the humerus in internal rotation, external rotation and neutral rotation. Also included are the axillary lateral and the supraspinatus outlet view. The external rotation view profiles the greater tuberosity and is the most useful view when templating the humerus. The radiographic findings in osteoarthritis include joint space narrowing, subchondral sclerosis and marginal osteophytes (Figure 1.1A and 1.1B). Rheumatoid arthritis is usually associated with symmetric joint space narrowing, osteopenia and subchondral erosions (Figure 1.2). Patients with RA of the shoulder may have medialization of the glenoid. This can be seen on the AP view. Various changes can be seen on both the humeral and glenoid side with AVN (Figure 1.3A and 1.3B) depending of the stage. Cuff tear arthropathy has classic radiographic signs of humeral head migration, erosion into the undersurface of the acromion and eburnation of the greater tuberosity (Figure 1.4). The supraspinatus outlet view in helpful in assessing the morphology of the acromion. It is extremely important to obtain an adequate axillary view to assess the glenoid vault, glenoid version, glenoid congruency as well as position of the humeral head.

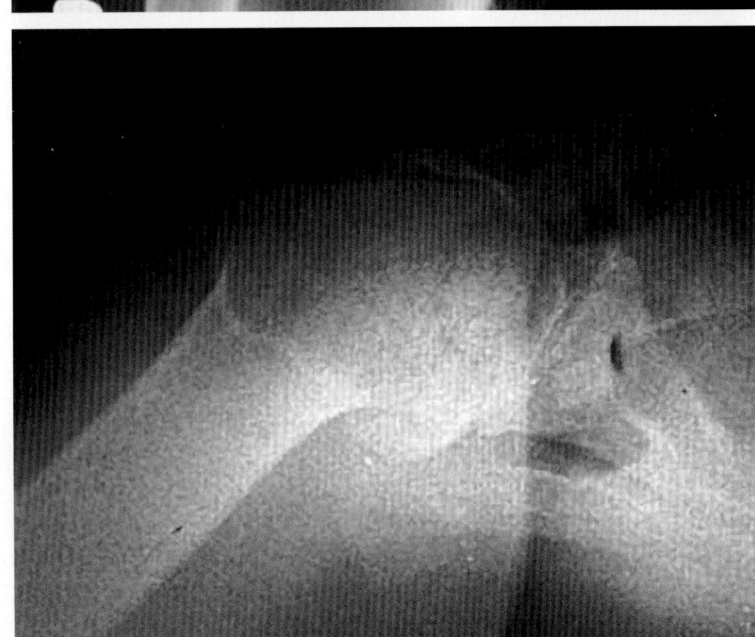

Figure 1.1. (A) AP radiograph of a patient's shoulder with osteoarthritis of the glenohumeral joint. Marginal osteophytes along both the humeral neck and glenoid can be visualized. Additionally present are subchondral sclerosis, subchondral cysts and narrowing of the joint line. **(B)** Axillary radiograph of a patient with osteoarthritis. Eccentric wear of the glenoid can be observed on this image, with moderate posterior wear.

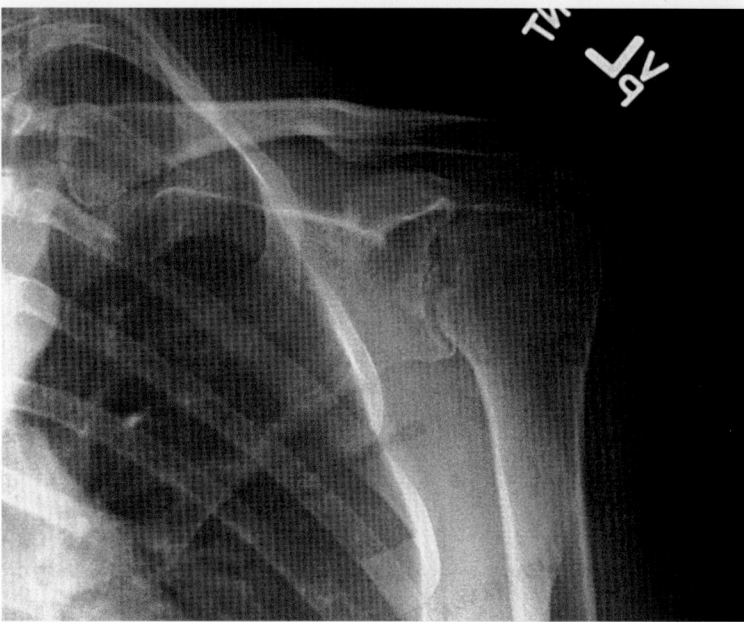

Figure 1.2. AP radiograph of a patient with rheumatoid arthritis. Medialization of the joint line can be noticed along with subchondral erosions, osteopenia and symmetric joint space narrowing. The maintenance of the humeral head to acromial distance is a good indication of a functional rotator cuff.

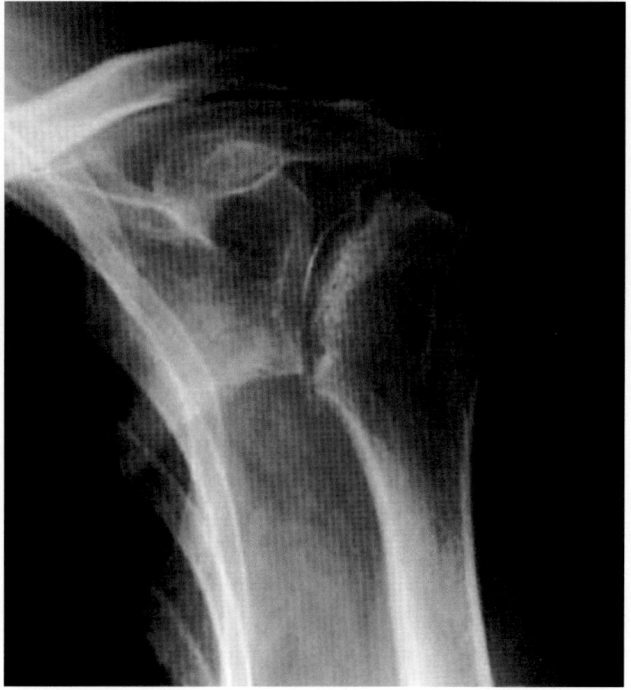

A

Figure 1.3. (A and B) AP and lateral radiograph demonstrating stage V AVN: humeral head collapse with involvement of the posterior glenoid.

(Continued)

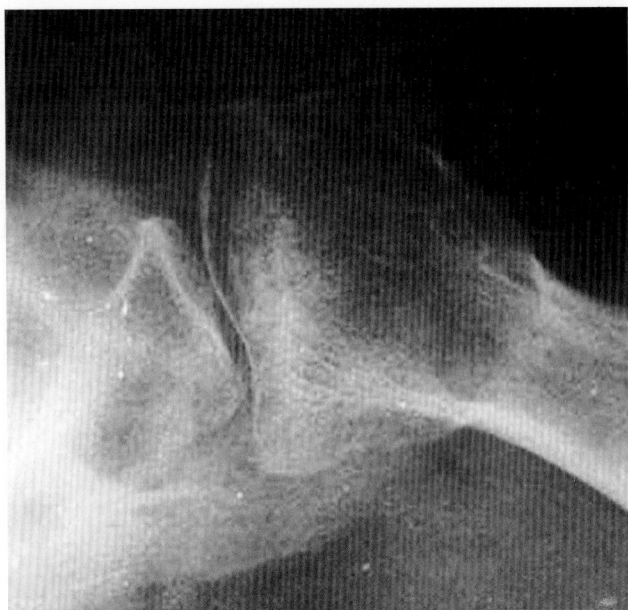

B

Figure 1.3. *Continued*

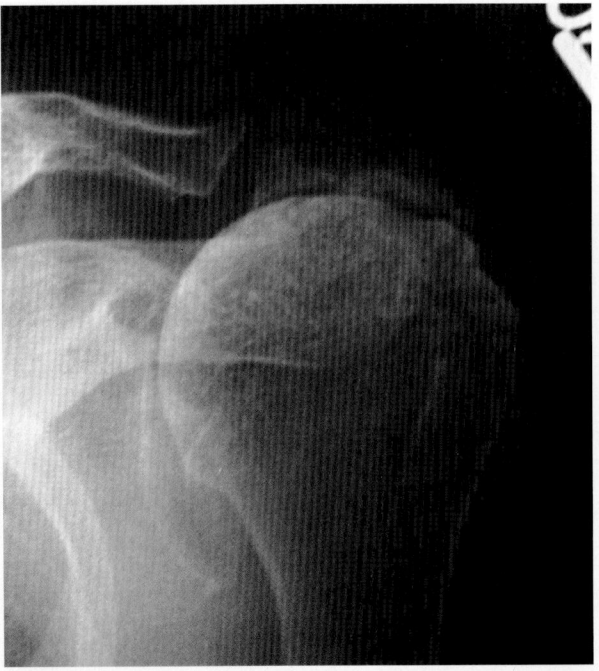

Figure 1.4. AP radiograph demonstrating cuff tear arthropathy. Note the superior migration of the humeral head, glenohumeral arthrosis, blunting of the greater tuberosity and *acetabularization* and almost complete erosion through the acromion.

Preoperative Templating

Restoration of function in shoulder arthroplasty is dependent on restoring soft tissue tension and reestablishing normal glenohumeral (GH) relationships. These relationships may be assessed in patients with preoperative radiographs and may guide the surgeon in sizing and positioning the implants. Preoperative measurements are performed using standard true AP and axillary radiographs. Size markers should be placed on the cassettes to normalize radiographic magnification. For the AP radiograph, the arm should be positioned in 20 to 30 degrees of external rotation for optimal evaluation of the greater tuberosity in relation to the articular surface. Measurements include humeral head diameter (HHD), humeral head height (HHH), acromio-humeral interval (AHI), humeral-tuberosity interval (HTI), lateral humeral offset (LHO), and glenoid joint line (JL) ([29]) (Figure 1.5A–D). From initial studies at Columbia University, the average humeral head dimensions in OA patients (HHD, HHH) were 47.9mm and 22.6mm, respectively, LHO was 49.4mm, HTI was 13.5mm while AHI averaged 7.5mm. Every effort should be made to reproduce these preoperative dimensions with prosthetic replacement [30].

Additional Studies

Nerve conduction studies and/or EMGs may be indicated for any patient with signs of radiculopathy, myelopathy, history of polyneuropathy, or any signs of weakness or asymmetry on physical examination. Patients with a history of instability repair, especially a Bristow or Laterjet, or patients who have a significant decrease in external rotation (less than 30 degrees), often will have excessive posterior wear of the glenoid. For these patients as well as those with inadequate axillary radiographs, it may be necessary to obtain a CT scan or MRI. CT scans are excellent at depicting glenoid and proximal humeral bony anatomy and usually provides superior assessment of osseous anatomy compared with MRI, although both modalities may provide useful information. Imaging in the axial plane is helpful in evaluating the glenoid vault for depth and wear (Figure 1.6). The MRI is also very informative when a rotator cuff tear is suspected, not only in identifying the tear but also in looking for atrophy of the rotator cuff muscle bellies. This is best seen on the medial sagittal images (Figure 1.7).

A careful preoperative history and physical examination should reveal significant comorbidities. If there is any question, the patient is referred to their primary care physician or cardiologist for a preoperative evaluation. Each preoperative laboratory evaluation includes CBC with differential, basic metabolic panel, ESR and coagulation profile. Any patient over the age of 40, or who has a history of smoking or lung disorder, receives a preoperative PA and lateral chest radiograph. A urinalysis is performed on any female, and any symptomatic male undergoing a TSA. Patients who are anemic, or those scheduled for extensive procedures are type and crossed appropriately.

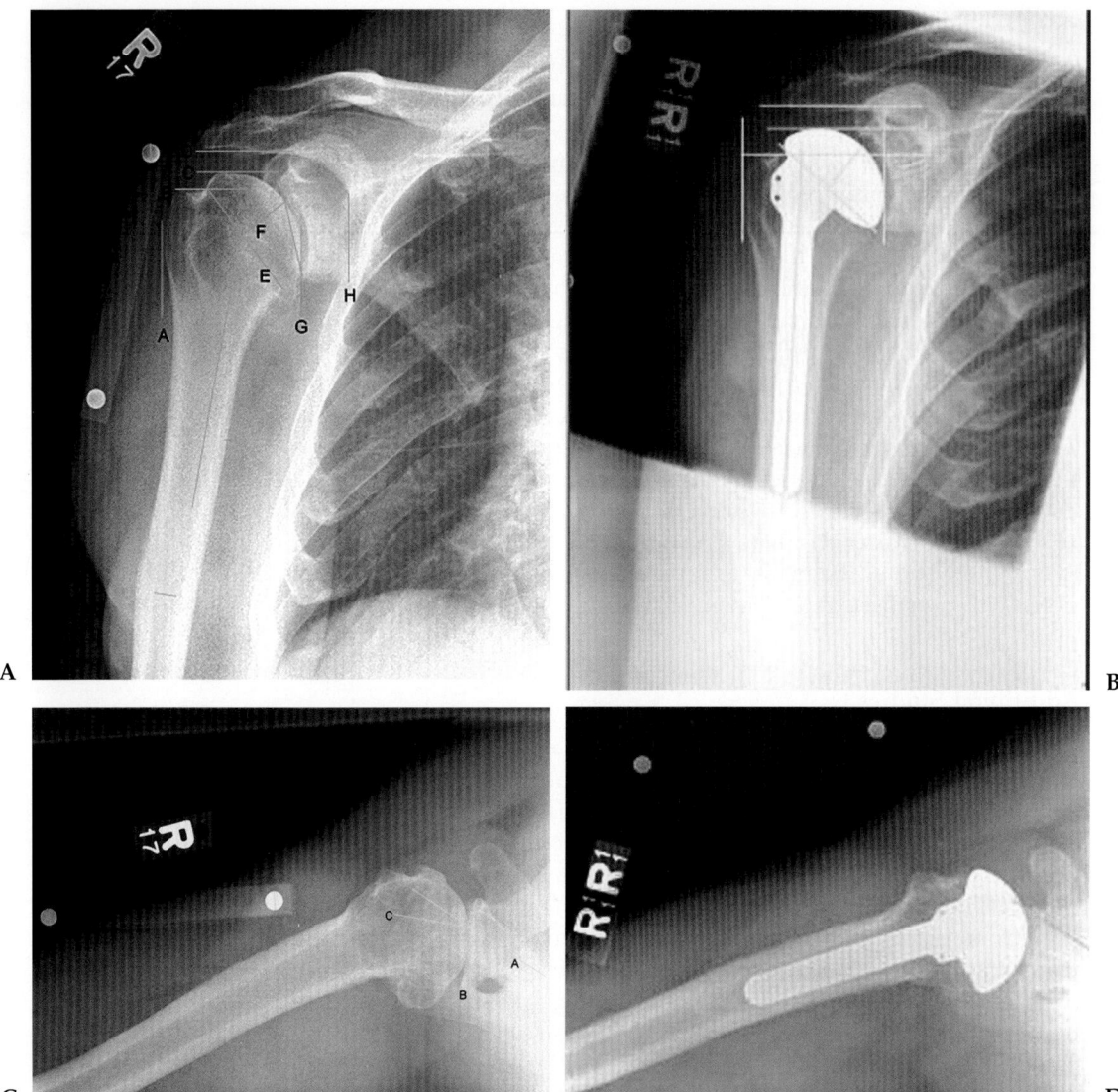

Figure 1.5. (A) Preoperative AP radiograph of a patient with osteoarthritis. Various measurements can be made: B–C represent the humeral-tuberosity interval; C–D the acromio-humeral interval; F, the humeral head height; E, the humeral head diameter; A–G, the lateral humeral offset; and G–H, the glenoid joint line. **(B)** Postoperative AP radiograph. Every effort should be made to reproduce these preoperative dimensions with prosthetic replacement. **(C and D)** Preoperative and postoperative axillary radiographs. Line C is perpendicular to line B, the angle between lines A and C is the glenoid version angle.

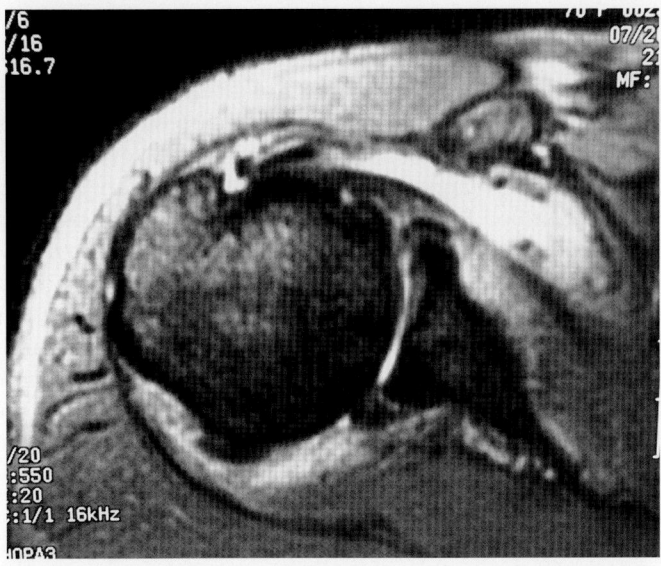

Figure 1.6. Axial MRI demonstrating both the size of the glenoid vault as well as the glenoid version.

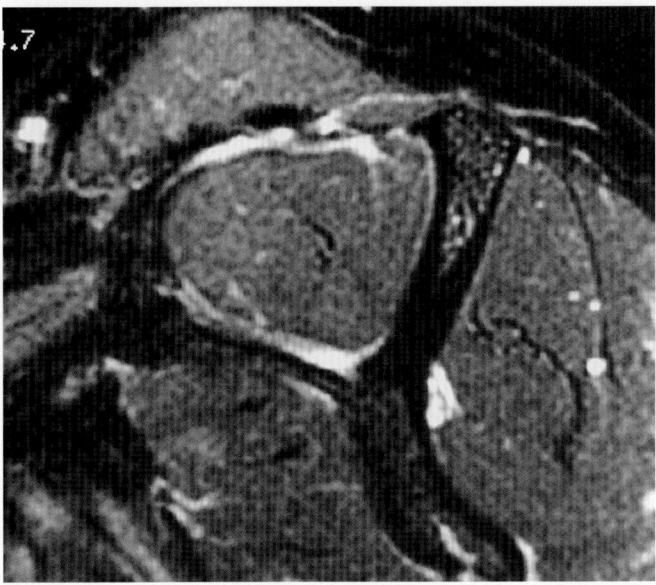

Figure 1.7. Sagittal oblique MRI indicating robust rotator cuff musculature without fatty infiltration.

Anesthesia and Patient Positioning

Unless it is necessary to rule out an indolent infection with operative frozen section and cultures, all patients receive preoperative antibiotics. A second-generation cephalosporin is preferred; however, if the patient is penicillin allergic, vancomycin or clindamycin can be used. The antibiotic is continued for 24 hours postoperatively. For postoperative pain control and immediate postoperative physical therapy, we prefer regional anesthesia. An interscalene block is placed before the patient is taken to the operating room. General anesthesia may be administered for an incomplete block or the desires of the patient and anesthetist. Often the block does not cover the T1 and T2 dermatomes and the block needs to be supplemented with local anesthesia at the inferior aspect of the wound. This is especially true if the less invasive axillary incision is used.

The patient is placed in the beach chair position. The hips and knees are flexed and the heels well padded. The head of the bed is elevated approximately 60 degrees. If an axillary approach is chosen, the head of the bed may be slightly lowered. The patient is shifted to the side of the bed corresponding to the shoulder that is being replaced. The arm should be able to hang freely without obstruction from the edge of the table. A short arm board is used and placed on the table just above the elbow. This along with a sterile bolster can be used to support the arm during the approach and glenoid preparation. The bolster can be removed and the short arm board slid distally, to allow adduction and extension of the humerus. This adduction and extension is necessary for humeral head removal and humeral shaft preparation. We use Ioban (3M, St. Paul, MN) for all arthroplasty procedures. Alternatively, an arm positioner can be used. Recently, we have used a hydraulic arm positioner (Tenet Medical, Calgary, Alberta, Canada) (Figure 1.8).

Approaches

Deltopectoral Approach

For routine primary TSA with an intact rotator cuff, the deltopectoral approach is used. The skin incision for the standard approach extends approximately 15 cm from just inferior to the clavicle, proceeds over the coracoid process and continues obliquely down the arm to the area of the deltoid insertion (Figure 1.9). Recently, we have employed a minimally invasive approach in certain patients in whom significant stiffness is not present and the patient can preoperatively externally rotate greater than 30 degrees. For the minimally invasive approach, a concealed axillary incision may be used. The concealed axillary incision begins approximately 3 cm inferior to the coracoid and extends inferiorly 7 cm into the axillary crease.

An additional minimally invasive incision has also recently been described by the senior author (TAB) that is centered just lateral to the coracoid and is 2 in. (5 cm) in length (Figure 1.10). At present, these limited incisions are only recommended for the most experienced of shoulder surgeons since exposure may be more difficult until mini-

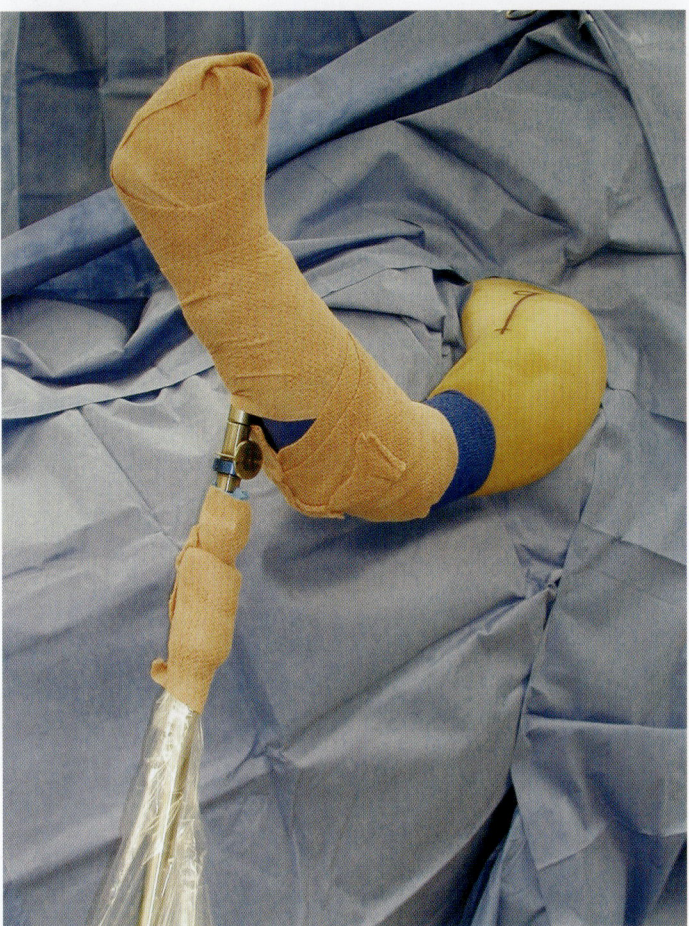

Figure 1.8. A hydraulic arm positioner (Tenet Medical) can be used to position the arm. This positioner allows the assistant to use both hands as the arm is fixed in position, yet can be moved simply by stepping on a foot pedal.

mally invasive shoulder instrumentation becomes available. Regardless of the incision, a needle-tipped Bovie is used to elevate full-thickness skin flaps medially and laterally. Dissection is also taken superior to the level of the clavicle and inferior to the pectoralis insertion. Two Gelpi retractors are placed and the deltopectoral interval identified (Figure 1.11). The cephalic vein should be identified and preserved whenever possible. Most often it is easier to dissect the vein medially and retract it laterally with the deltoid, as it has less contributories from the pectoralis from the medial side. Less bleeding is encountered if the vein remains laterally with the deltoid. The undersurface of the deltoid is then identified. In the vast majority of primary TSA the subdeltoid space is easily identified. However, in the shoulder that has undergone previous surgery or in the revision setting, this interval may not be obvious. Not properly identifying this space using an elevator to find the space raises the possibility of delaminating the deltoid muscle or injuring the axillary nerve. A fairly simple way to identify this space is

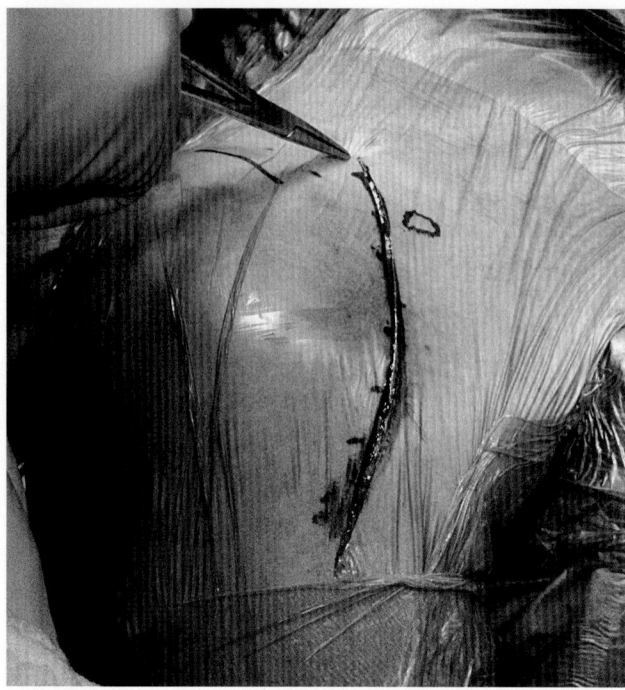

Figure 1.9. Clinical photograph of our standard skin incision for total shoulder arthroplasty.

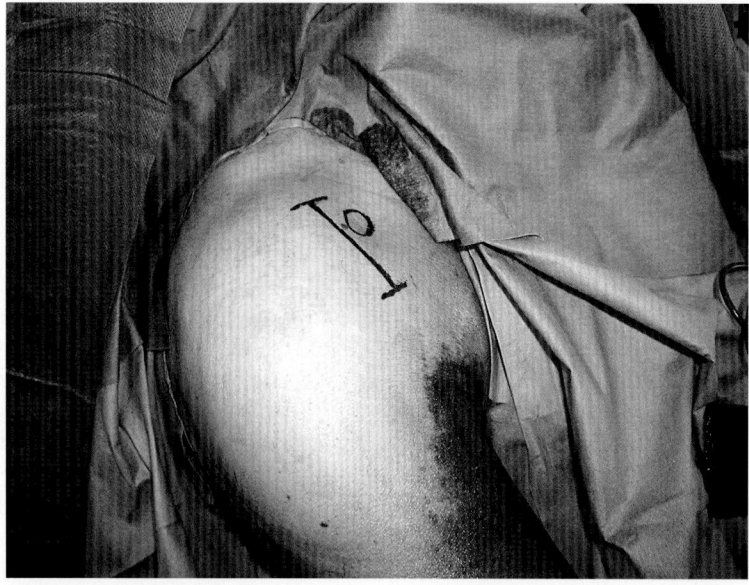

Figure 1.10. Minimal incision is centered just lateral to the coracoid approximately 5 cm in length. It is made proximal enough to allow both adequate exposure to the glenoid and a straight shot at the humeral canal. This incision is used in selected patients.

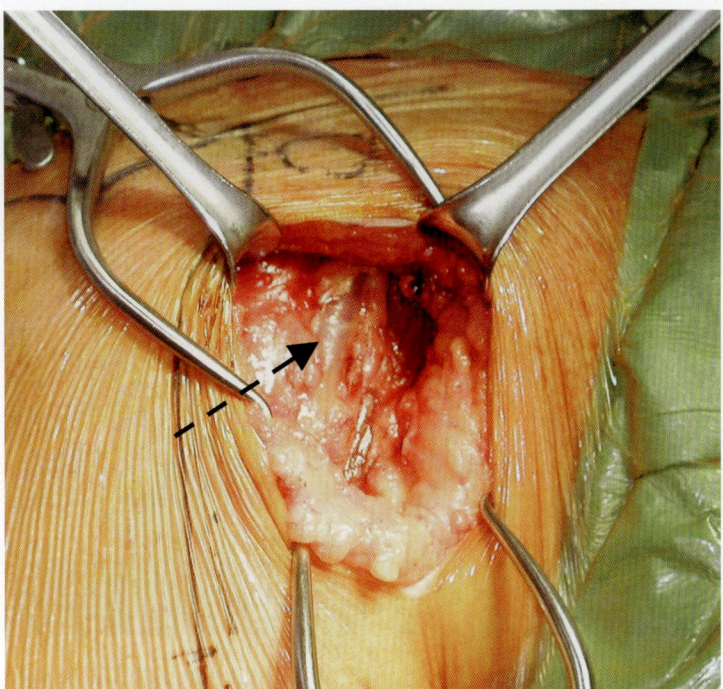

Figure 1.11. The deltopectoral interval is identified. The dashed arrow is pointing to the cephalic vein encased in its fat pad. This is a fairly reliable way to identify the proper interval.

to find the subacromial space. Once identified, an elevator can be used to enter the subdeltoid interval, which is contiguous with the subacromial space. A Richardson retractor can be placed deep to the deltoid once this space has been properly identified. The superior aspect of the pectoralis major tendon is identified. If additional exposure is necessary or for patients with limited external rotation, the upper $1/2$—1 cm of the pectoralis tendon is tagged and released. This is anatomically repaired at the end of the procedure. A Richardson retractor is then placed deep to the pectoralis major retracting it inferior and medial. The clavipectoral fascia is then incised lateral to the conjoint tendon. It is important to recognize that distally, the muscle belly of the short head of the bicep is more lateral than the tendon. Care should be taken not to enter this plane when dissecting lateral to the conjoint tendon. A medium Richardson can then be used to retract the conjoint tendon medially. The coracoid and the coracoacromial ligament are then identified. The leading edge of the CA ligament is then resected improving superior exposure (Figure 1.12). A metal finger or narrow Darrach can be used to help expose the proximal humerus by placing it deep to the deltoid and gently levering the humeral head anteriorly. A complete anterior bursectomy is then performed. This allows excellent exposure of the subscapularis. The upper border of the subscapularis is identified by finding the rotator interval. The lower border is identified by

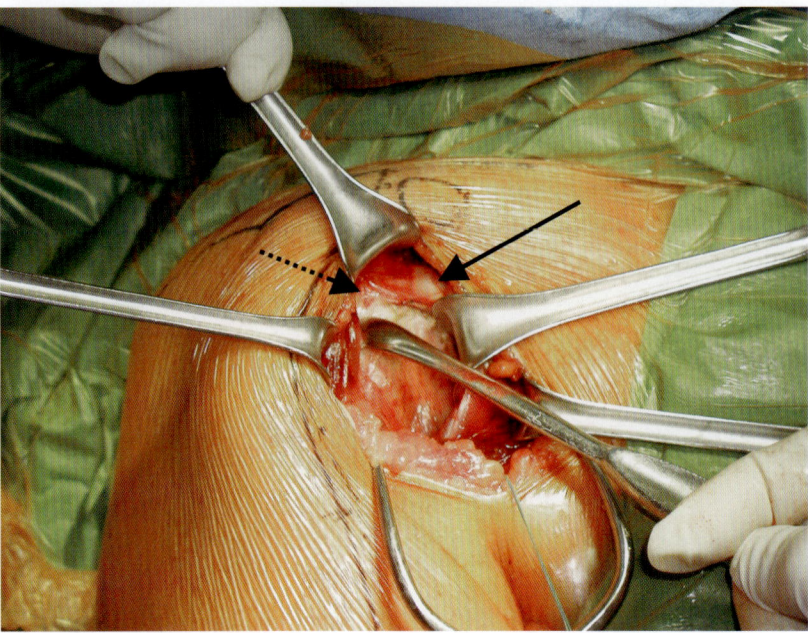

Figure 1.12. The coracoid (*solid arrow*) and anterior lateral edge of the cora-coacromial ligament is identified (*dotted arrow*). Resection of this edge improves superior exposure.

the anterior circumflex artery and its two venae comitantes. These vessels are then coagulated using the needle-tipped Bovie, or tied depending on their girth. Since every centimeter of length gained for the subscapularis repair allows for 10 to 15 degrees of external rotation achieved, to maximize length the subscapularis is removed from the humerus just medial to the bicep tendon. The subscapularis is removed with the anterior capsule as a single unit. This is done to preserve length. An anterior capsulectomy is later performed to correct the anterior soft tissue contracture (Figure 1.13). For severe anterior soft tissue contractures, especially if the tendon has been shortened previously for and instability repair, the subscapularis and anterior capsule as a unit can be Z-lengthened. If this proves to be inadequate, a pectoralis transfer may be used for a deficient subscapularis. This is discussed in Chapter 6. Once the anterior soft tissue is released a Darrach retractor can be placed posterior to the head, the arm can be externally rotated and the head dislocated anteriorly (Figure 1.14). Preparation of the humerus is covered in Chapter 2.

Extensile Approach

More often in the revision setting rather than the primary setting, an extended approach may be necessary to gain access to the proximal humerus. The technique for the removal of a humeral stem in the revision setting is discussed in Chapter 3. If more access to the humerus is necessary, the deltopectoral incision can be extended. Proximally, the interval is developed between the deltoid and the pectoralis (axillary nerve and the medial/lateral pectoral nerves). The skin incision is the same as for the deltopectoral approach, but extends down the arm along the lateral edge of the biceps. Distally, the interval between the biceps and the brachialis is identified. The fascia is then split protecting the cephalic vein, and the biceps retracted medially. This exposes the brachialis. Secondary to its dual innervation, the brachialis can be split longitudinally down the midline. Care must be taken to protect the radial nerve, which pierces the intramuscular septum approximately 10 cm proximal from the articular surface [31, 32]. The periosteum over the anterior humerus can then be split longitudinally and subperiosteal dissection performed to avoid injury to the radial nerve laterally, and the ulnar nerve medially. It should also be noted that if exposure of the distal humerus is necessary, the lateral antibrachial cutaneous nerve should be identified and protected. The nerve is easiest identified in the interval lateral to the distal bicep tendon.

Anterosuperior Approach and Combined Approach

This approach may become necessary when there is inadequate proximal exposure from the deltopectoral approach to expose and repair a deficient rotator cuff. Usually, this approach is performed in combination with the deltopectoral approach using the same skin incision and performing subcutaneous dissection with a lateral skin flap. The vascularity of the shoulder is typically ample enough to allow healing of

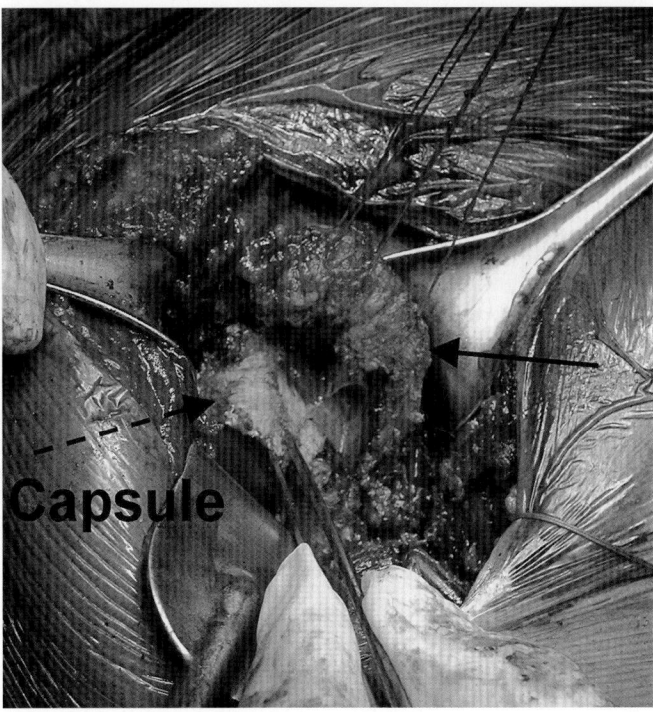

Figure 1.13. The contracted anterior capsule (*dashed arrow*) is carefully excised from the undersurface of the tagged subscapularis. We have found that, although a circumferential subscapularis is often necessary, this release significantly mobilizes the subscapularis tendon.

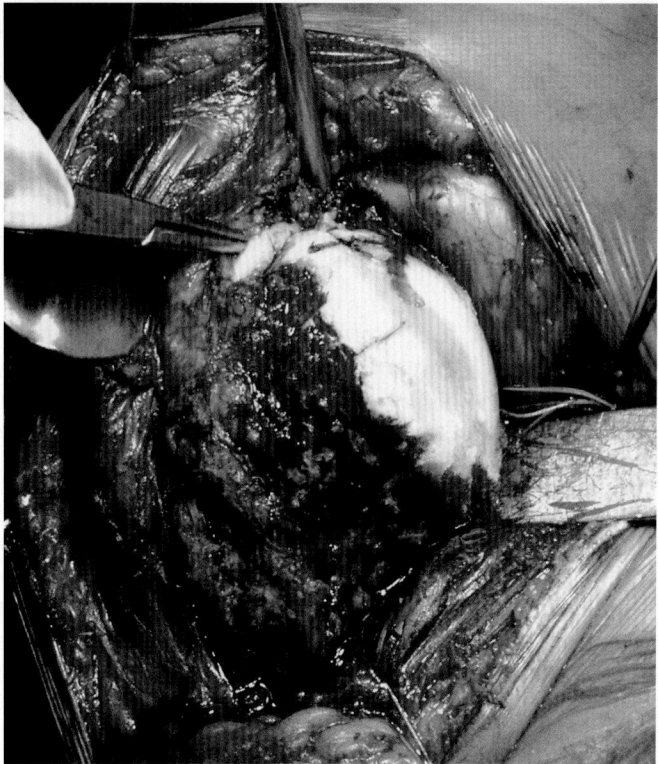

Figure 1.14. With external rotation and adduction of the humerus, retractors can be placed posterior to gently lever the humeral head anteriorly, delivering it from the wound and granting excellent exposure. Once delivered and after removal of osteophytes, removal of the anterior retractor and internal rotation can often provide enough exposure to the posterior superior rotator cuff such that repair may be possible without removal of the deltoid.

this flap. If it is anticipated preoperatively that this approach may be required, the skin incision may be planned slightly more lateral than normal with the more proximal extent aimed at the acromion rather than the coracoid. Except in the most severe of cases, deltoid detachment from the lateral acromion is avoided due to the potential complication of operative deltoid rupture—a complication for which there is no reliable salvage. Once subcutaneous dissection is complete, the deltopectoral interval is identified and entered as described previously. For the combined approach, the anterosuperior portion of the approach is performed by incising the strong fascial attachment of the anterior deltoid to the anterior acromion curving laterally around the anterolateral corner of the acromion and followed by a longitudinal split through the fibers of the middle deltoid. This split is continued approximately 3 cm to 4 cm past the lateral tip of the acromion. A stay stitch may be placed at the distal end of the split to help prevent extension of the split. The axillary nerve generally runs 5 cm to 6 cm distal to the lateral tip of the acromion. It is important to leave an adequate portion of the deltoid origin remaining attached to the acromioclavicular joint and distal clavicle to avoid intraoperative deltoid pull-off. The deltoid origin is preserved as a 5 cm to 10 mm cuff of stout tissue is left on the anterior aspect of the acromion. This facilitates repair of the deltoid at the end of the procedure.

The proximal edges of the incised anterior deltoid are tagged and retracted posteriorly. This affords excellent exposure of the greater tuberosity and posterior rotator cuff. This exposure can be improved with extension and internal rotation of the humerus. When the humeral head is removed and retracted posteriorly with a Fukuda retractor, the combined approach allows excellent exposure of the posterior glenoid. Great care must be taken to remain cognizant of the axillary nerve as it resides on the undersurface of the deltoid just distal to the deltoid split. Just as important as the careful removal of the deltoid leaving adequate tissue for reattachment, the deltoid needs to be meticulously repaired. We prefer to use no. 2 nonabsorbable sutures in a figure of eight fashion to repair the deltoid back to the anterior cuff of tissue. The lateral split in the middle deltoid is also repaired. If there is any question regarding the quality of repair to the anterior cuff of tissue, the deltoid should be repaired to the clavicle and acromion through drill holes.

References

1. Hill JM. Total Shoulder Arthroplasty: Indications. In Total Shoulder Arthroplasty, LA Crosby, Editor. Rosemont, IL: AAOS, 2000;17–25.
2. Barrett WP, Franklin JL, Jackins SE, et al. Total shoulder arthroplasty. J Bone Joint Surg Am 1987;69(6):865–872.
3. Hawkins RJ, Bell RH, Jallay B. Total shoulder arthroplasty. Clin Orthop 1989;242:188–194.
4. Cofield RH. Total shoulder arthroplasty with the Neer prosthesis. J Bone Joint Surg Am 1984;66(6):899–906.
5. Figgie HE 3rd, Inglis AE, Goldberg VM, et al. An analysis of factors affecting the long-term results of total shoulder arthroplasty in inflammatory arthritis. J Arthroplasty 1988;3(2):123–130.
6. Kelly IG, Foster RS, Fisher WD. Neer total shoulder replacement in rheumatoid arthritis. J Bone Joint Surg Br 1987;69(5):723–726.
7. McCoy SR, Warren RF, Bade HA, et al. Total shoulder arthroplasty in rheumatoid arthritis. J Arthroplasty 1989;4(2):105–113.
8. L'Insalata JC, Pagnani MJ, Warren RF, et al. Humeral head osteonecrosis: clinical course and radiographic predictors of outcome. J Shoulder Elbow Surg 1996;5(5):355–361.
9. Cruess RL. Steroid-induced avascular necrosis of the head of the humerus. Natural history and management. J Bone Joint Surg Br 1976;58(3):313–317.
10. Cruess RL. Corticosteroid-induced osteonecrosis of the humeral head. Orthop Clin North Am 1985;16(4):789–796.
11. Cruess RL. Osteonecrosis of bone. Current concepts as to etiology and pathogenesis. Clin Orthop 1986;208:30–39.
12. Marra G, Wiater JM, Levine WL, Pollock RG, Bigliani LU. Shoulder Arthroplasty for Avascular Necrosis. In Total Shoulder Arthroplasty, LA Crosby, Editor. Rosemont, IL: AAOS, 2000.
13. Blaine TA, Marra GN, Park JY, Flatow EL, Pollack RG, Bigliani LU. Shoulder Arthroplasty for Avascular Necrosis of the Humeral Head. In Total Shoulder Arthroplasty, LA Crosby, Editor. Rosemont, IL: AAOS, 2000.

14. Neer CS II, Kirby RM. Revision of humeral head and total shoulder arthroplasties. Clin Orthop 1982;170:189–195.
15. Bigliani LU, Kelkar R, Flatow EL, et al. Glenohumeral stability. Biomechanical properties of passive and active stabilizers. Clin Orthop 1996;330: 13–30.
16. Neer, CS II, Craig EV, Fukuda H. Cuff-tear arthropathy. J Bone Joint Surg Am 1983;65(9):1232–1244.
17. Gartsman GM, Roddey TS, Hammerman SM. Shoulder arthroplasty with or without resurfacing of the glenoid in patients who have osteoarthritis. J Bone Joint Surg Am 2000;82(1):26–34.
18. Orfaly RM, Rockwood CA Jr, Esenyel CZ, et al. A prospective functional outcome study of shoulder arthroplasty for osteoarthritis with an intact rotator cuff. J Shoulder Elbow Surg 2003;12(3):214–221.
19. Edwards TB, Kadakia NRE, Boulahia A, et al. A comparison of hemiarthroplasty and total shoulder arthroplasty in the treatment of primary glenohumeral osteoarthritis: results of a multicenter study. J Shoulder Elbow Surg 2003;12(3):207–213.
20. Rodosky MW, Bigliani LU. Indications for glenoid resurfacing in shoulder arthroplasty. J Shoulder Elbow Surg 1996;5(3):231–248.
21. Smith KL, Matsen FA III. Total shoulder arthroplasty versus hemiarthroplasty. Current trends. Orthop Clin North Am 1998;29(3):491–506.
22. Connor PM, Flatow EL. Surgical Considerations of Bony Deficiency in Total Shoulder Arthroplasty. In Complex and Revision Problems in Shoulder Surgery, JJ Warner, Iannotti JP, Gerber C, Editors. Philadelphia: Lippincott-Raven, 1997;339–354.
23. Hayes P, Flatow EL. Steps for Reliable Glenoid Exposure and Preparation in Shoulder Arthroplasty. Tech Shoulder Elbow Surg 2000;1(4):209–219.
24. Field LD, Dines DM, Zabinski SJ, et al. Hemiarthroplasty of the Shoulder for rotator Cuff Arthropathy. J Shoulder Elbow Surg 1997;6(1):18–23.
25. Connor PM, Bigliani LU. Prosthetic Replacement for Osteoarthritis: hemiarthroplasty versus total shoulder replacement. Semin Arthroplasty 1997;8: 268–277.
26. Flatow EL. Prosthetic Replacement in the Rotator Cuff Deficient Shoulder. In Surgery of the Shoulder, M Vastamaki, Jalovaara P, Editors. Amsterdam: Elsevier, 1995;335–345.
27. Franklin JL, Barrett WP, Jackins SE, et al. Glenoid loosening in total shoulder arthroplasty. Association with rotator cuff deficiency. J Arthroplasty 1988;3(1):39–46.
28. Ibarra C, Dines DM, McLaughlin JA. Glenoid replacement in total shoulder arthroplasty. Orthop Clin North Am 1998;29(3):403–413.
29. Iannotti JP, Gabriel JP, Schneck SL, et al. The normal glenohumeral relationships. An anatomical study of one hundred and forty shoulders. J Bone Joint Surg Am 1992;74(4):491–500.
30. Blaine TA, Kim P, Ogwonali, O, Heyworth, B, Choi, C, Levine WL, Bigliani LU. Radiographic Assessment of Glenohumeral Relationships in Patients with Osteoarthritis Pre and Post-Arthroplasty. In ASES Focus Meeting. 2003. Las Vegas.
31. Siegel DB, Gelberman RH. Radial nerve: applied anatomy and operative exposure. In Operative Nerve Repair and Reconstruction, RH Gelberman, Editor. Philadelphia: Lippincott, 1991;393–407.
32. Uhl RL, Lasora JM, Sibeni T, Martino LJ. Posterior Approaches to the Humerus: when Should You Worry about the Radial Nerve? J Orthop Trauma 1996;10(5):338–340.

Chapter 2

Total Shoulder Replacement: Humeral Component Technique

William N. Levine and Steven Aviles

Shoulder arthroplasty reliably relieves pain and improves function in the majority of patients with painful arthritic shoulders. However, with modern prosthetic designs, improved anatomical understanding, and continued emphasis on proper rehabilitation, our goals of restoring near-normal function are more often realized. This chapter reviews our approach to proper preparation of the humerus in helping to achieve these patient-oriented goals.

Preoperative Considerations

Preoperative Templating

Most shoulder arthroplasty systems have preoperative templates, and they can be of significant value in the preoperative preparation and the intraoperative implementation of the procedure. We prefer to use a dedicated marker on the preoperative true AP radiograph to assure reproducible magnification (Figure 2.1). Templating has been discussed in Chapter 1.

Humeral Fixation: Press-Fit or Cement?

Prosthetic designs allow for both press-fit and cemented humeral components, and both systems have had their advocates over time. Decision-making factors to consider include the patient's age, quality of bone stock, previous arthroplasty, associated disease entities (i.e., avascular necrosis (AVN); rheumatoid arthritis (RA)), presence of fracture, presence of rotator cuff tear, and surgeon's experience. While humeral loosening is rare in osteoarthritis, it occurs with a much higher incidence in rheumatoid arthritis [1, 2] so we routinely recommend cemented prostheses in these patients.

Typically, patient factors such as age at time of implant (especially less than 60 years of age) and excellent bone quality may guide the surgeon to press fit the humeral component. However, the press-fit technique is not recommended in proximal humerus fractures. Without

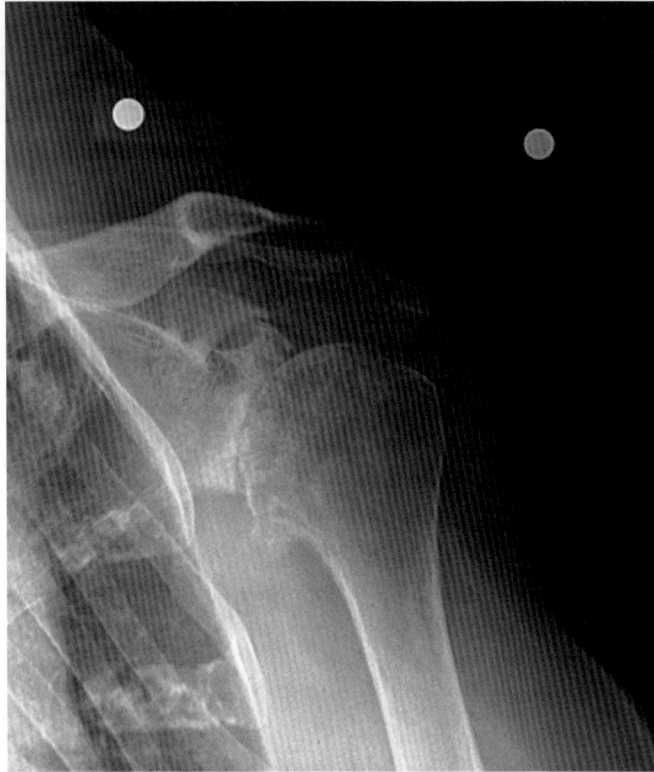

Figure 2.1. Preoperative template with commercially available radiographic marker to assist in assessment of magnification.

the greater tuberosity in position, there is less rotational control and higher risk of prosthetic loosening.

Press-fit components are available with and without porous ingrowth. Ingrowth contributes to more stable fixation; however, it may make revision surgery more difficult. Therefore, it may be an unnecessary burden.

Press fitting the humeral component is faster since the surgeon does not need to wait for cement to cure; however, it may be more technically challenging because there is less room for error in positioning. Furthermore, press-fit prostheses may be predisposed to loosening. A recent study showed that there is increased rotational motion when press-fit prostheses are placed in cadavers [3]. In addition, Torchia et al. demonstrated radiographic shifting in 49% of the press-fit humeral components compared with none with cemented components after 15 years [4]. The clinical significance of this remains unclear, however, since none of these patients were symptomatic. More recently, Matsen et al. have shown radiolucencies comparable with cementing techniques and no shifting in position of press-fit prostheses after two-year follow-up with newer press-fit designs [5].

Neer, as well as other authors, have shown that the incidence of humeral loosening is low (0%–2.5%) with the use of cemented humeral stems [4, 6]. Given this success with long-term follow-up, cementing is the authors' preference in the majority of older patients for humeral stem placement. Options include full cementation or proximal cementing. Proximal cementation involves placing cement on the proximal fins and shaft of the prosthesis before insertion. Two cadaveric studies have shown that there was no difference in fixation between fully cemented and proximally cemented prostheses [5, 7].

Proximal cementing can also make revision easier. However, there is currently no long-term or in vivo data to support this technique. Neer et al. recommended full cementing of the humeral stem, which involves finger packing or the use of a 60-ml syringe for application of cement into the humerus [6]. A cement restrictor is used as well to prevent distal migration of cement. We currently perform a proximal humeral cementing technique and do not use any pressurization during insertion of the cement.

Components

Nearly all components today are modular, allowing the surgeon a great deal of intraoperative flexibility in decision-making with respect to humeral head height, humeral prosthetic version, head-tuberosity interval, offset, and head and stem size. The original Neer prosthesis was a fixed monopolar device with either a 15-mm or 22-mm head with 3 stem sizes. All of today's prostheses have evolved from Neer's original prosthetic designs.

Modularity

Monoblock stems, or stems with humeral heads as already placed may have advantages to their use; however, they do not provide the greater choice of head radius with curvature and thickness that is seen with modular systems. With greater diversity of head size, adjustments can be made to properly establish soft tissue tension. Given the importance of soft tissue balancing, modular humeral components are preferred.

There are disadvantages to a modular system. Wear can occur from either a standard or reverse morse taper. Furthermore, component dissociation may occur. This is rare (1:1000); however, it is still a possibility [8]. It is usually associated with contamination by fluids (as little as 0.5 ml), which can decrease forces necessary for dissociation. Dissociation tends to occur more often when fluid is trapped in a reverse morse taper [8]. Therefore, a standard morse taper is recommended with meticulous cleaning of the interface.

Humeral Head

The native head should be replaced with a prosthetic head of the same height, diameter, and offset. Typically, the head size should allow passive translation of the prosthesis of approximately 50% of the glenoid width in the superoinferior and anteroposterior planes as well as restore distance between the greater tuberosity and glenoid to provide an adequate fulcrum for raising the arm. The preoperative radiographs should be templated to determine the head size and this can be adjusted intraoperatively as necessary. The variables associated with determining head size include the following ones.

Thickness (Height)

On average, the humeral height is 18.5 mm and the radius is 23.8 mm in cadaveric studies [9, 10]. An increase in height can result in humeral head translation on the prosthetic glenoid. It can also lateralize the center of axis of the humeral head. One must be careful not to place a humeral head that is too thick, which would result in *overstuffing* (see complications).

Radius of Curvature

The average radius is 22.0 mm to 25.3 mm and it directly correlates to head thickness [9–13]. Normal radii of curvature of humeral heads and glenoid are essentially equal, within 2 mm in 88% of cases and within 3 mm in all cases [14]. However, the prosthesis is designed with a mismatch in the curvature to limit constraints of the prosthesis.

Head Tuberosity Interval

Maintaining a distance between the superior edge of the head and the greater tuberosity greater than 8 mm safely prevents impingement between the tuberosity and the acromion [11]. This is critical to restore normal range of motion and function for patients postoperatively.

Offset

In an attempt to match the proximal humeral anatomy more closely, offset humeral heads have been designed. This may be necessary because the center of rotation of the humeral shaft and the head do not coincide. While the concept makes intuitive sense, there is no study documenting that offset humeral heads result in better outcome. A relatively recent study by Pearl indicated that humeral offset designs resulted in better replication of anatomy in cadavers [13]. One potential problem for concentric heads is that they may protrude too anteriorly placing increased tension on the subscapularis. Trial reductions with concentric and offset heads should be performed to determine the final implant.

Patient Positioning

Interscalene regional anesthesia is preferred since it is safe and effective and provides excellent postoperative analgesia. However, general anesthesia may be added as an adjunct as well, especially in muscular patients in whom paralysis will be necessary for exposure. Intravenous antibiotics should be given before the incision and are continued for 24 to 48 hours postoperatively.

The patient is placed in the beach chair position with the operating table semi-reclined to approximately 45 to 60 degrees. The operative shoulder should be positioned over the lateral edge of the table to properly allow extension and better exposure. The patient's head should be secured to a soft cushioned head rest to avoid rotation or cervical spine hyperextension. A short arm side board should be attached at the mid aspect of the humeral shaft and can be shifted distally later to allow for arm extension. Two folded towels are placed under the ipsilateral scapula to minimize movement of the shoulder blade and deliver the glenoid more anteriorly. The arm is then draped free to allow the to flexion, extension and rotation without restrictions.

Approach

A standard deltopectoral approach is the most common incision for this procedure, although more recently minimally invasive incisions have been introduced. The deltopectoral skin incision begins just inferior to the clavicle, extends lateral to the coracoid, directed toward the insertion of the deltoid (Figure 2.2). The cephalic vein and deltopectoral interval are identified by a fat stripe. Retract the cephalic vein medially or laterally to avoid stretching and tearing as it traverses the clavipectoral fascia. There is a deep branch of the cephalic vein that is encountered proximally. It usually needs to be ligated for proper exposure. Incise the clavipectoral fascia lateral to the coracobrachialis and release any adhesions and bursal tissue. Retract the pectoralis medially with the conjoined tendon gently to avoid neurapraxia. The musculocutaneous nerve penetrates the lateral coracobrachialis muscle anywhere from 3.1 cm to 8.2 cm distal to the coracoid [15]. The deltoid should not be detached from either its origin or insertion in primary shoulder arthroplasty. There are some situations in revision surgery

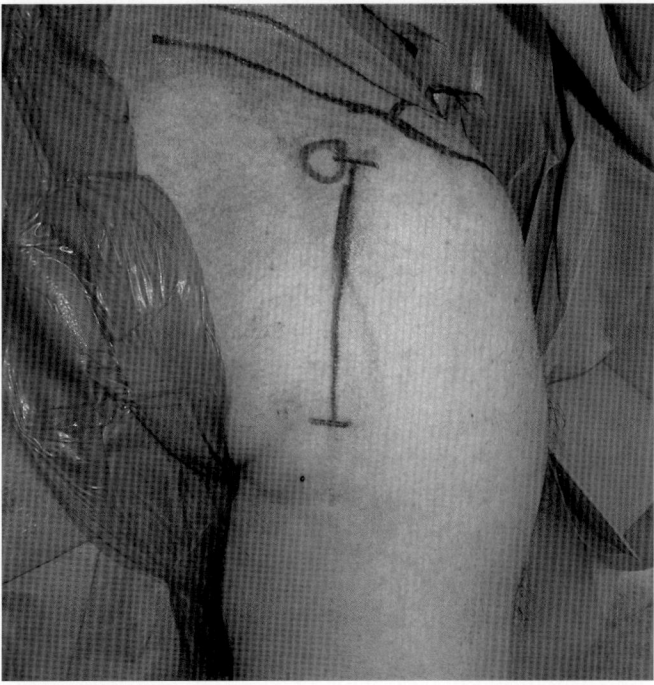

Figure 2.2. Deltopectoral incision drawn from coracoid to lateral deltoid insertion.

in which detachment of some or all of the deltoid may become necessary.

Once exposure is obtained, release any adhesions between the deltoid and coracoacromial ligament. The anterior humeral circumflex artery and its two veins are located at the inferior edge of the incision (just inferior to the subscapularis) and are either ligated or cauterized. The coracoacromial ligament should be preserved in most cases, especially in patients with rotator cuff tears since it is the only structure preventing superior migration. However, if it markedly limits exposure or external rotation, partial or complete excision may be necessary. In most cases, the pectoralis major does not require release. However, in extremely tight shoulders, the proximal 2 cm of pectoralis tendon can be released and repaired at the conclusion of the case. Care should be taken to avoid the long head of the biceps beneath the pectoralis major. Next, the rotator cuff should be exposed and bursal adhesions can be excised.

Attention can then be turned to the subscapularis by externally rotating the arm. Excise the subscapularis bursa to adequately visualize the tendinous insertion onto the lesser tuberosity. The rotator interval marks the superior extent of the tendon while the anterior humeral circumflex vessels identify its inferior extent. There are several options for subscapularis detachment depending on patient factors and surgeon choice.

Severe Loss of External Rotation (<0 Degrees with the Arm at the Side)

In patients with severe loss of external rotation, we prefer to take the subscapularis off as far laterally as possible to maximize length and restore motion postoperatively.

Normal External Rotation (i.e. Avascular Necrosis)

In most patients, we prefer to take the tendon off by leaving a stump on the lesser tuberosity for later repair.

Poor Tendon Quality (i.e. Prior Subscapularis Surgery)

In patients who have had prior instability surgery (Bankart, capsular shift, Magnuson-Stack), the subscapularis tendon may be of poor quality. In these rare cases, we prefer to take the tendon in its entirety as lateral as possible. Alternatively, in some instances, the entire tendon may be taken off with a small piece of bone as this may improve the strength of the repair.

The subscapularis routinely has severe contractures and should be released of these to allow proper mobilization and return of motion postoperatively. Preservation of the biceps tendon has become a controversial topic. There are some surgeons who recommend routine sacrifice of the biceps tendon to improve visualization and exposure [16–18]. We do not routinely resect the biceps tendon in all patients but instead make an individual decision in each patient based on quality of the tendon, visualization, and need for improved exposure. However, it is more common to perform a biceps tenodesis in recent years.

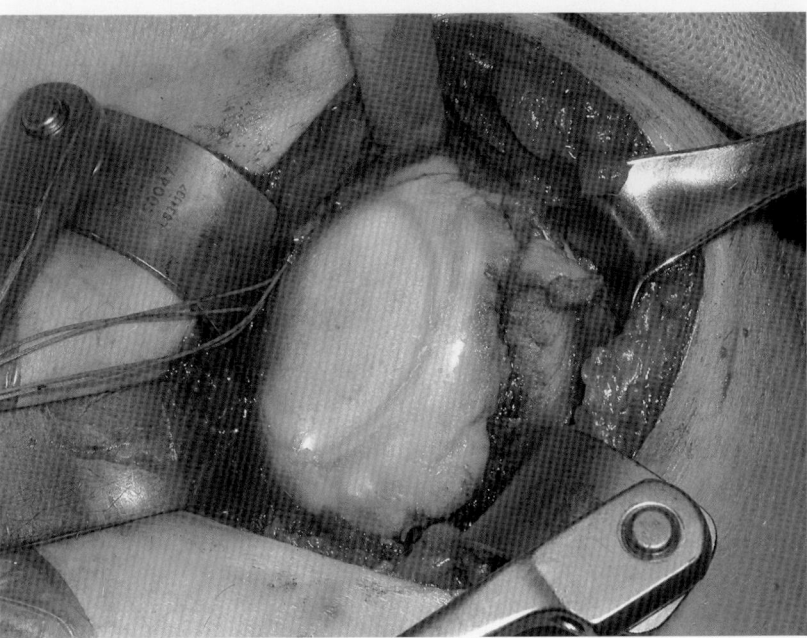

Figure 2.3. The humerus is delivered into the wound with extension, adduction, and external rotation. Excessive osteophyte formation has obscured the surgical neck area.

Next, the capsule should be released anteriorly and inferiorly. The posterior capsule is not released in the majority of patients as this may contribute to postoperative instability. Take caution to avoid the axillary nerve by externally rotating and flexing the arm. Release the capsule to at least 6 o'clock. Be sure to take down all of inferior capsule or exposure will be limited. The axillary nerve is always identified and protected at the inferior aspect of the capsular anatomy. We routinely perform a capsulectomy of the inferior and anterior capsule to allow for proper visualization and preparation of the glenoid component in total shoulder arthroplasty (TSA) (see Chapter 3).

The humerus can now be dislocated anteriorly with extension, adduction, and external rotation (Figure 2.3). This is facilitated by placing a metal finger superiorly in back of the biceps and a blunt elevator anteriorly and inferiorly to lever the head out.

Humeral Preparation

Once the humeral head has been properly exposed and osteophytes removed, the starting point for canal reaming is 3 mm to 5 mm posterior and 6 mm medial to the bicipital groove (Figure 2.4). The humeral canal center of axis is anterior and lateral to the center of axis for the humeral head. This places the entry point to ream down the center of the canal in the posterolateral corner of the humeral head cut. However, one should be careful with using the bicipital groove as a landmark.

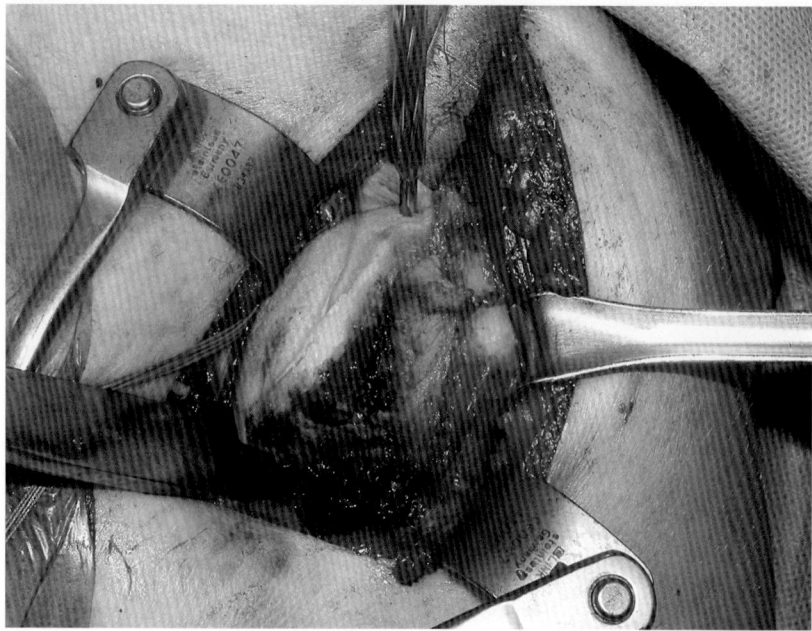

Figure 2.4. Starting point for humeral canal reaming medial and posterior to the bicipital groove.

While the bicipital groove is directly correlated with humeral head version, there is a fair amount of variability and in its relative geography and in its width [19]. Therefore, it is better to use the bicipital groove as a rough guideline more than an absolute landmark.

Reamers should be narrower at the tip and wider proximally given the tapering of the humerus in the coronal plane. Care is taken to avoid perforation of the canal by constantly orienting the reamer with the longitudinal axis of the humeral canal. Sequential reaming is done until mild resistance is met and there is a snug cortical fit.

Humeral Head Cut

Use a smooth metal finger to retract the biceps and rotator cuff posteriorly and another wide retractor to protect the glenoid. The use of a commercially available arm positioner greatly facilitates the exposure to allow gentle distraction and fixed position of the extremity.

The humeral head cut needs to take into account the neck shaft angle, which ranges from 30 to 50 degrees and varies directly with head size [11]. Neck shaft angle is predetermined by the prosthetic design. It should be noted that a shorter neck decreases the arc of motion. Shortening it 5mm would decrease the range of motion from 160 to 136 degrees [20].

Errors in neck cuts have important implications. Decreased cut angles can result in leaving articular cartilage laterally or resection of medial calcar. This results in a varus alignment and overstuffing of the joint secondary to an inferior and often medialized stem. Cutting at a higher neck shaft angle results in a valgus alignment and superior placement of the head [12]. While this could be corrected with head selection, proper recreation of anatomy is the priority.

The height of the cut is determined by the supraspinatus tendon insertion, typically it is 8 mm ± 3.2 mm cephalad to the superior edge of the greater tuberosity [11]. An overaggressive head cut results in greater tuberosity impingement on the acromion. On the other hand, however, undercutting will result in *overstuffing*, leading to increased soft tissue tension, increased load on the glenoid, decreases motion, and pain.

Before the humeral head is cut, excise all osteophytes surrounding the articular surface that might alter the perception of the true neck of the humerus. This aids in preventing a varus or valgus cut (Figure 2.5). The system we use relies on an intramedullary guide for making the humeral head cut. When the largest reamer is felt to be of good fit (determined by cortical *chatter* and rotational control), the handle is removed, the reamer left in the canal, and the cutting jig is then applied. Before cutting, proper retroversion needs to be assessed by using the transepicondylar axis or special version instrumentation (Figure 2.6).

The normal range of retroversion is 20 to 40 degrees. Retroversion is crucial for prosthetic stability and motion. It also allows normalization of soft tissue tension and proper articulation with the prosthetic glenoid. Originally, the trend in humeral stem placement was to standardize the retroversion. However, several authors have indicated that study of the version of the proximal humerus is difficult and highly variable [9, 21, 22]. For this reason, the current emphasis is to adjust version to match each patient's own shoulder's retroversion. Retro-

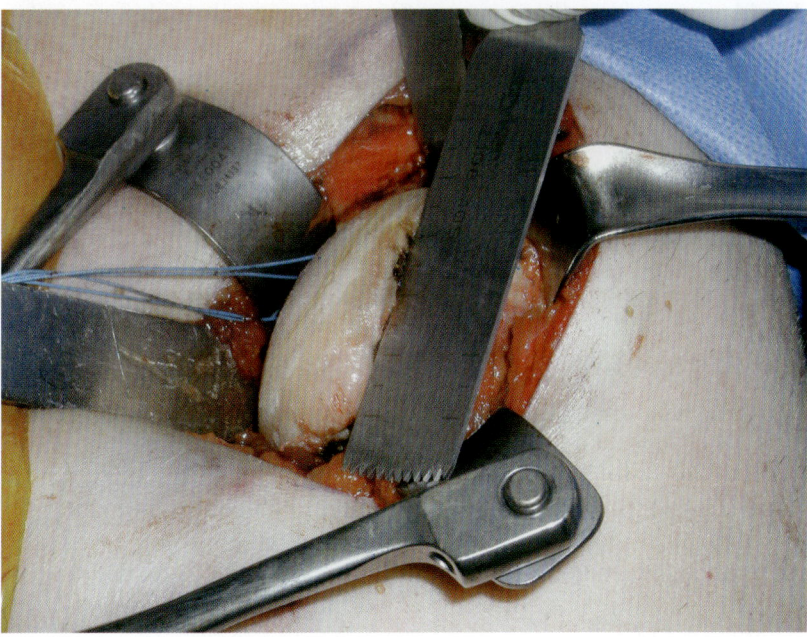

Figure 2.5. If osteophytes are not removed, incorrect humeral head cuts can easily be performed.

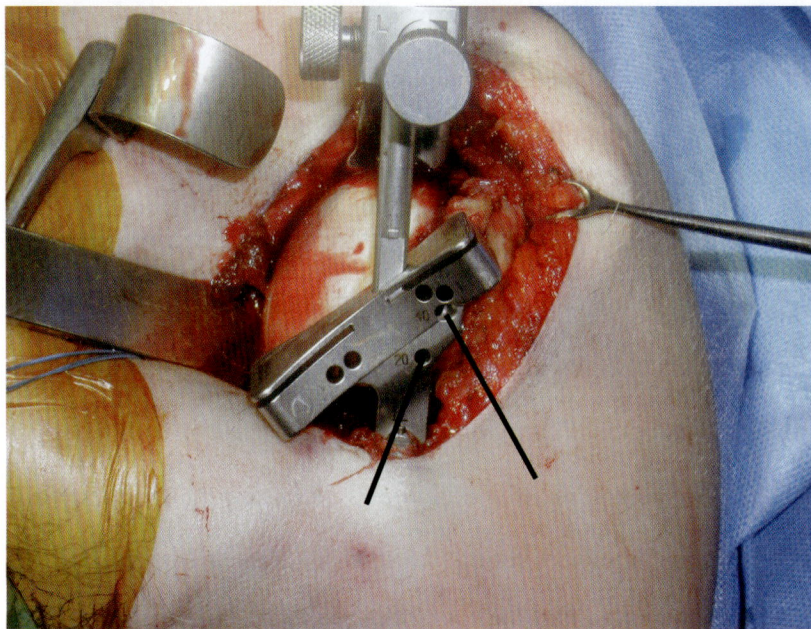

Figure 2.6. Humeral cutting jig applied to reamer with version rods in place.

version may need to be decreased accordingly in shoulders with significant posterior glenoid wear to avoid posterior instability. Of course, glenoid component placement is also critical in the ultimate decision-making of the overall version of the two components. Conversely, in shoulders in which there is significant anterior glenoid wear, more humeral component retroversion may be necessary to avoid anterior instability.

After confirmation of proper head height and retroversion, the head cut is made with an oscillating saw. Care is again taken at this step to protect against inadvertent injury to the rotator cuff. A trial implant (same size as final reamer) is then placed in the previously determined retroversion (and confirmed with the version rods or the transepicondylar axis).

Humeral Head Trial

Trial prosthetic heads are then placed to match the patient's anatomy. Preoperative templating should be used to help determine the proper head. We recommend routine radiographs of the contralateral shoulder (if it is not pathological) to try and recreate the normal head height. In addition, the resected humeral head is measured and compared with the available prosthetic heads on the back table. It is important to measure only the head height and not any osteophytes or involved metaphyseal bone.

The proper head size allows approximately 50% translation in all planes with the subscapularis provisionally tensioned to mimic the final repair situation. When a decision between two sizes occurs, we recommend choosing the smaller of the two sizes to avoid over-stuffing of the joint.

Final decision-making involves choosing between concentric and off-set heads. As mentioned previously, there are currently no clinical series to support the superiority of offset heads, but they do seem to better replicate the anatomy and therefore have increased in popularity over the last decade (Figure 2.7A and 2.7B).

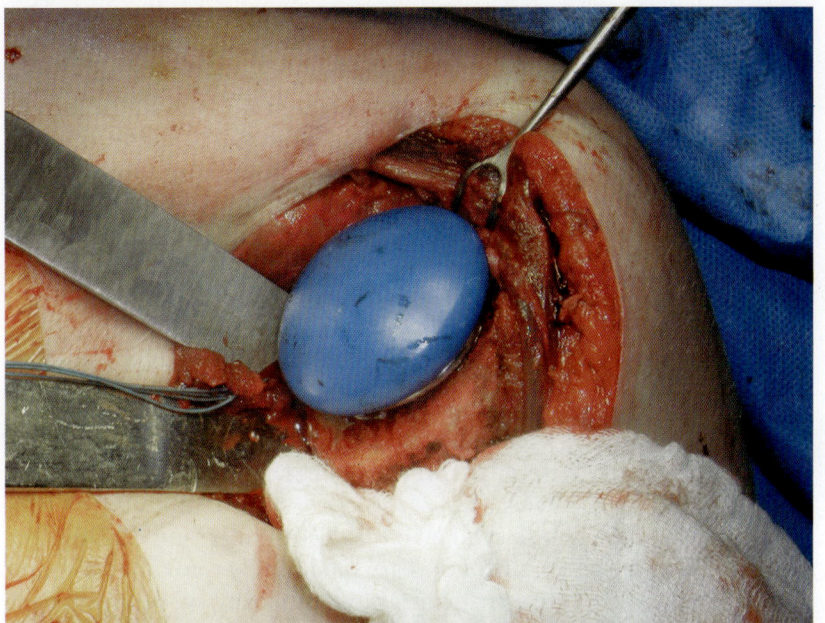

A

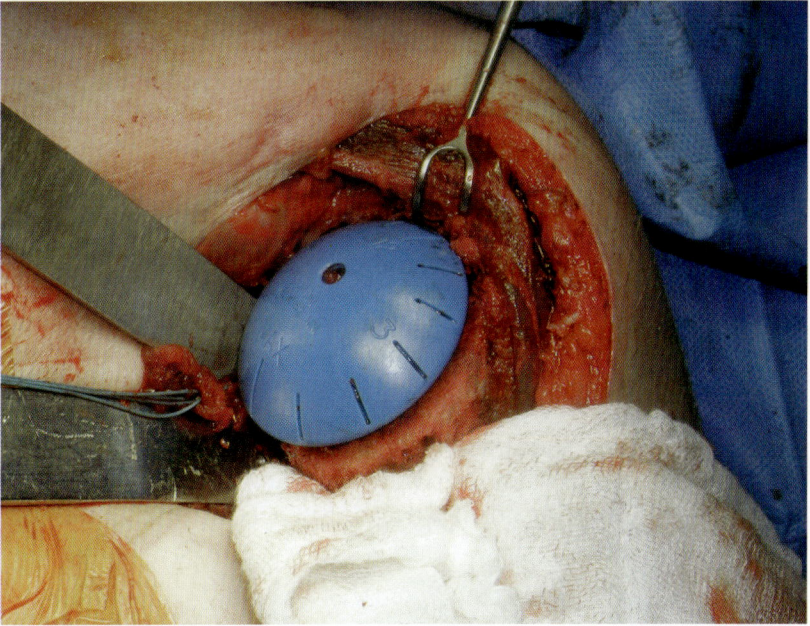

B

Figure 2.7. The humeral trial is in position with a **(A)** concentric head and an **(B)** eccentric head.

The head should be stable anteriorly in 60 degrees of external rotation relative to the scapular plane and posteriorly in the adducted, internally rotated position. After trialing is performed, a calcar planer is used to level the humeral osteotomy and ensure circumferential contact with the collar of the prosthesis.

Stem Size

The medullary canal is shaped like a champagne flute on the anteroposterior radiograph and like a stove pipe on the lateral radiograph. This makes it difficult to obtain intimate contact between the prosthesis and bone. Distally, there is improved cortical bone and stem contact can be achieved in this region. Typically, shaft diameters range from 6 mm to 20 mm, requiring a wide variety of stem sizes. Stem size can be assessed by preoperative radiographs and templating from the diameter of the distal cortical bone. Proximally, prostheses are designed with fins that can be cut into slots in the bone to control rotational stability [23].

The optimal length for the humeral stem is six times the diameter of the humerus. This allows for proper distribution of stress. Prostheses that are too long can lead to *windshield wiping* and associated bone resorption, while short prostheses may not provide adequate fixation [24].

Preparation for Subscapularis Repair

If the subscapularis has been taken off its lesser tuberosity insertion (as far laterally as possible), drill holes are made in the proximal humeral shaft prior to humeral prosthetic insertion. Typically, we recommend 5 drill holes and placement of heavy (either no. 2 or 5) nonabsorbable braided sutures for the tendon repair.

If a stump of subscapularis was left for repair, then several additional bone sutures are used as an adjunct to the soft-tissue repair (i.e., tendon to tendon repair). If the lesser tuberosity has been osteotomized then wire or heavy (either no. 2 or 5) nonabsorbable sutures are used.

Stem Insertion

Decision-making on press-fit versus cementation remains controversial. We prefer to use patients' age, bone quality, and humeral canal type in each case to determine the type of fixation. In patients who are young (<60) with good bone quality and appropriate bone-prosthetic contact, we prefer press-fit fixation. However, in older patients with poorer bone quality and stove-pipe type proximal anatomy, we prefer cement fixation. In most patients with rheumatoid arthritis we recommend cement fixation as detailed previously.

Press-Fit

Reaming is performed up to the proper size as determined by cortical chatter, rotational control and preoperative templating. In the system

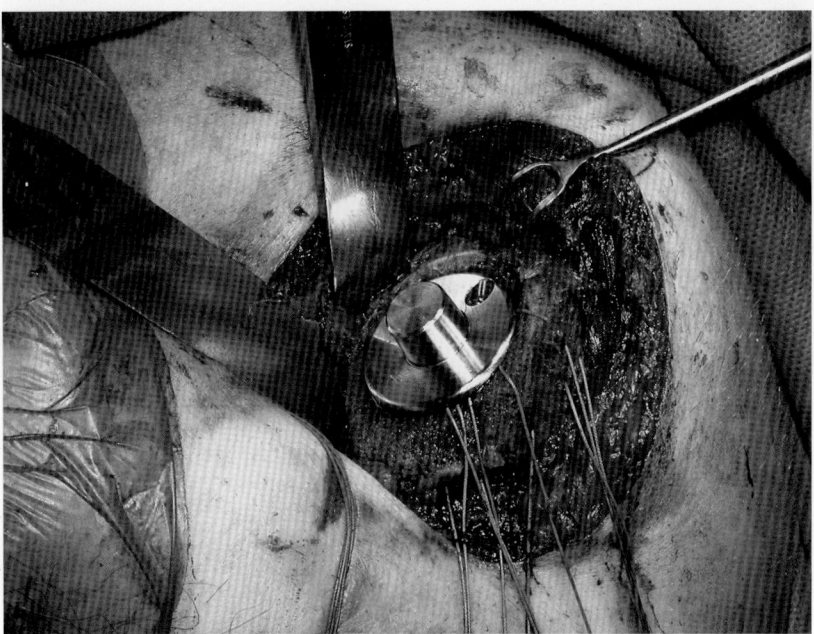

Figure 2.8. Humeral prosthesis in final position with subscap sutures previously placed.

we use, the same size final implant is then chosen (i.e., 10-mm trial and a corresponding 10-mm prosthesis). When the trial is placed, rotate the entire inserter/trial device. If the trial rotates, the press-fit technique may not be advisable. In this setting, either ream up one size or convert to a cemented implant. The final implant is placed on the humeral inserter and final version can again be confirmed. The implant is then gently tapped into final position and the insertion device is removed (Figure 2.8).

Cement Fixation

A cement restrictor is placed 1 cm distal to the final resting position of the prosthesis to assist in cement containment. The cement restrictor is typically the same size as the final reamer size. The medullary canal is then properly prepared by pulse saline irrigation with a commercially available system, followed by thrombin-soaked gauze dressings to minimize bleeding. A large dressing is placed into the glenoid to protect it from extruded cement. One package of polymethyl-methacrylate cement is then mixed and placed into a 60-ml syringe. When the cement achieves a doughy consistency, it is injected into the medullary canal. Pressurizing the cement (as is performed in hip arthroplasty) is not necessary and may lead to humeral shaft fracture, especially in osteoporotic bone. Remove any excess cement from the surrounding soft tissues and hold the prosthesis in position to prevent rotation and movement into malposition. Ideally, we like to use a minimal amount of cement, as the humeral component should be reamed closely to the inside diameter of the humeral canal.

Finally, place the real humeral head prosthesis on in the previously determined position (if an off-set head is chosen) and gently tap into position. Reduce the humerus and repair the subscapularis with the previously placed heavy nonabsorbable sutures. The rest of the wound is then closed in layers over a drain and a subcuticular suture is placed to close the wound. A dry sterile dressing and a sling with the arm in neutral position is then applied.

Complications

Overstuffing

A medialized stem or an oversized head may lead to increased volume within the glenohumeral joint. This places increased tension on the capsule and rotator cuff, which can lead to decreased joint motion and possible rupture of the subscapularis repair. Avoid this with preoperative templating and testing the stability as well as the motion prior to committing to the final prosthesis.

Humeral Loosening

Natural progression of development in long bones is to develop wider diaphyseal canals over time. Torchia et al. reported 49% asymptomatic loosening in press-fit stems and none in cemented components [4]. While this may occur in cemented or press-fit stems, it is more likely in press-fit stems, especially in osteoporotic bone. Therefore, the best prevention of this complication is to cement the humeral prosthesis in some cases, especially when bone quality and shape are of concern. Revision to a cemented stem is indicated when symptomatic humeral loosening occurs.

Posterior Subluxation

Posterior capsular stretching and posterior glenoid wear provide the basis for the most common instability pattern associated with TSA. Patients with degenerative arthritis often lose external rotation leading to contracture of the anterior capsule, thus pushing the humeral head posteriorly. Increased posterior pressure creates this wear pattern and stretching of the posterior capsule. Intraoperative assessment of this potential complication is critical. The following technical pointers are provided to avoid this complication:

1. Use the offset (eccentric) head to correct for potential posterior instability. While a posterior offset head may recreate anatomy, it can also lead to posterior instability because the head is less anterior to the central axis of the humeral head. Avoid the temptation to use a larger head size to correct for prosthetic instability as this may only overstuff the joint and lead to a global loss of motion. We recommend increasing the head size as a last resort if all other techniques mentioned fail to gain appropriate stability.

2. Retroversion can be altered to improve stability. This should be taken into consideration at the beginning of the case, for example, in patients with extreme posterior wear identified on preoperative radiographs and/or CT scan. In these cases, choose a decreased retroversion angle to make the humeral cut and thereby decrease the likelihood of posterior instability. Take care not to change retroversion too much as this can create anterior instability and place tension on the subscapularis repair.

3. Soft tissues should be balanced. If instability persists, posterior capsular imbrication can be performed with suture to achieve optimal capsular tension. Best results are achieved when imbrication is preformed close to the glenoid surface with an *inside-out technique*. A second incision is not necessary and this can always be performed from the anterior deltopectoral incision.

Anterior Instability

This is an uncommon problem. It is usually associated with anterior glenoid deficiency. Again, this can be corrected with adjustment of head offset. Increasing retroversion no more than 5 degrees may assist and should be determined before the humeral head cut. Tightening of the subscapularis is a final option to consider; however, it should be done judiciously to avoid restricting external rotation.

Impingement

This complication is best avoided of course by proper placement of the humeral prosthesis within the canal. Maintenance of proper humeral tuberosity interval, head height, size, and appropriate humeral neck shaft cuts all play a significant role in preventing this complication.

If impingement does occur, carefully scrutinize the placement of the prosthesis. If it is only minimally inferiorly situated, an acromioplasty may be all that is needed to correct the problem. However, if there is significant component malposition, it is appropriate to consider revision of the humeral prosthesis to restore the appropriate anatomic relationships and avoid the impingement.

References

1. Kelly IG. Unconstrained shoulder arthroplasty in rheumatoid arthritis. Clin Orthop 1994;307:94–102.
2. Stewart MP, Kelly IG. Total shoulder replacement in rheumatoid disease: 7- to 13-year follow-up of 37 joints. J Bone Joint Surg Br 1997;79(1):68–72.
3. Harris TE, Jobe CM, Dai QG. Fixation of proximal humeral prostheses and rotational micromotion. J Shoulder Elbow Surg 2000;9(3):205–210.
4. Torchia ME, Cofield RH, Settergren CR. Total shoulder arthroplasty with the Neer prosthesis: long-term results. J Shoulder Elbow Surg 1997; 6(6):495–505.
5. Matsen FA III, Iannotti JP, Rockwood CA Jr. Humeral fixation by press-fitting of a tapered metaphyseal stem: a prospective radiographic study. J Bone Joint Surg Am 2003;85-A(2):304–308.

6. Neer CS II, Watson KC, Stanton FJ, Recent experience in total shoulder replacement. J Bone Joint Surg Am 1982;64(3):319–337.

7. Peppers TA, Jobe CM, Dai QG, et al. Fixation of humeral prostheses and axial micromotion. J Shoulder Elbow Surg 1998;7(4):414–418.

8. Blevins FT, Deng X, Torzilli PA, et al. Dissociation of modular humeral head components: a biomechanical and implant retrieval study. J Shoulder Elbow Surg 1997;6(2):113–124.

9. Boileau P, Walch G. The three-dimensional geometry of the proximal humerus. Implications for surgical technique and prosthetic design. J Bone Joint Surg Br 1997;79(5):857–865.

10. Pearl ML, Volk AG. Coronal plane geometry of the proximal humerus relevant to prosthetic arthroplasty. J Shoulder Elbow Surg 1996;5(4):320–326.

11. Iannotti JP, Gabriel JP, Schneck SL, et al. The normal glenohumeral relationships. An anatomical study of one hundred and forty shoulders. J Bone Joint Surg Am 1992;74(4):491–500.

12. Pearl ML, Kurutz S. Geometric analysis of commonly used prosthetic systems for proximal humeral replacement. J Bone Joint Surg Am 1999; 81(5):660–671.

13. Pearl ML, Kurutz S, Robertson DD, et al. Geometric analysis of selected press fit prosthetic systems for proximal humeral replacement. J Orthop Res 2002;20(2):192–197.

14. Soslowsky LJ, Flatow EL, Bigliani LU, et al. Articular geometry of the glenohumeral joint. Clin Orthop 1992;285:181–190.

15. Flatow EL, Bigliani LU, April EW. An anatomic study of the musculocutaneous nerve and its relationship to the coracoid process. Clin Orthop 1989; 244:166–171.

16. Boileau P, Avidor C, Krishnan SG, et al. Cemented polyethylene versus uncemented metal-backed glenoid components in total shoulder arthroplasty: a prospective, double-blind, randomized study. J Shoulder Elbow Surg 2002;11(4):351–359.

17. Edwards TB, Kadakia NR, Boulakia A, et al. A comparison of hemiarthroplasty and total shoulder arthroplasty in the treatment of primary glenohumeral osteoarthritis: results of a multicenter study. J Shoulder Elbow Surg 2003;12(3):207–213.

18. Walch G, Boileau P. Prosthetic adaptability: a new concept for shoulder arthroplasty. J Shoulder Elbow Surg 1999;8(5):443–451.

19. Kummer FJ, Perkins R, Zuckerman JD. The use of the bicipital groove for alignment of the humeral stem in shoulder arthroplasty. J Shoulder Elbow Surg 1998;7(2):144–146.

20. Jobe CM, Iannotti JP. Limits imposed on glenohumeral motion by joint geometry. J Shoulder Elbow Surg 1995;4(4):281–285.

21. Flatow EL. Prosthetic design considerations in total shoulder arthroplasty. Semin Arthroplasty 1995;6(4):233–244.

22. Tillet E, Fulcher M, Shanklin J. Anatomic determination of humeral head retroversion: the relationship of the central axis of the humeral head to the bicipital groove. J Shoulder Elbow Surg 1993;2:255–256.

23. Neer CS II. Replacement arthroplasty for glenohumeral osteoarthritis. J Bone Joint Surg Am 1974;56(1):1–13.

24. Orr TE, Carter DR. Stress analyses of joint arthroplasty in the proximal humerus. J Orthop Res 1985;3(3):360–371.

Chapter 3

Glenoid Component Preparation and Soft Tissue Releases

Kevin J. Setter, Ilya Voloshin, and Christopher S. Ahmad

In 1974, Charles Neer reported his early results of shoulder hemiarthroplasty for the treatment of glenohumeral arthritis and concluded that a properly performed hemiarthroplasty could relieve pain, halt joint deterioration, and withstand normal use [1]. More recently, reports of shoulder osteoarthritis treated with hemiarthroplasty have demonstrated deterioration of good initial results with longer term follow-up [2]. Several studies have compared the outcome of total shoulder replacement to hemiarthroplasty for degenerative shoulder conditions and have demonstrated improved pain relief and satisfaction with glenoid resurfacing compared with humeral head replacement alone [3–7]. In the past decade, there has been an increasing number of shoulder arthroplasties performed in the United States, with more than 20,000 arthroplasties implanted each year. Approximately half of these arthroplasties are total shoulder arthroplasties (TSAs) [8]. Still, many surgeons find replacing the glenoid technically demanding and time consuming and fear eventual glenoid component loosening. Successful glenoid resurfacing requires a thorough understanding of both glenoid bony pathology and adjacent soft tissue pathology to achieve exposure, proper implantation, and soft tissue balancing.

Indications and Contraindications

The most common etiologies leading to TSA include primary degenerative arthritis, inflammatory arthritis, osteonecrosis, posttraumatic arthritis, and arthritis following instability procedures [9], with degenerative osteoarthritis accounting for approximately 60%. Patient factors required for successful glenoid replacement include a functioning rotator cuff, functioning deltoid, and adequate glenoid bone stock to support the component. Rotator cuff dysfunction permits superior migration of the humeral head causing eccentric loading of the glenoid component and early loosening [3, 10–13]. Similarly, a dysfunctional deltoid can result in instability of the humeral component relative to the glenoid component, resulting in glenoid loosening. Loosening may also occur if the glenoid bone stock is not large enough to support the periphery of the component or the keel or pegs of the implant within the glenoid vault.

Rotator cuff tears are found in approximately 5% of patients undergoing shoulder arthroplasty for degenerative arthritis [14]. Glenoid replacement is still recommended if the tear is repairable. For patients with rheumatoid arthritis (RA), rotator cuff pathology is observed in 10% to 50% of patients [12, 15–18]. In addition, extensive central erosion of the glenoid may occur. Therefore, for RA patients with either nonfunctional rotator cuffs, irreparable cuff tears, or severe glenoid erosion, TSA is contraindicated and hemiarthroplasty is recommended. For patients with arthritis after instability repair, several studies have also indicated better results with TSA compared with hemiarthroplasty [19, 20]. Special issues with these patients involve young age and unbalanced soft tissues. For patients with osteonecrosis, TSA is preferred to hemiarthroplasty when the glenoid is damaged [21]. Arthroplasty should be avoided in neuropathic arthropathy of the shoulder, the most common cause being syringomyelia [22]. The sensation and proprioception deficits that result in joint destruction will also cause early component loosening.

Preoperative Evaluation

Preoperative planning has been described in Chapter 1; however, several points related to glenoid preparation are emphasized. Standard radiographs must be used to assess degree of both glenoid arthrosis and glenoid wear pattern. The AP radiograph should assess humeral head position with superior migration indicating rotator cuff dysfunction or medialization indicating decreased glenoid vault volume. An axillary view is necessary to assess glenoid vault volume, extent of posterior glenoid wear, and alterations in glenoid version. If plain radiographs do not inadequately visualize the glenoid, a CT or MRI should be obtained. Both MRI and CT scan clearly delineate bony changes while the MRI adds additional information on the integrity of the rotator cuff.

Patient history and physical examination can predict technical difficulty of glenoid replacement and assist with preoperative planning. History of previous instability procedures suggests excessive anterior soft tissue tightening and contractures. On physical examination, loss of passive external rotation, especially when limited to less than 20 degrees, indicates anterior soft contractures and potentially excessive posterior glenoid wear that would need to be addressed for adequate glenoid exposure and proper implantation.

Technique

Positioning

Regional anesthesia is preferred when possible for better postoperative pain control and enhanced recovery [23]. Proper patient positioning is important with a table that supports the scapula. The patient must be positioned lateral enough on the table to allow the operative extremity to be adducted, extended, and externally rotated without being hindered by the side of the table. To prevent scapular retraction, two folded towels are placed under the medial border of the scapula. The patient is placed in the beach chair position with the thorax at 45 degrees. A headrest is used to support the neck in neutral position.

Approach

Exposure of the glenoid requires adequate soft tissue releases as well as proper retractor selection and placement. Without proper exposure, glenoid resurfacing can be time consuming, frustrating, and poorly performed. Traditionally, we have employed a standard deltopectoral incision. More recently, a more cosmetic hidden axillary incision has been used in selected patients (Figure 3.1). It is contraindicated for patients with excessive stiffness, passive external rotation less than 20 degrees, excessive posterior wear, or severe bony deformity.

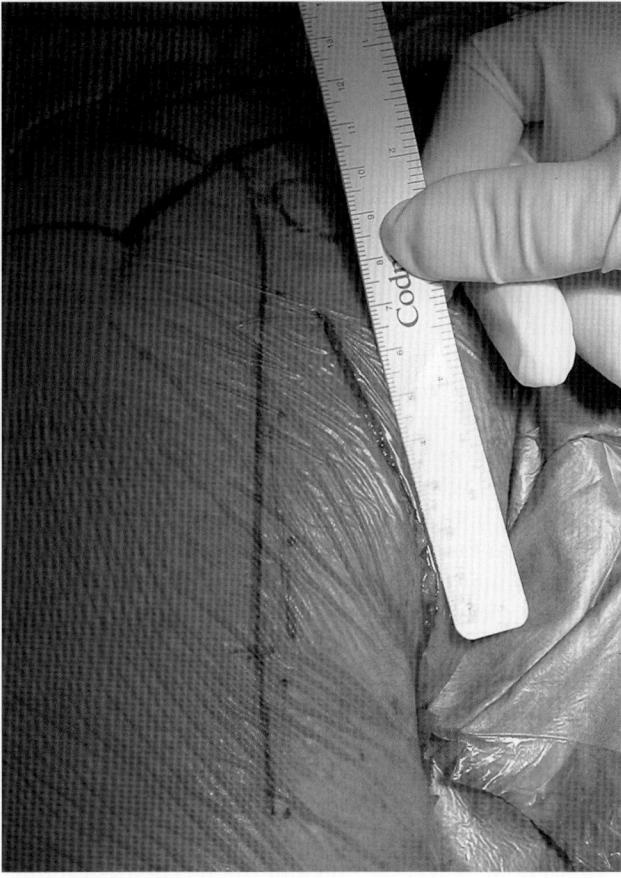

Figure 3.1. Hidden axillary incision (approximately 7 cm) adjacent to ruler used in selected patients. The skin incision for the standard deltopectoral approach is marked more laterally (right shoulder).

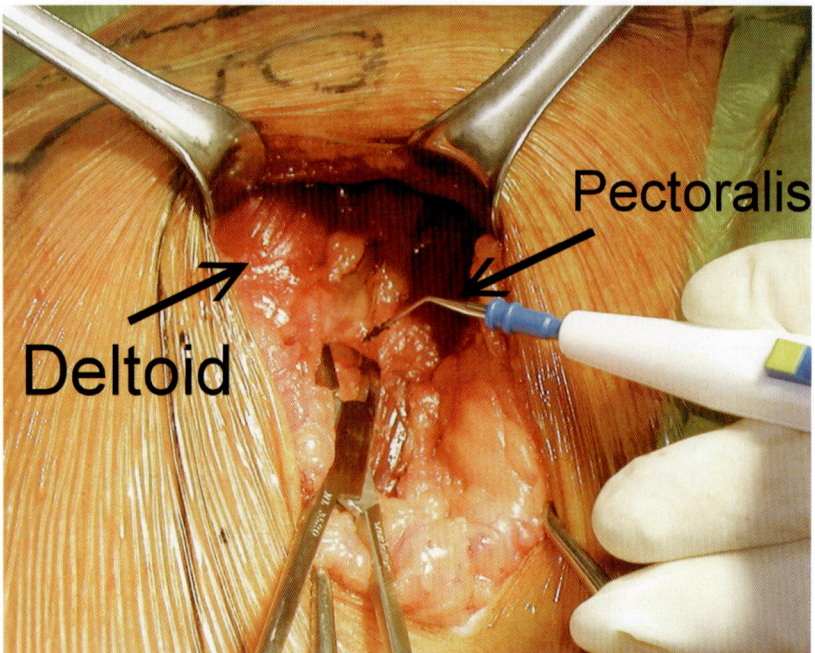

Figure 3.2. Full-thickness skin flaps are developed with mobilization in all directions. The deltopectoral interval is identified, finding the cephalic vein.

With either incision, full-thickness skin flaps are raised medially and laterally. The deltopectoral interval is identified. Often it is easiest to find the interval by looking for the triangular fat streak proximally. The cephalic vein is unroofed in the interval (Figure 3.2) and branches are cauterized or ligated. Large cross-over branches are often found superiorly at the fat triangle near the coracoid. The vein is preferentially retracted laterally as we have noted fewer branches from the pectoralis major. The upper .5 cm to 1 cm of pectoralis major tendon is then identified, tagged, and released, taking care to avoid injury to the long head of the bicep tendon, which lies deep to the pectoralis tendon (Figure 3.3). This increases both inferior exposure as well as external rotation.

The clavipectoral fascia is exposed and incised lateral to the strap muscle tendons, identified at their insertion on the coracoid. It should be recognized that distally, the muscle belly of the strap muscles are more lateral than the tendon. Care should be taken not to enter this plane when dissecting lateral to the conjoint tendon. Blunt finger dissection under the strap muscles facilitates safe placement of a Richardson retractor for medial retraction. The anteriolateral leading edge of the coracoacromial ligament is identified and resected to increase superior exposure (Figure 3.4). A finger or an elevator is then used to free adhesions beneath the deltoid and acromion to develop the subacromial and subdeltoid space. This facilitates placement of retractors with less injury to the deltoid muscle. With a large Richardson retractor under the deltoid, a bursectomy of the subdeltoid space is performed. This more clearly exposes the superior and inferior borders of the subscapularis. The lower border is heralded by the anterior circumflex

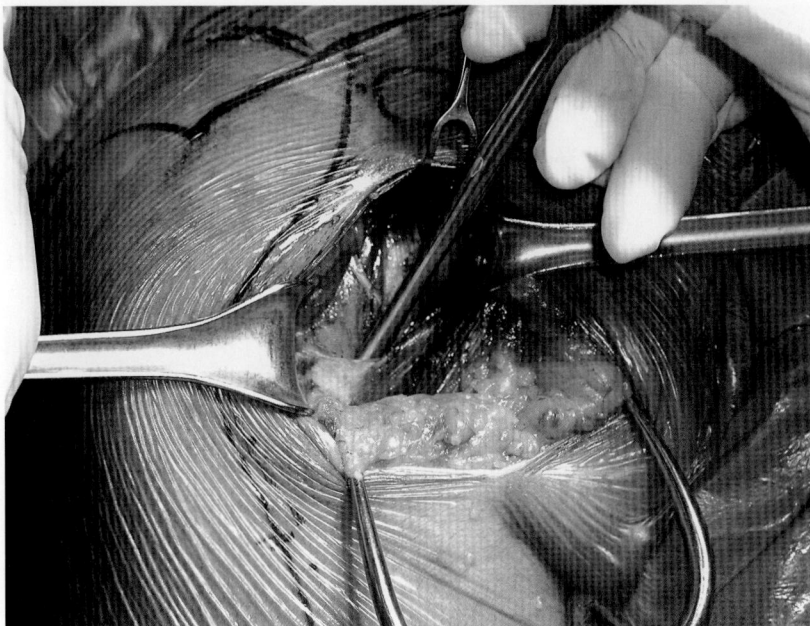

Figure 3.3. The pectoralis insertion is identified, tagged, and released. It is anatomically repaired at the conclusion of the procedure. This release improves inferior exposure and external rotation.

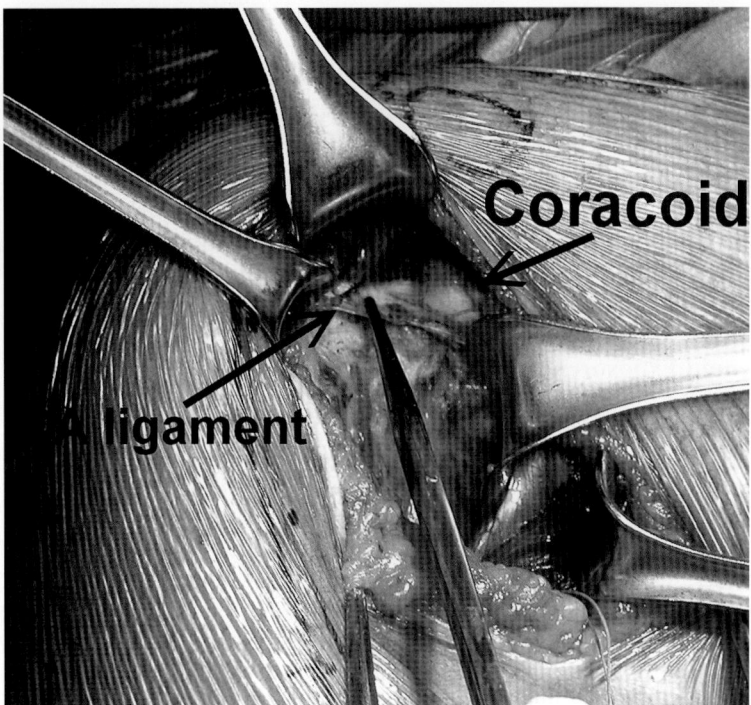

Figure 3.4. The clavipectoral fascia has been incised laterally and a Richardson retractor placed for medial exposure. With the clavipectoral fascia incised, the coracoacromial (CA) ligament is identified and the anterolateral leading edge is excised improving superior exposure.

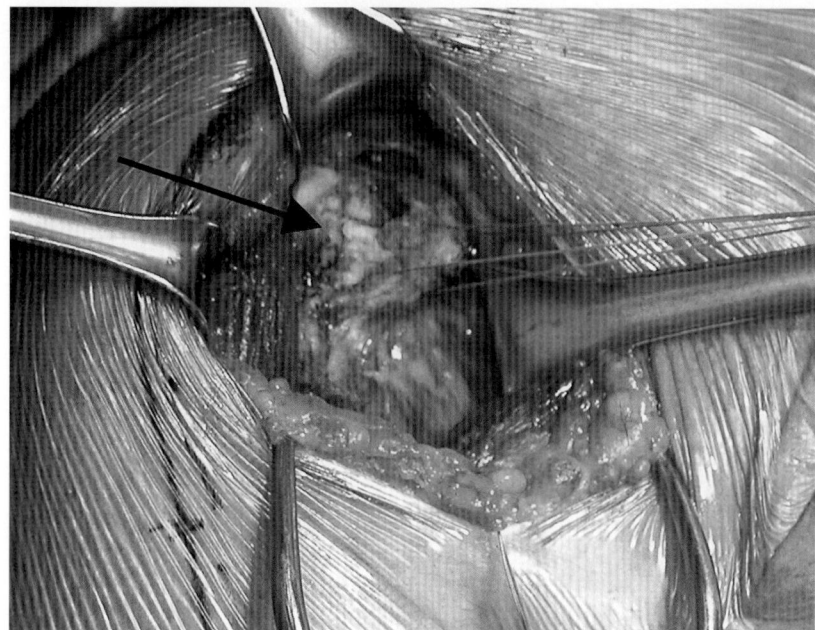

Figure 3.5. The subscapularis and anterior capsule are released laterally off the lesser tuberosity (just medial to the bicep tendon, *arrow*) for maximum length.

vessels, which are coagulated or ligated. The upper border can be identified by visualizing or palpating the rotator interval. The subscapularis and confluent anterior capsule are detached as one layer from the lesser tuberosity just medial to the bicipital groove as shown in Figure 3.5. The inferior capsule is released from the humerus to the 6 o'clock position with the humerus held in abduction and external rotation to move the axillary nerve away from the dissection. The capsular release from the neck of the humerus can be extended to the 9 o'clock position if necessary for increased exposure or osteophyte removal. The humerus is dislocated anteriorly and prepared as described in Chapter 2.

Glenoid Exposure

The provisional humeral stem component is kept in place to protect the humerus from retractors placed during glenoid exposure. A Fukuda retractor is hooked behind the posterior glenoid rim and retracts the humerus posteriorly (Figure 3.6). Slight flexion and abduction of the humerus to approximately 70 degrees reduces soft tissue tension facilitating placement of the Fukuda retractor. Other types of retractors that are more malleable that hook the posterior glenoid and posteriorly depress the shaft can also be used. Often we place both retractors and choose the retractor that affords the best exposure. The proper choice of posterior retractor for the best exposure is dictated by the patient's anatomy. A metal finger retracts the deltoid superiorly, exposing the superior glenoid. Hypertrophic synovial tissue surrounding the glenoid is removed using a Bovie cautery. The contracted anterior

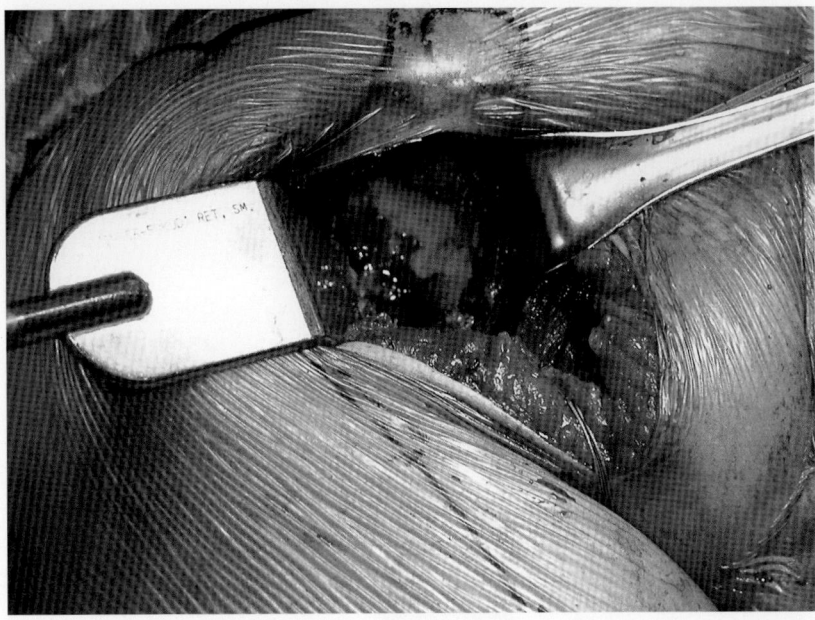

Figure 3.6. Care must be taken when dissecting the capsule off the inferior neck as the axillary nerve is in close proximity. A Darrach retractor can be used inferiorly to protect the axillary nerve. A Fukuda retractor is used to retract the humerus posteriorly.

capsule is then removed from the under surface of the subscapularis. The anterior capsulectomy assists with mobilization of the contracted subscapularis (Figure 3.7). Care must be taken not to button hole through the tendon or injury the axillary nerve. A spiked Darrach can be placed on the anterior glenoid neck for anterior exposure.

Glenoid Preparation

Following adequate glenoid exposure, glenoid preparation begins with removing remaining cartilage from the glenoid down to subchondral bone using a scraping instrument (Figure 3.8). The center of the glenoid must then be accurately determined and is often distorted by osteophytes. A rongeur can be used to carefully remove marginal osteophytes with care to avoid inadvertent detachment of the posterior capsule that could lead to posterior instability.

The glenoid size is matched against the largest trial that does not allow overhang. Most total shoulder systems include a choice of sizes that allow flexibility to conform to individual patient anatomy. For example, the system we use has three choices for size and curvature: 40 mm, 46 mm, and 52 mm. The glenoid-centering guide is placed and the glenoid center marked with Bovie cautery through the guide. The centering guide is then removed and the glenoid is visually inspected to ensure the accurate positioning of the centering hole before drilling (Figure 3.9). The centering guide is then reinserted and a finger is placed along the anterior glenoid neck to determine the proper angle

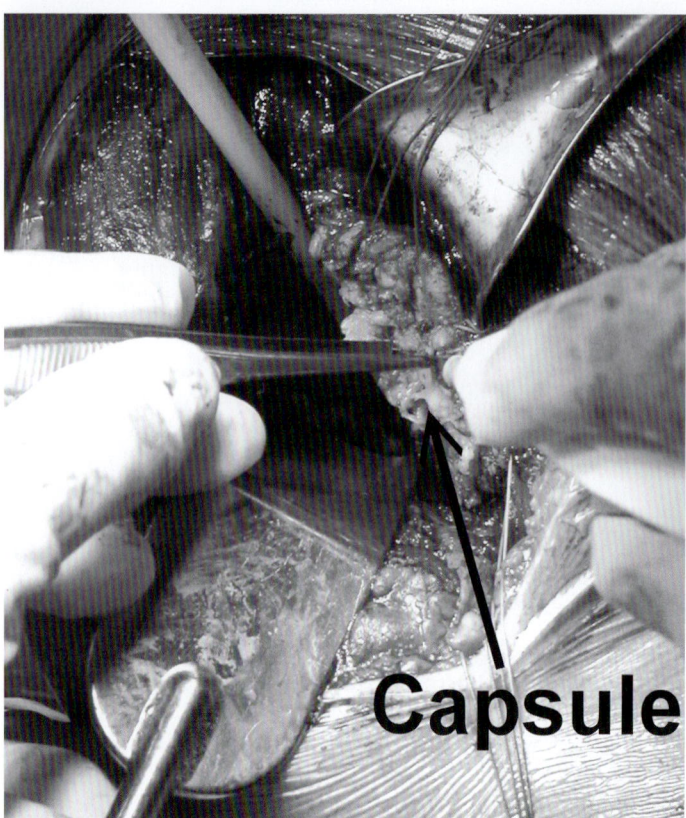

Figure 3.7. The contracted anterior capsule (*arrow*) is carefully excised from the undersurface of the subscapularis.

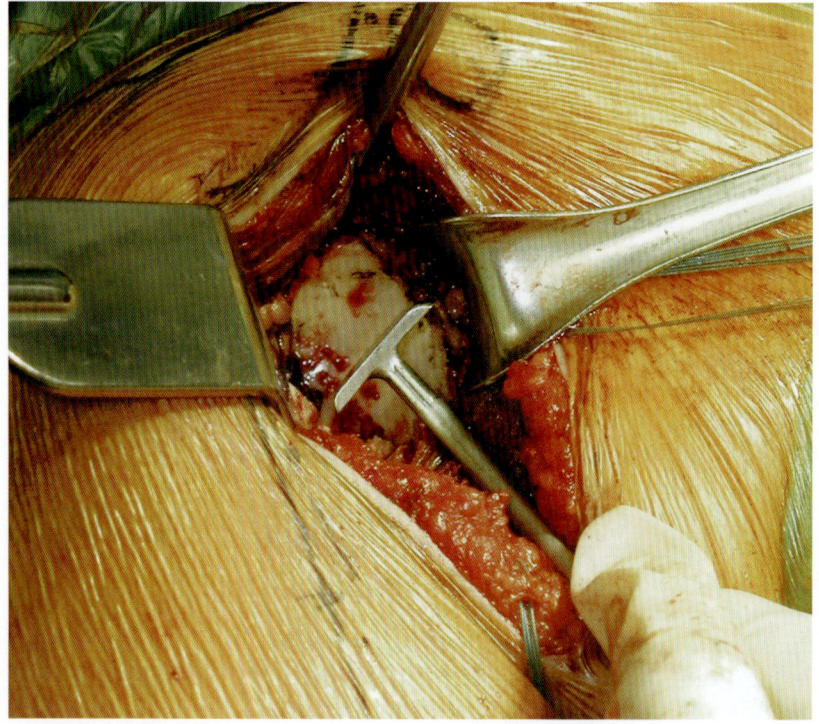

Figure 3.8. Remaining cartilage is removed from the glenoid surface with a scraper.

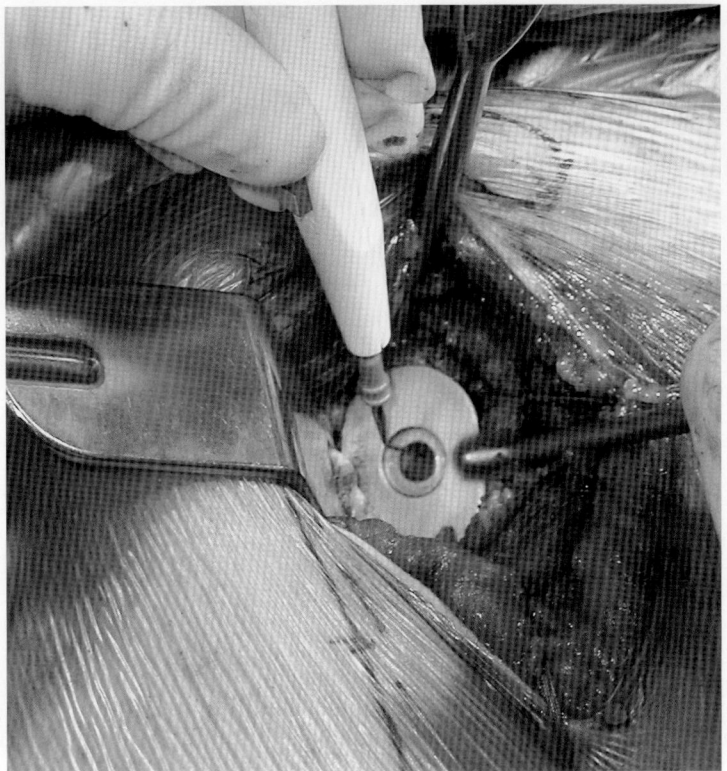

Figure 3.9. The sizing and centering guide is used to mark the center of the glenoid.

of the glenoid vault. The centering hole is then drilled. A probe can be used to ensure the centering hole is contained within the vault. Glenoid surface reaming is then performed with attention to maintaining or correcting glenoid version. Visualization of both the direction and amount of bone being reamed is improved with an open-faced reamer (Figure 3.10). When posterior glenoid wear exists, glenoid version is corrected by selectively removing anterior bone.

The science regarding pegged versus keeled glenoids is discussed later in this chapter. The appropriate guide for the component selected is inserted into the centering hole. For a pegged glenoid, the superior and inferior holes are drilled. Once the superior hole is drilled, a derotation pin can be placed through the superior hole to ensure good positioning of the inferior hole (Figure 3.11A and 3.11B). For a keeled glenoid, the three holes are drilled in a similar manner. Then a slotted guide is inserted and a 5-mm burr is used to create a vertical slot in the subchondral bone of the glenoid. To decrease the risk of anterior or posterior cortical penetration, a curette, rather than the burr, is used to deepen the slot to the vault apex. A pegged or keeled pressurizer is then malleted into the slot to impact any remaining bone within the holes (Figure 3.12).

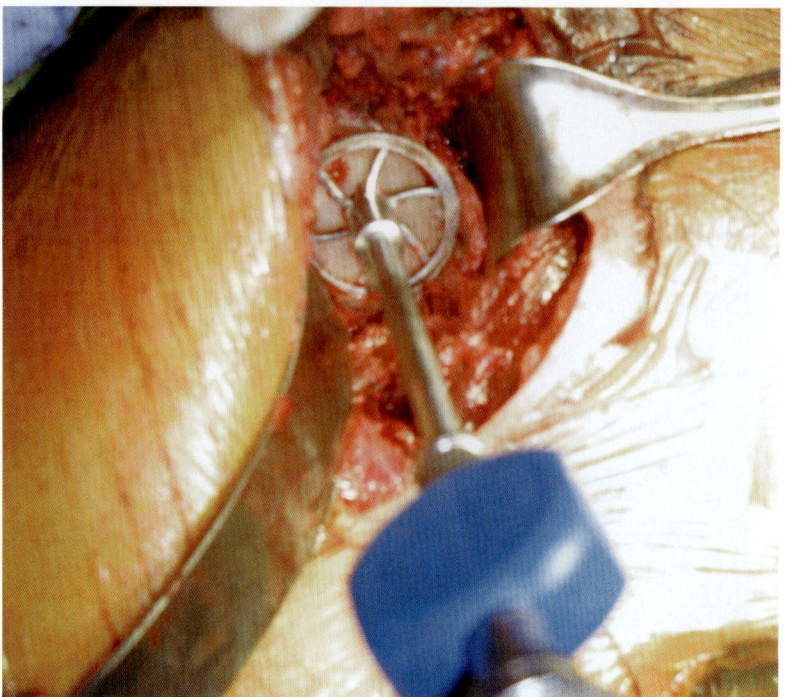

Figure 3.10. An open-faced reamer is preferred to allow better assessment of glenoid surface anatomy during the reaming process.

A provisional glenoid prosthesis is placed (Figure 3.13) and assessed for uniform seating and stability to rocking stresses in all planes. If the provisional glenoid is unstable, a burr and or reamer can be used to further contour the glenoid surface to be concentric. The glenoid component should not overhang or be unsupported by the periphery of the glenoid.

Once satisfied with the sizing and stability of the trial prosthesis, the glenoid vault is prepared for cementing. High-pressure pulse lavage is used to irrigate the prepared glenoid. Thrombin soaked sponges are cut into strips to fit either the peg holes or keel in the glenoid and inserted in place until the cement is ready for implantation. The cement is mixed on the back table and placed into a 60-ml Toomey syringe. Once the cement attains a dough-like consistency, the thrombin-soaked sponges are removed and the glenoid holes suctioned. The cement is pressurized into the holes using the Toomey syringe and an impactor is used to further pressurize the cement (Figure 3.14). Any excess cement is removed from the glenoid surface and the process is repeated two more times. Marra has shown the effectiveness of pressurization on cement penetration into the glenoid vault: it increases the depth of cement penetration (Marra G. Personal communication, 1998). The glenoid component is then implanted and held in place under finger pressurization while the cement cures. Cement should only be placed in the glenoid vault and not on the glenoid surface. Excess cement will

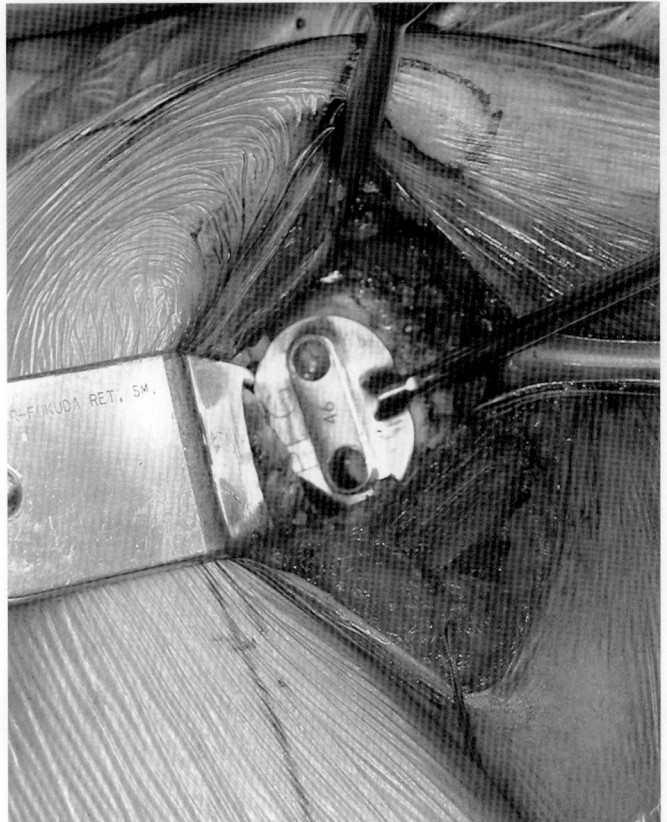

A

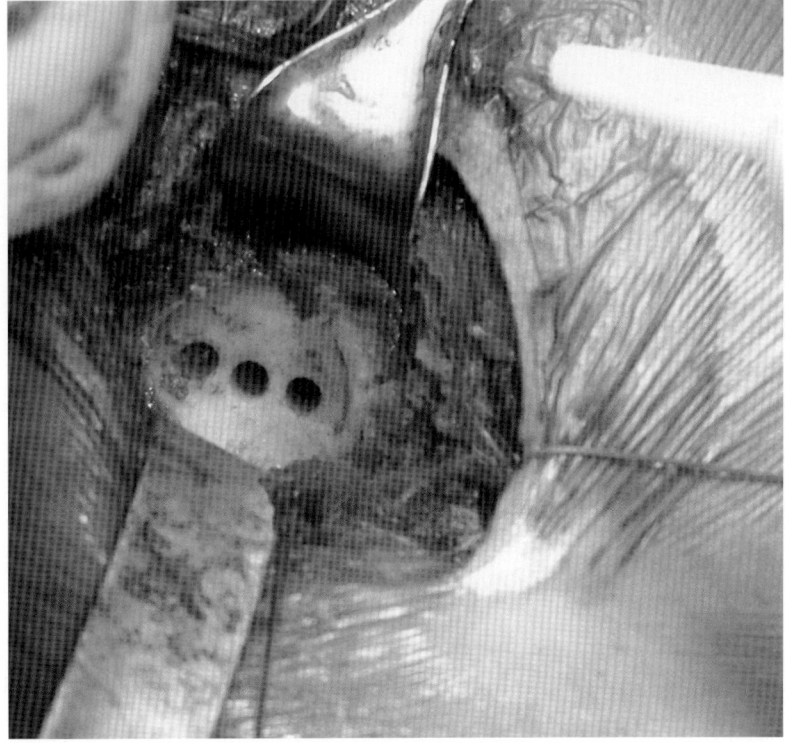

B

Figure 3.11. (A and B) The three holes for the pegged glenoid component are drilled using the guide.

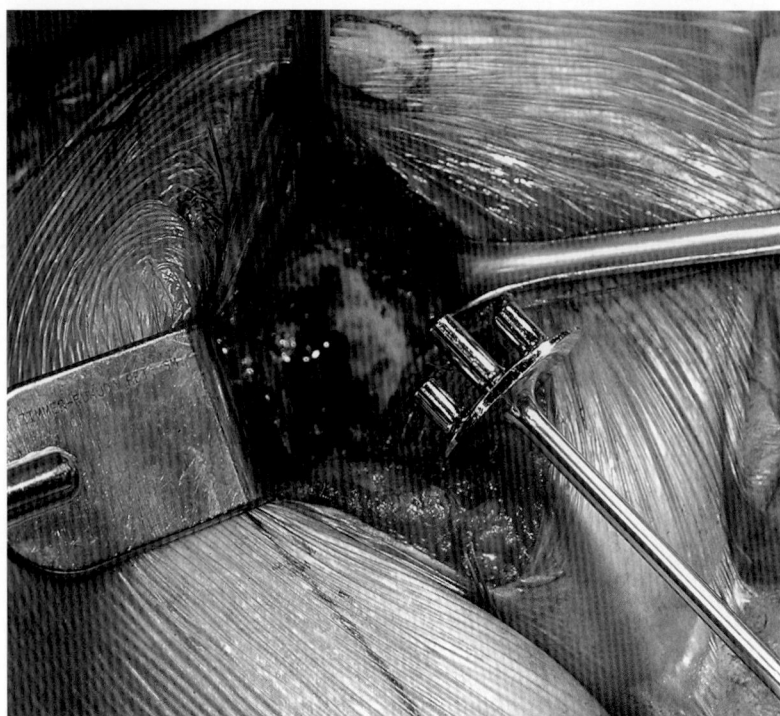

Figure 3.12. An impactor is used to remove any remaining bone to facilitate full seating of the glenoid component.

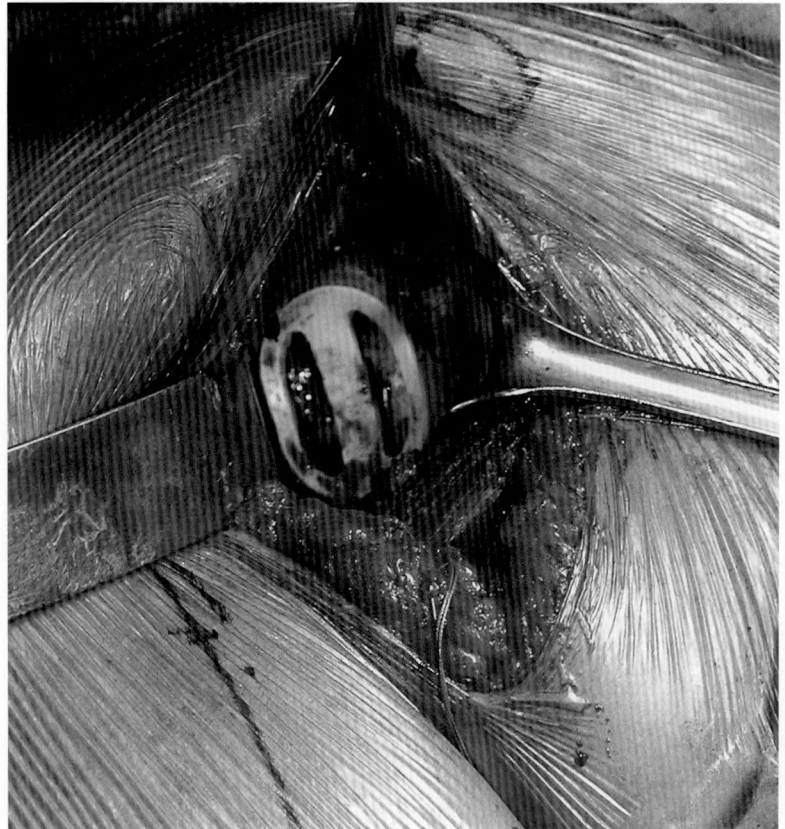

Figure 3.13. The open-faced trial glenoid is inserted, which allows easier assessment of the component fit. The trial should be stressed in all planes to ensure there is no rocking.

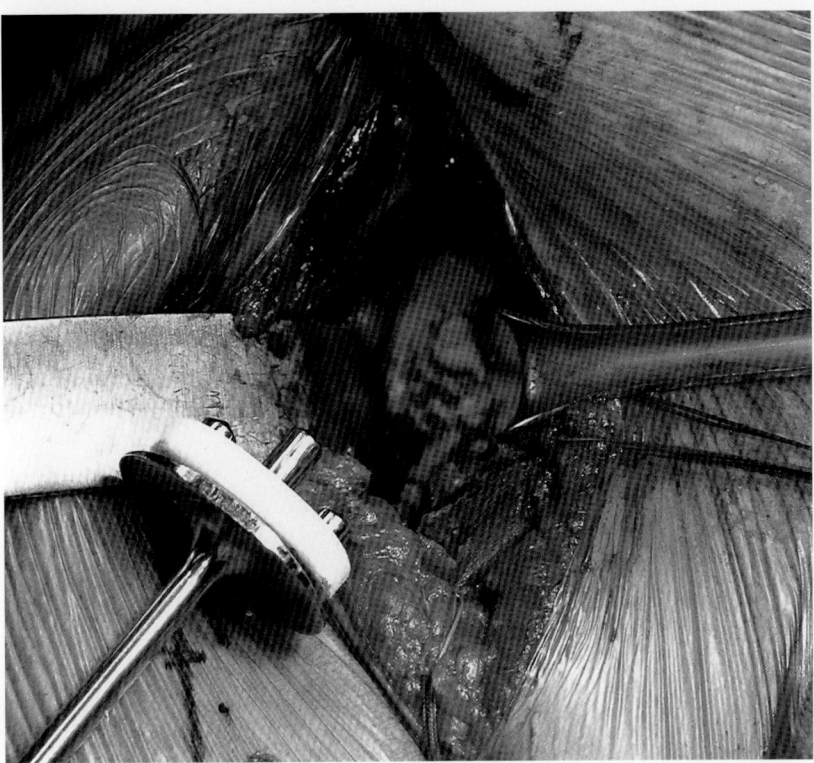

Figure 3.14. After thorough irrigation of the peg holes, thrombin-soaked sponges are inserted for hemostasis. Cement is then pressurized into the holes for optimal penetration into the cancellous bed of the vault.

flow out during pressurization and implantation of the glenoid component and should be removed with a small curette (Figure 3.15).

Anterior Soft Tissue Release

Once the glenoid has been implanted, attention is turned to soft tissue balancing. Most patients with osteoarthritis of the shoulder have limited external rotation secondary to a contracted anterior capsule and subscapularis tendon. As mentioned, the anterior capsulectomy mobilizes the subscapularis. Superficially, the subscapularis may be adherent to the under surface of the strap muscles. It can be released sharply from the conjoint tendon laterally, but medially, blunt dissection is necessary to avoid injury to the musculocutaneous nerve. Superiorly, the rotator interval and coracohumeral ligament are released down to the base of the coracoid to further mobilize the subscapularis. Inferiorly the subscapularis is often adhered to latissimus dorsi, which can be addressed with blunt dissection using a peanut or elevator.

The axillary nerve should be identified or palpated before subscapularis releases are performed. A narrow Darrach retractor placed along the anterior inferior glenoid neck retracts the nerve from the operative field. Once the subscapularis muscle has been completely

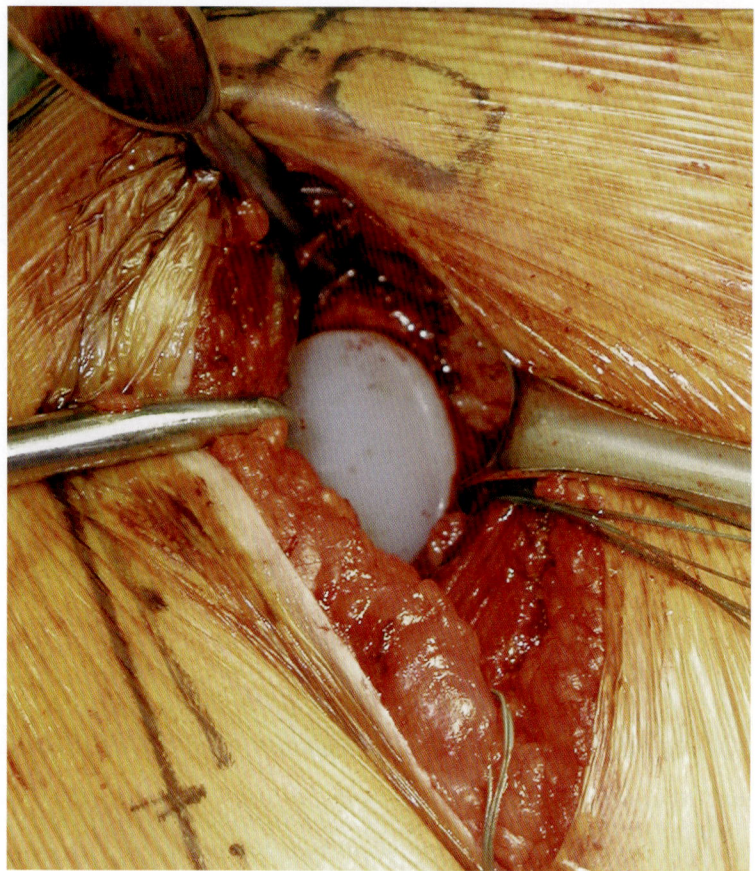

Figure 3.15. The glenoid component should be held in place with finger pressurization while the cement cures. After that it is inspected for loose cement.

released, attention is turned to repair of the subscapularis tendon back to the humerus. The Fukuda, Darrach, and metal finger retractors are removed. The humerus is externally rotated and extended. A Darrach retractor is placed anterior and deep to the humeral shaft, delivering the proximal humerus from the wound. The provisional humeral stem is then removed from the humerus using the extractor. Anchoring holes are drilled in the proximal neck of the humerus. Number 2 nonabsorbable sutures are then placed and the subscapularis is repaired to the humerus. A sturdy subscapularis repair is critical to allow postoperative rehabilitation without risk of failure of the repair. The sutures should be placed with large bone bridges to ensure a wide contact area for healing and secure fixation (Figure 3.16A and 3.16B). The pectoralis is then repaired anatomically and the wound closed in layers over a drain (Figure 3.17).

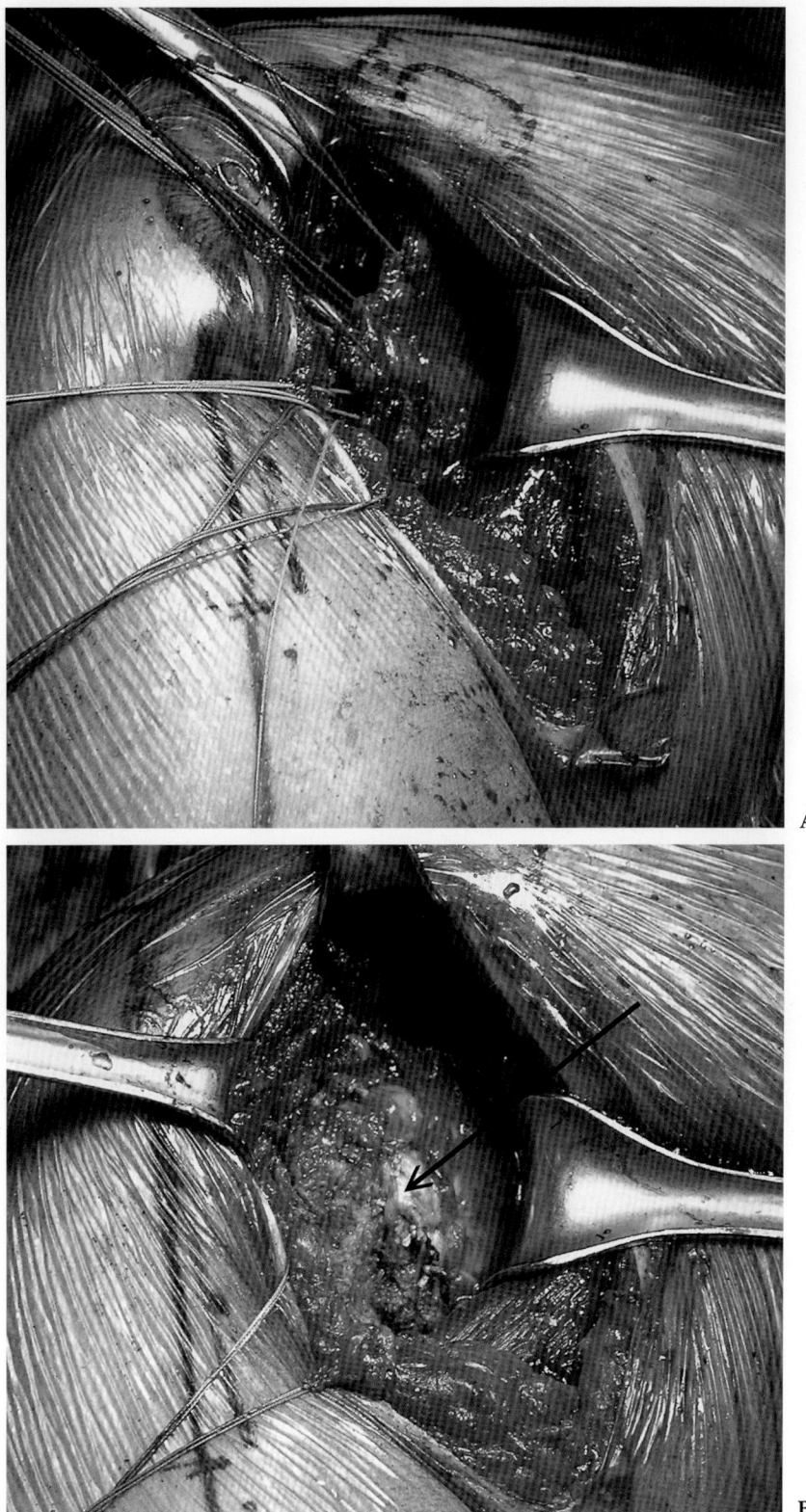

Figure 3.16. The entire circumference of the subscapularis is mobilized **(A)** and securely repaired to the humerus **(B)**.

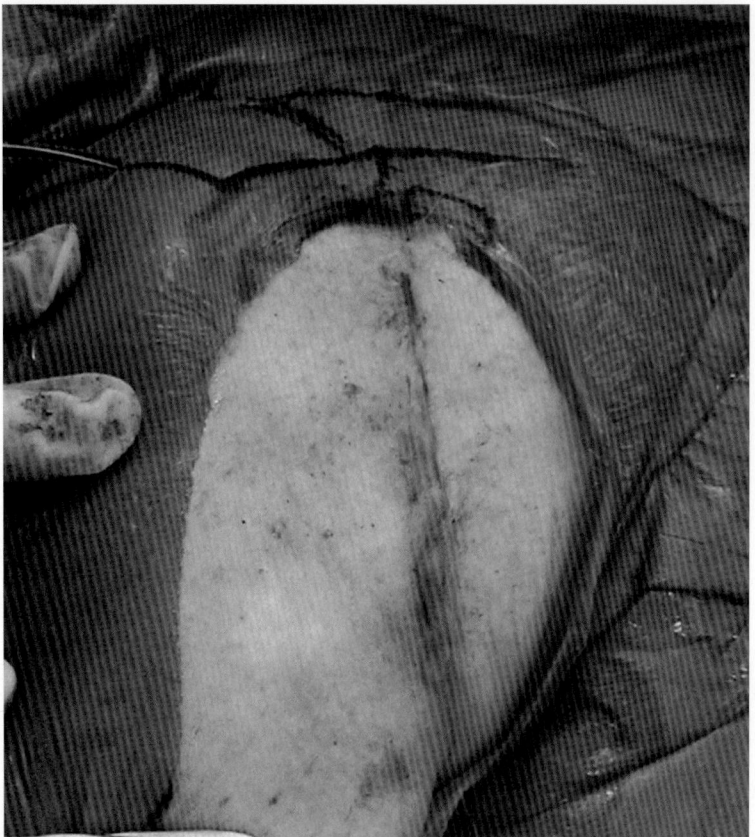

Figure 3.17. The pectoralis tendon is repaired anatomically and the wound closed in layers over a drain.

Special Considerations

This stepwise technique should help the surgeon become comfortable and proficient at exposing and implanting the glenoid for routine primary total shoulder arthroplasty (TSA). Three situations may be encountered that deserve special attention: glenoid placement and soft tissue releases in the young patient, a poorly exposed glenoid despite routine releases, and the glenoid with peripheral or central bone deficiencies. Exposure, decision making, and implantation of the glenoid component during revision TSA are addressed in Chapter 6.

The Young Patient

Fear of early glenoid loosening in the young patient is a relative contraindication of glenoid resurfacing. For such patients who elect to undergo hemiarthroplasty, we consider the use of biological resurfacing of the glenoid. Our early results with interpositional meniscal allograft have been encouraging. This necessitates adequate exposure of

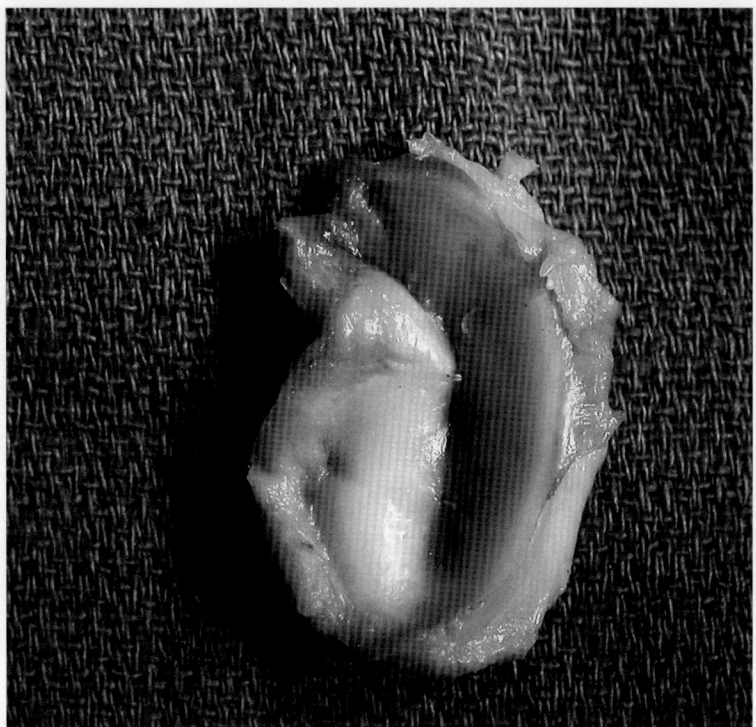

Figure 3.18. A lateral meniscal allograft is fashioned to fit the surface of the glenoid.

the glenoid. A lateral meniscal allograft is fashioned to fit the glenoid face (Figure 3.18). Four bioabsorbable anchors are place in the glenoid, one in each quadrant; anteriosuperior, anteroinferior, posterosuperior, and posteroinferior. Any remaining peripheral rim of labrum can also be used for improved fixation. All sutures are passed through the allograft, and the allograft is then slid down the sutures into position (Figure 3.19). Once satisfied with the position of the allograft, the sutures are then tied (Figure 3.20).

Higher demands on the shoulder are expected when selecting glenoid replacement in the younger patient; therefore, improved fixation is extremely desirable. With short-term success, we have recently began using a new trabecular metal-backed glenoid (Implex, Allendale, NJ) that achieves a cementless bond to the native bone. Certain technical considerations need to be made when implanting a metal-backed glenoid component. First, excellent exposure of the glenoid must be achieved because the metal-backed component must be impacted with perfect alignment. The prosthesis requires meticulous bone preparation to achieve a press fit. After the center of the glenoid is defined, a small, 2-mm drill is placed through a centering guide and the center hole is drilled. This pilot hole is then inspected; if the surgeon is satisfied this hole is in the center of the glenoid, the standard 6-mm centering hole is made. The superior and inferior glenoid drill holes are then made in the same manner as mentioned for the cemented

Figure 3.19. Suture anchors in the glenoid vault and sutures placed around the peripheral rim of the glenoid are used to secure the allograft to the face of the glenoid. All sutures are passed through the allograft, corresponding to their placement on the prepared glenoid surface. The allograft is slid down the sutures to the glenoid surface. This facilitates proper seating of the allograft.

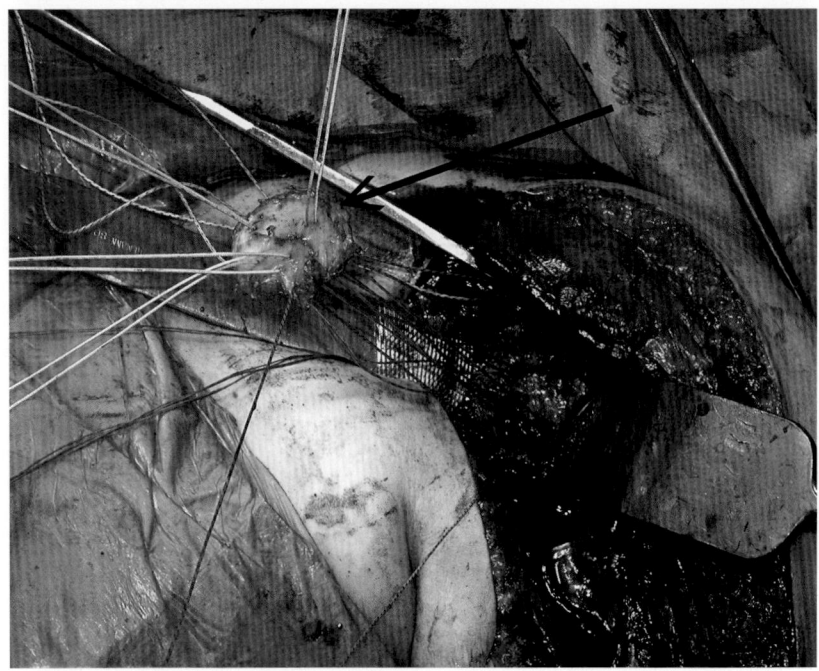

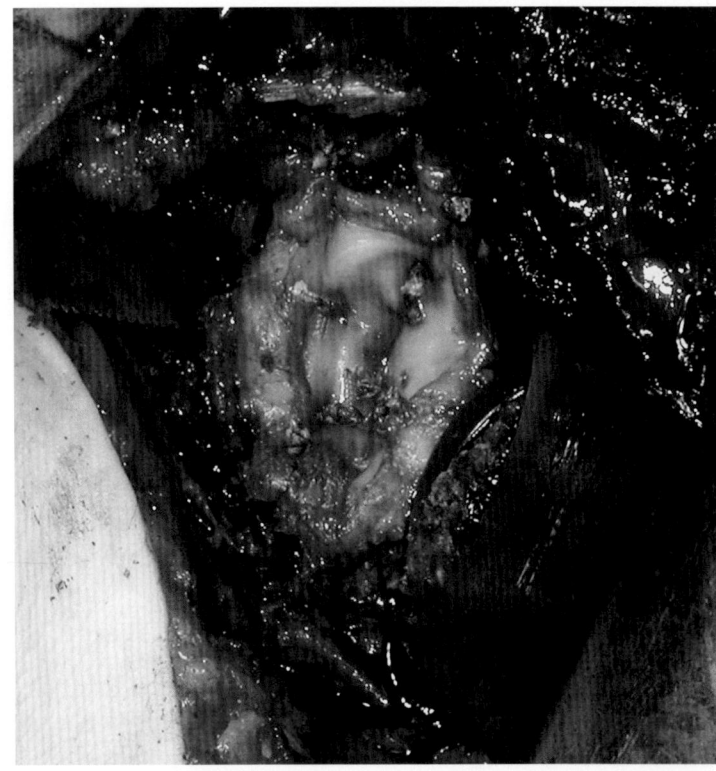

Figure 3.20. One satisfied with the position of the allograft, it is secured into place.

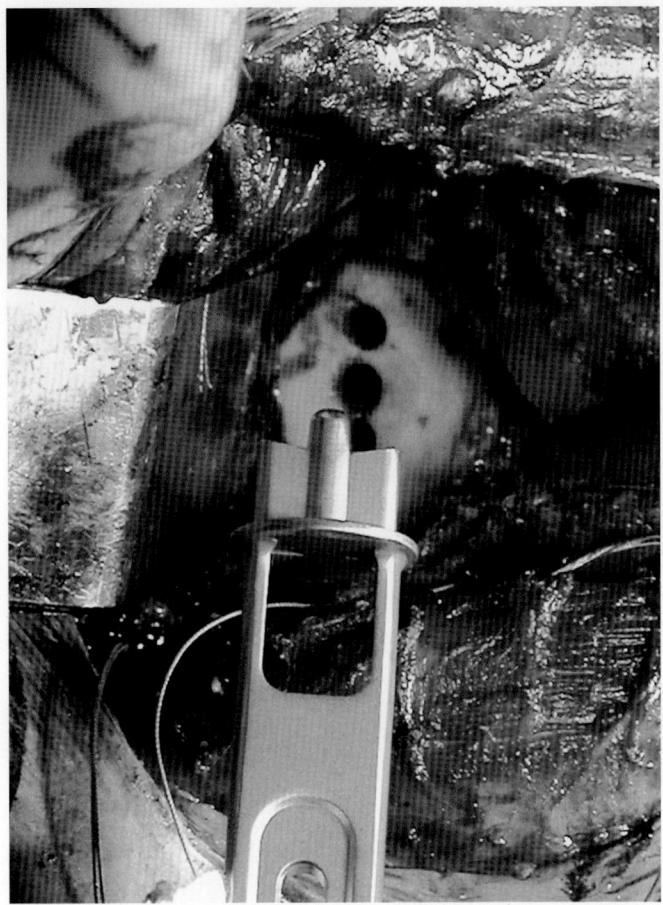

Figure 3.21. A glenoid chisel is used to prepare the surface for the component.

glenoid. A glenoid chisel is used to finish the preparation of the glenoid (Figure 3.21). This chisel is slightly smaller than the component to produce a press fit on insertion. The provisional glenoid component is inserted and its stability assessed. Once again, if unstable, a burr or reamer can be used to make the surface conform with the prosthesis so it is well seated. The trabecular metal-backed glenoid can then be press fit into place once satisfied with the provisional stability (Figure 3.22).

Excessive Soft Tissue Contractures

Soft tissue contractures are generally the cause of a glenoid that is difficult to expose. Many of these contractures can be addressed with a careful and methodological exposure as well as properly placed retractors. If exposure of the glenoid remains poor, the previous steps need to be reassessed for their accuracy and completion. Unaddressed humeral/glenoid osteophytes or an inappropriate humeral neck cut can hinder exposure of the glenoid. Assuring complete release of the anterior capsule off the humerus, from the rotator interval to beyond the 6

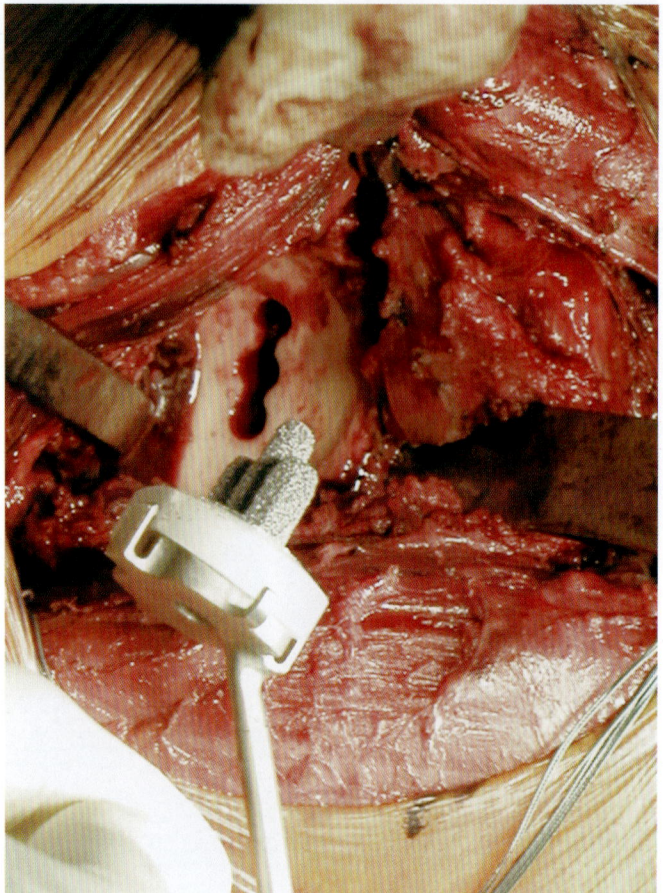

Figure 3.22. The component is press fit in place.

o'clock position inferiorly, and appropriate release of the subdeltoid and subacromial spaces may also improve exposure. If the superior .5 cm to 1 cm of the pectoralis has not been released, this can be performed with anatomic repair at the conclusion of the procedure. Additionally, although unnecessary for routine cases, proximal release of the long head of the biceps tendon, with subsequent tenodesis, improves glenoid exposure. If, despite this, exposure of the glenoid is still inadequate, the capsule can be released from the glenoid superiorly to the 12 o'clock position, as well as inferiorly to the 6 o'clock position as needed.

When planning soft tissue releases to address inferior contractures, the axillary nerve must be protected. Working from inside the capsule and using a Darrach inferiorly to retract the axillary nerve helps keep the nerve safe. We have found posterior contractures rarely to be a problem. Care must be taken not to release the posterior capsule unnecessarily as this can cause posterior prosthetic instability.

Glenoid Bone Deficiency

Both subchondral and cancellous bone stock available for implantation are important considerations for successful glenoid resurfacing. To help stabilize eccentric forces, the glenoid component needs to be supported by subchondral bone. High-quality and quantity of glenoid vault cancellous bone provides a stable lattice for the component cement mantle. Peripheral bone deficiency, especially posterior glenoid erosion, is more commonly associated with osteoarthritis and capsulorraphy arthritis. Medialization of the humeral head with central glenoid erosion is commonly associated with rheumatoid arthritis. Superior wear of the glenoid along with superior migration of the humeral head and an *acetabularized* coracoacromial arch is the pattern seen with cuff tear arthropathy.

To accurately determine the true version of the glenoid intraoperatively, peripheral osteophytes need to be removed. For mild to moderate posterior glenoid wear, a burr or reamer can be used to resect the anterior *high* side. Alternatively, the reamer can be used after a shallow centering hole has been drilled to eccentrically ream the anterior glenoid. Eccentric reaming of the glenoid can diminish the size of the glenoid vault volume and depth preventing proper glenoid placement. If there is any question, the provisional glenoid prosthesis should be reinserted after reaming to assess its seating against the glenoid. If necessary, the peg holes may need to be redrilled to ensure the correct depth has been achieved. The technique of placing a component on built up cement without adequate bone support can lead to cement fragmentation and loosening [20]. A comprehensive component sizing option enables the surgeon to address component mating issues. For example, if version needed to be corrected with eccentric reaming, and this reaming rendered the glenoid capable of only fitting a 40-mm glenoid, but the desired humeral head size was 46 mm, there would be a component mismatch. Either the head would need to be undersized or the glenoid oversized. A system that provides a variety of sizing and component pairing options allows surgical flexibility. For the patient, this translates into a more anatomic fit. A system with the versatility of placing glenoid components of different radii of curvature (Figure 3.23) (on the internal and external glenoid component surfaces) to better match size of the humeral head component is preferred.

For the patient with significant posterior wear, it must be remembered that eccentric reaming or burring down the high side makes the glenoid vault both more narrow and shallow, rendering implantation of a component more difficult or impossible. Additionally, excessive reaming removes the subchondral plate, which may weaken bone support for the component. Few data exist on how much reaming is safe and how much residual retroversion is acceptable. We have tried to limit high-side resection to less than 5 mm to 6 mm and are willing to accept approximately 20 degrees of retroversion. Instability has been unusual using these criteria. Resurfacing is not recommended if the glenoid neck has less than 1 cm remaining [24].

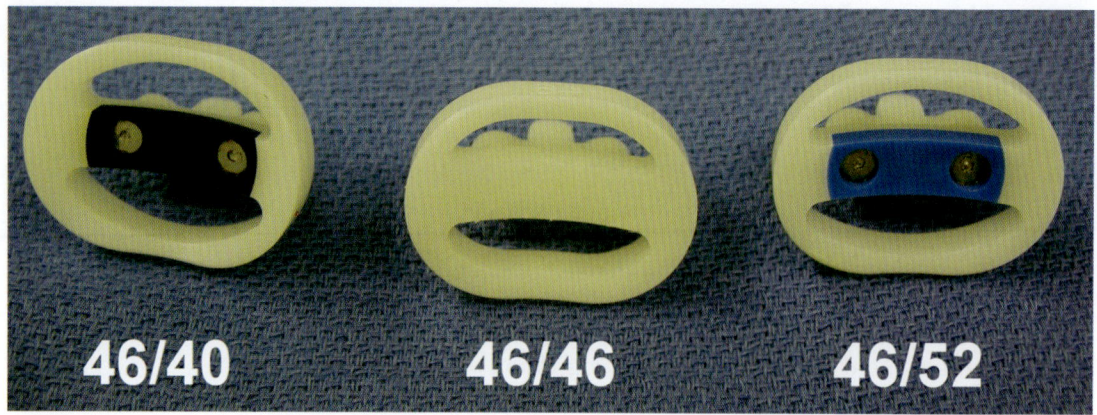

Figure 3.23. The inner and outer glenoid surfaces have different radii of curvature. Different colors represent different sizes. The outer curvature as denoted by the color of the central bar on the provisional glenoid should match the curvature of the humeral head. This affords the surgeon more versatility. For example, if eccentric reaming is necessary and results in decreasing the size of the glenoid vault, a smaller outer diameter (white, 46mm) may be used to fit the prepared surface, while maintaining the size necessary to properly fit the curvature of the humeral head (blue, 52mm) (Zimmer, Warsaw, IN).

The version of the humeral stem can also be altered to help with posterior glenoid wear. Less retroversion of the humeral head places the functional ROM of the shoulder in a better zone. A retroverted glenoid could cause the posterior instability of the shoulder with internal rotation. Placing a humeral component with less retroversion would favorably alter the patient's functional range of motion (ROM), requiring more internal rotation to cause instability. The majority of our humeral components are place in approximately 30 degrees of retroversion. For patients with excessive posterior wear, the humeral component retroversion can be decreased by as much as 10 degrees, but should not go below 20 degrees of retroversion.

Posterior bone grafting can be considered to alter glenoid version. A peripheral graft can preserve a vault large enough to accept a component. Glenoid bone grafting is rarely necessary. If necessary, use of a tricortical iliac crest autograft is preferred. The graft is shaped to fit the deficit and is held in place with two K-wires. The graft is then fixed using two small (3.5mm) cortical screws. The screws are countersunk to prevent interference with the polyethylene glenoid component.

Patients with posterior wear often have anterior capsular contractures, loss of external rotation, and posterior capsular laxity. Once the glenoid has been inserted, a provisional head can be inserted and stability assessed. If it is thought that there is too much posterior laxity, greater than 50% translation, nonabsorbable sutures are placed in the posterior capsule. The stitch is placed in a north-south direction, decreasing the posterior capsular volume. This is similar to what we have described as the barrel stitch for anterior inferior capsular shifts [25].

For the patient with an excessive amount of glenoid retroversion, such that altering the version would render the vault unacceptably small to accept an implant, a hemiarthroplasty may be the only option. In this case the remaining glenoid should be reamed anteriorly to both correct the version and provide a concentric articulation for the hemiarthroplasty. Levine et al. have shown patients with a concentric hemiarthroplasty have significantly better results than those with non concentric [2].

Unlike patients with osteoarthritis, those affected with rheumatoid arthritis often present with central glenoid bone deficiencies. Patients with mild central deficiencies generally have an intact peripheral glenoid rim. Mild central deficiency does not extensively decrease the volume of the glenoid vault, rendering it able to accept a prosthesis. For small contained defects methacrylate bone cement can be used to fill the defect. If large, the central defect can be bone grafted with cancellous bone from the resected humeral head. Severe central erosion may preclude placement of a glenoid and necessitate the use of hemiarthroplasty.

Decision-Making

Choosing a glenoid design should be based on knowledge of the biomechanics of glenoid component design. With respect to glenohumeral arthroplasty, two concepts must be considered: constraint and conformity. *Conformity* relates to how concentric, or how similar the curvature is between the glenoid and humeral components. A prosthesis with high conformity can lead to rim loading, polyethylene deformation and potentially, early loosening [26]. A prosthesis with low conformity distributes the load through a smaller contact area, thus increasing contact stresses. *Constraint* refers to the surface area of the glenoid relative to that of the humeral head [26]. A component with high constraint would have added stability by limiting glenohumeral subluxation. However, the forces needed to prevent such subluxation would be concentrated toward the periphery of the component. This could lead to edge loading and potentially early loosening. What is the proper balance between conformity and constraint? We chose to use a component with variable conformity. The central conforming zone maximizes contact area, therefore minimizing contact stresses when the component is centered. The nonconforming peripheral zone minimizes edge loading and wear debris while providing resistance to instability [26]. Lo et al. have shown that contact area is more centered and evenly distributed with a variable conforming implant [26]. For the conforming glenoid component, eccentric loading caused more posterior stresses.

The decision to use a pegged versus keeled prosthesis depends on surgeon preference, exposure, and patient age. When exposure permits, a pegged component is preferred. While some still consider keeled components the gold standard, no good clinical studies have compared the two. Success of the cementing technique is in part dependent on the quality and quantity of cancellous bone within the vault. The pegged technique removes less bone, leaving more for a stable bone-cement interface. Use of the keeled component removes more bone from the glenoid, raising the concern for a potential problem if a revision becomes necessary. The ideal glenoid component would replicate the normal stresses on the glenoid bone. Recent studies have suggested that pegged glenoids provide more favorable glenoid stress distribution considering glenoid body stresses, surface contact stresses, cement mantle stresses, and stress shielding. [27] In two situations a keeled prosthesis is preferred. A glenoid with a small dimension in the superior to inferior direction may preclude the placement of a pegged component. The superior and inferior pegs may not fit within the vault, whereas the keeled prosthesis is beveled and more conforming. Second, for cases with extremely difficult exposure, the keeled prosthesis is somewhat easier to insert as there is more tolerance fitting the keel into a slot as opposed to three pegs through holes.

Whether or not to remove the biceps tendon during routine TSA remains controversial. Our indications for biceps tenodesis are extensive pathology of the tendon or difficulties with exposure. The use of meticulous technique during exposure should prevent the need for taking the biceps in routine TSA. We believe the long head of the biceps has function and should not be sacrificed if it is not diseased or compromising to the exposure. We have observed minimal problems with biceps-related pain after TSA. If the biceps needs to be released, we advocate a tenodesis as opposed to a tenotomy. The long head of the biceps is tagged pulled distally and amputated from its insertion on the labrum. It is then *tenodesed* to the soft tissue adjacent to the bicepital groove. Tenotomy is avoided secondary to the potential for cosmetic deformity as well as cramping biceps pain.

Summary

Perhaps the most common reasons to perform a hemiarthroplasty instead of a TSA remain fear of glenoid component failure and difficulty exposing the glenoid. Numerous reports in the literature support the superiority of TSA to hemiarthroplasty for shoulder arthritis [4, 7, 13, 28]. Advocates of hemiarthroplasty use the argument than glenoid components fail; they are difficult to revise; and hemiarthroplasty can be later converted to TSA if necessary. Although some alarming papers on glenoid lucency have been reported, the rate of revision TSA secondary to glenoid failure remains low [6, 14, 29, 30]. It has been reported that primary TSA provides significantly better results than conversion of hemiarthroplasty to TSA [31]. Third, hemiarthroplasty can cause glenoid erosions that could potentially be difficult to handle during TSA. We firmly believe that glenoid replacement performed with meticulous attention to technique, including the approach, retractor placement, soft tissue balancing, and cement technique can lead to a successful and enduring solution for the arthritic shoulder.

References

1. Neer CS II. Replacement arthroplasty for glenohumeral osteoarthritis. J Bone Joint Surg Am 1974;56(1):1–13.
2. Levine WN, Djurasovic M, Glasson JM, et al. Hemiarthroplasty for glenohumeral osteoarthritis: results correlated to degree of glenoid wear. J Shoulder Elbow Surg 1997;6(5):449–454.
3. Connor PM, Bigliani LU. Prosthetic Replacement for Osteoarthritis: hemiarthroplasty versus total shoulder replacement. Semin Arthroplasty 1997;8:268–277.
4. Edwards TB, Kadakia NR, Boulahia A, et al. A comparison of hemiarthroplasty and total shoulder arthroplasty in the treatment of primary glenohumeral osteoarthritis: results of a multicenter study. J Shoulder Elbow Surg 2003;12(3):207–213.
5. Orfaly RM, Rockwood CA Jr, Esenyel CZ, et al. A prospective functional outcome study of shoulder arthroplasty for osteoarthritis with an intact rotator cuff. J Shoulder Elbow Surg 2003;12(3):214–221.
6. Rodosky MW, Bigliani LU. Indications for glenoid resurfacing in shoulder arthroplasty. J Shoulder Elbow Surg 1996;5(3):231–248.
7. Smith KL, Matsen FA III. Total shoulder arthroplasty versus hemiarthroplasty. Current trends. Orthop Clin North Am 1998;29(3):491–506.
8. AAOS. Arthroplasty and Total Joint replacement Procedures: 1991–2000. AAOS, 2004.
9. Friedman RJ. Total Shoulder Arthroplasty. Orthop Clin North Am 1998;29.
10. Field LD, Dines DM, Zabinski SJ, et al. Hemiarthroplasty of the Shoulder for rotator Cuff Arthropathy. J Shoulder Elbow Surg 1997;6(1):18–23.
11. Flatow EL. Prosthetic Replacement in the Rotator Cuff Deficient Shoulder. In Surgery of the Shoulder, M Vastamaki, Jalovaara P, Editors. Amsterdam: Elsevier, 1995;335–345.
12. Franklin JL, Barrett WP, Jackin SE, et al. Glenoid loosening in total shoulder arthroplasty. Association with rotator cuff deficiency. J Arthroplasty 1988;3(1):39–46.
13. Ibarra C, Dines DM, McLaughlin JA. Glenoid replacement in total shoulder arthroplasty. Orthop Clin North Am 1998;29(3):403–413.
14. Norris TR, Iannotti JP. Functional outcome after shoulder arthroplasty for primary osteoarthritis: a multicenter study. J Shoulder Elbow Surg 2002;11(2):130–135.
15. Cofield RH. Degenerative and Arthritic Problems of the Glenohumeral Joint. In The Shoulder, CA Rockwood, FA Matsen III, Editors. Philadelphia: WB Saunders, 1990;678–749.
16. Figgie HE III, Inglis AE, Goldberg VM, et al. An analysis of factors affecting the long-term results of total shoulder arthroplasty in inflammatory arthritis. J Arthroplasty 1988;3(2):123–130.
17. Collins D. Inflammatory Arthritis of the Shoulder. In Orthopedic Knowledge Update: Shoulder and Elbow 2, T Norris, Editor. Rosemont, IL: AAOS, 2002;251–256.
18. Stewart M, Kelly IG. Total Shoulder Replacement in Rheumatoid Disease: 7 to 13 year followup of 37 joints. J Bone Joint Surg Br 1997; 79:68–72.
19. Brems J. Arthritis of Dislocation. Orthop Clin North Am 1998;29(3):453–466.
20. Bigliani LU, Weinstein DM. Glenohumeral arthroplasty for arthritis after instability surgery. J Shoulder Elbow Surg 1995;4(2):87–94.
21. Marra G, Wiater JM, Levine WL, Pollock RG, Bigliani LU. Shoulder Arthroplasty for Avascular Necrosis. In AAOS. 2000. Orlando, Fl.

22. Hayes PR, Flatow EL. Steps for Reliable Glenoid Exposure and Preparation in Shoulder Arthroplasty. Techniques Shoulder Elbow Surg 2000; 1(4):209–219.

23. Wu CL, Chen JM, Miller RJ. Comparison of Postoperative Pain in Patients Receiving Interscalene Block or General Anesthesia for Shoulder Surgery. Orthopedics 2002;25(1).

24. Klepps S, Hazrati Y, Flatow E, May LPW. Management of Glenoid Bone Deficiency During Shoulder Replacement. Techniques Shoulder Elbow Surg 2003;4(1):4–17.

25. Ahmad CS, Freehill MO, Blaine TA, et al. Anteromedial capsular redundancy and labral deficiency in shoulder instability. Am J Sports Med 2003; 31(2):247–252.

26. Lo I, Bishop JY, Wang VM, Flatow EL. Biomechanics Of Glenoid Component Design. Techniques Shoulder Elbow Surg 2003;4(3):110–120.

27. Connor PM. Glenoid Design- Pegs are better than Keels. In 18th Annual Vail Symposium. 2003. Vail, CO.

28. Gartsman GM, Roddey TS, Hammerman SM. Shoulder arthroplasty with or without resurfacing of the glenoid in patients who have osteoarthritis. J Bone Joint Surg Am 2000;82(1):26–34.

29. Boileau P, Avidor C, Krishnan SE, et al. Cemented polyethylene versus uncemented metal-backed glenoid components in total shoulder arthroplasty: a prospective, double-blind, randomized study. J Shoulder Elbow Surg, 2002; 11(4):351–359.

30. Boyd AD Jr, Wilber JH. Total shoulder arthroplasty versus hemiarthroplasty. Indications for glenoid resurfacing. J Arthroplasty 1990;5(4): 329–336.

31. Carroll R, Izquierdo R, Levine WN, Blaine TA, Bigliani LU. Glenoid Arthrosis after Hemiarthroplasty: Results of Conversion to Total Shoulder Arthroplasty. In AAOS. 2003. New Orleans.

Chapter 4

Glenohumeral Inflammatory Arthritis: Special Issues

Ian G. Kelly and Angus D. MacLean

The inflammatory conditions affecting the shoulder include rheumatoid arthritis, juvenile chronic arthritis, and the seronegative spondyloarthropathies—a group of interrelated conditions including ankylosing spondylitis, psoriatic arthropathy, Reiter's disease, and the intestinal arthropathies. Shoulder involvement in the seronegative spondyloarthropathies is uncommon, with the acromioclavicular joint being most commonly affected. This chapter concerns itself principally with the surgical considerations in the rheumatoid patient and particularly the technique of glenohumeral arthroplasty in the rheumatoid shoulder.

Rheumatoid disease, with a prevalence estimated to be between 1% and 3% in Western Europe and North America, is by far the most common of the inflammatory arthropathies to affect the shoulder joint complex. It is a systemic illness requiring a multidisciplinary approach because of the nonarticular facets of the disease. The polyarticular involvement requires a methodical assessment of the patient as a whole in addition to specific assessment of the shoulder joint complex, which may be involved in one or more of its parts.

Pathology and Patterns of Disease

The rheumatoid disease process involves synovitis, vasculitis, and secondary changes such as anemia. As far as the shoulder is concerned, the synovitis is probably the most significant factor. The initial changes are confined to the soft tissues, and it has been suggested that it is the synovial sheath of the intraarticular portion of the long head of biceps that is first involved. It appears that the process commences with vascularization followed by hyperplasia of the synovium and formation of a pannus. Pannus is an abnormal synovium secreting hyaluronase, collagenase, proteolytic enzymes, proteoglycan proteases, and other regulatory agents that contribute to joint destruction. As the disease progresses there is continuing cellular infiltration, mainly small lymphocytes, and proliferation of blood vessels and fibroblasts resulting in a thickened membrane with multiple villi.

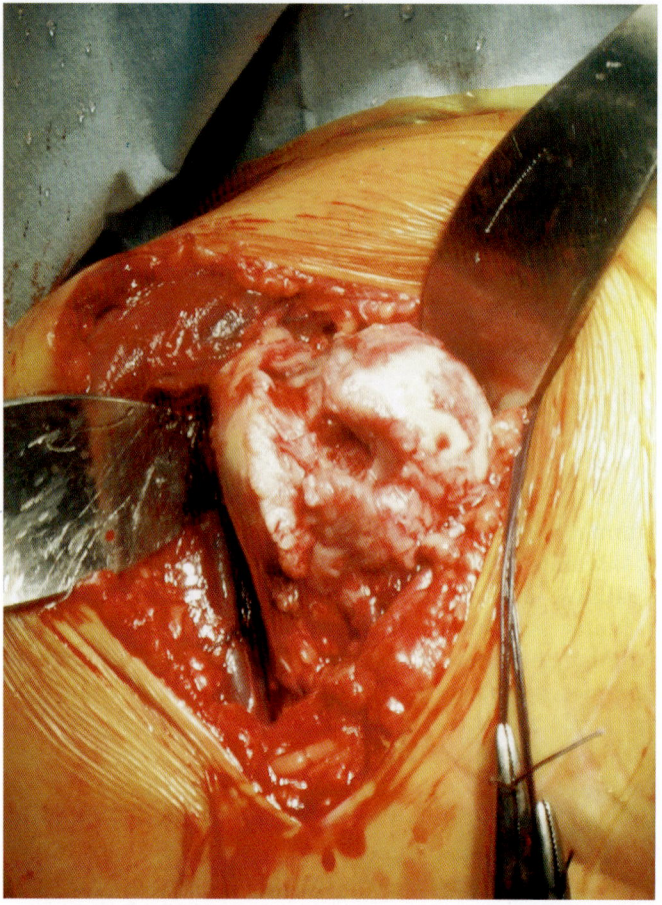

Figure 4.1. A *wet* rheumatoid shoulder. Note the marginal cystic erosion from penetrating synovium and joint surface damage.

At the eroding front of the pannus, where it contacts the articular cartilage, the synovium both penetrates deep into the cartilage producing marginal erosions and also spreads over its surface. Cartilage destruction is also seen remote from the pannus and may be the result of proteolytic enzymes in the synovial fluid (Figure 4.1). When the inflammatory process involves the tendon sheaths it is in a confined area and may infiltrate the tendon to a variable degree. The rotator cuff tendons do not have a synovial sheath but the subacromial bursa is intimately connected to the superior surface of the supraspinatus tendon, which is always involved when there is a bursitis. If invasion of the tendon is marked, fibrinoid necrosis and nodule formation may be seen and rupture of the tendon may ensue.

In addition to producing bony erosions, the rheumatoid process stimulates osteoclast activity through the secretion of prostaglandins and cytokines, which in turn contributes to the osteopenia commonly seen in these patients.

The wide variety of pathological processes involved in rheumatoid disease is reflected in the diverse clinical presentations with different aspects dominating in different patients.

Little has been written about the natural history of the rheumatoid shoulder but an understanding of this is essential to determine the most appropriate form of therapy. Petersson [1] has suggested that rheumatoid shoulders progress toward joint destruction at varying rates, with failure of the rotator cuff occurring at a late stage. The sub-acromial bursa and the acromioclavicular joint may be affected early. Petersson related his account of the natural history to the Larsen grading system [2], which is widely used amongst rheumatologists and rheumatoid surgeons (Figure 4.2). This classification identifies 6 groups at the glenohumeral joint with grade 0 being normal, grade 3 having

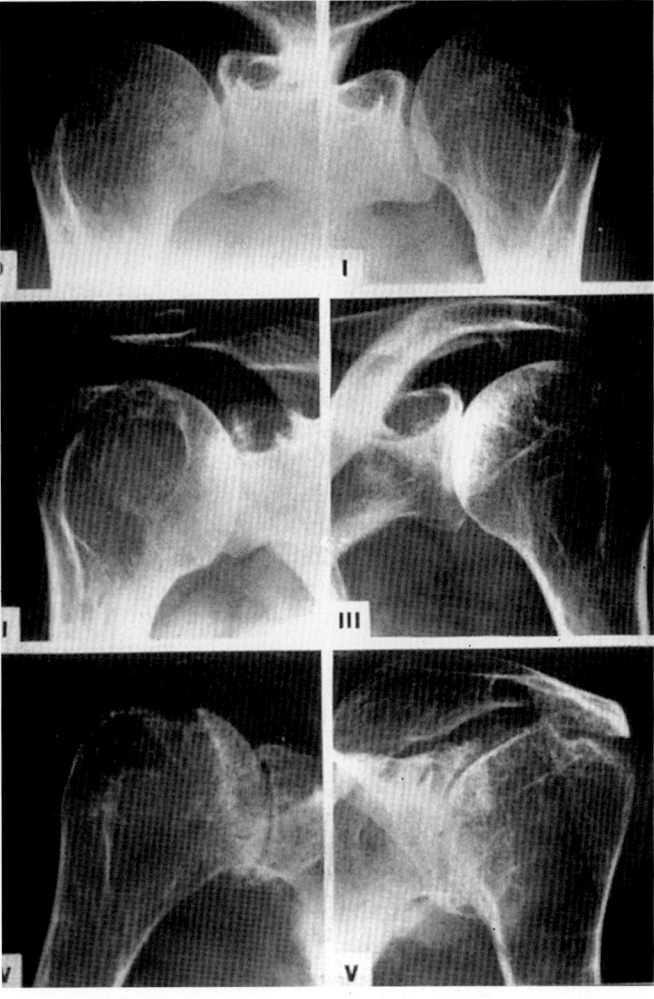

Figure 4.2. The radiological grading system of Larsen, Dale, and Eek (1977) for the rheumatoid glenohumeral joint. Higher grade disease is characterised by diminished bone stock. (Courtesy of Larsen, University of Lund, Sweden; by permission of Kelly I, Trends in Orthopaedics, 2003.)

loss of joint space, and grade 5 being total destruction of the gleno-humeral joint. Larsen has also produced a grading system for the acromioclavicular joint.

We have found a great variety of pathology at the time of surgery in our rheumatoid patients and feel that although the rate of progression is variable, there are different patterns of pathology.

Neer described four radiological patterns in the rheumatoid shoulder [3]. These are wet, dry, resorptive, and end stage (Figure 4.3A–D). The *wet* form is characterized by periarticular erosions. The *dry* form shows many features of osteoarthritis, with subchondral sclerosis and osteo-phytes. The *resorptive* form is associated with considerable bone loss and little in the way of bone reaction. The *end stage* joint shows extensive destruction of the glenoid and humeral head such that the inferior pole of the glenoid articulates with the humeral shaft. Neer used these terms in a purely descriptive way and did not relate them to pathology or identify any difference in natural history.

We applied these terms to the preoperative radiographs of 104 shoulders undergoing arthroplasty [4]. We found the wet shoulder was more likely to have a cuff rupture than other patterns and this could occur at an early stage, before there was a significant amount of bony damage. By contrast the dry pattern appeared to protect the rotator cuff while the resorptive form was usually associated with a thin but intact cuff. It must be remembered that all of these patients were at an advanced stage of disease.

Hirooka and colleagues [5] have reported five radiological patterns of disease in the rheumatoid shoulder in a group of 83 patients (133 shoulders) followed for 5 to 23 years (mean 14 years). The first type was non-progressive and therefore normal. The second type was *erosive* and in this group the articular surface was well preserved until 10 years after the onset of the disease, after which joint destruction progressed slowly. The *collapse* pattern was the most common and these shoulders developed osteopenia rapidly with associated cysts. This progressed to collapse of the subchondral bone and advanced joint destruction within 5 to 10 years. The arthrosis group showed osteophytes and subchondral sclerosis with the joint structure being well preserved for a long time. Finally the mutilans group showed extensive and rapid bone resorption.

Hirooka's patterns match those of Neer very closely, wet corresponding to erosive, dry to arthritic and resorptive to collapsing, but the former has defined and charted the progress of the patterns more carefully. Our own study relates the soft tissue changes to these patterns and, used together with Hirooka's data, it provides some indication of the likely rate and type of progression of glenohumeral disease in the rheumatoid shoulder. The propensity for cuff rupture in the wet or erosive shoulder before there is very much bone destruction has resulted in us regarding this type of shoulder as a *shoulder at risk*.

Indications

The indications for shoulder arthroplasty in the rheumatoid patient are persistent glenohumeral joint pain, unresponsive to nonoperative

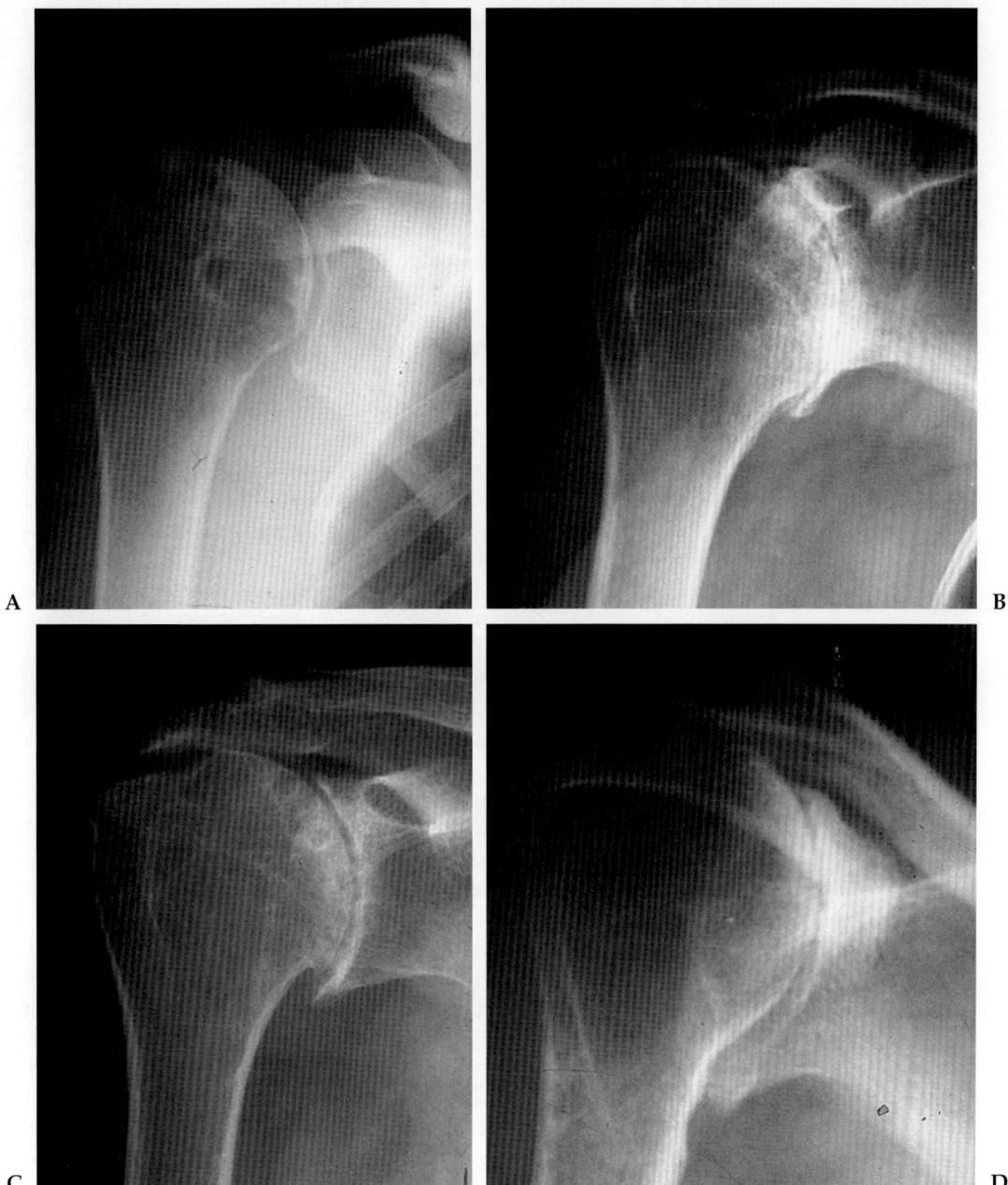

Figure 4.3. (A) The *erosive* or wet pattern of disease showing marked periarticular erosions. Note the superior subluxation and the preservation of the glenoid bone and glenohumeral joint space. **(B)** The *resorptive* or *collapsing* pattern. Note the osteopenia and marked medialization of the joint. **(C)** The *dry* or *arthrotic* pattern. Bone quality is usually good and the rotator cuff usually healthy. **(D)** The *end stage* or *mutilating* pattern. There is gross destruction of bone and, usually, the rotator cuff.

measures and associated with significant functional impairment and radiographic evidence of joint destruction.

Before undertaking glenohumeral joint replacement, it is necessary to establish that the glenohumeral joint is the source of the patients' pain. This may not be a problem in the patient with osteoarthritis, but can be difficult in the polyarthritic rheumatoid patient. Radiographic involvement alone does not provide sufficient basis and local tenderness is a poor guide to the site of the pain. It is often necessary to use local anesthetic injection testing [6] to locate the source of the pain in the rheumatoid shoulder and it is surprising how often this process reveals the acromioclavicular joint or subacromial space as the unexpected source of the pain. We have also found that if humeral head sphericity is maintained, then an extra glenohumeral source of pain is likely, even with obliteration of the joint space (Larsen grades 3 and 4). Although restriction of external rotation usually indicates a glenohumeral problem, the medialization of the joint in this condition often results in limitation of external rotation as the result of subacromial disease. This type of restriction is reversed by injection of local anesthetic into the subacromial bursa.

Much has been made of the timing of shoulder arthroplasty in the rheumatoid patient. Rheumatologists have been accused of referring patients too late in the disease process when significant rotator cuff disease or glenoid bone loss may compromise arthroplasty results. There is at present no good evidence to support this view although intuitively early arthroplasty would be technically easier. Many rheumatoid patients with significant shoulder pathology do not present to any physician until they have reached an advanced stage of disease. Patients tend to present when motion is restricted such that function is impeded or pain becomes constant. Shoulder pain in inflammatory disease is often intermittent with a stepwise decline in range of motion occurring with exacerbations or *flares* of disease.

Close collaboration between rheumatologist and surgeon is essential. A number of reports have given conflicting opinions on the need to stop Methotrexate before surgery. A prospective randomized trial of 388 RA patients undergoing orthopedic procedures [7] found that continuation of Methotrexate treatment increased neither the risk of infection or surgical complication. However, they also demonstrated that other drugs used to treat RA such as penicillamine, cyclosporin hydroxychloroquine, and prednisolone all did increase the risk of problems. Anti-TNF alpha agents may have implications for surgery, but experience with these agents is limited. We routinely stop these agents several weeks prior to surgery, although evidence based practice is not available at present.

Polyarthritic involvement frequently means that several joints require surgical treatment at any one time. Shoulder arthroplasty should never be carried out without consideration of the state of the other joints and the overall function of the patient. There is little point in replacing a diseased shoulder if ipsilateral wrist and hand problems preclude useful function of the limb. In such instances hand surgery should take precedence. Whether to operate on the elbow or shoulder first is controversial. It would seem reasonable to be guided by the patients' wishes and symptoms although bearing in mind that a painful or unstable elbow interferes with shoulder rehabilitation. Simultaneous shoulder and elbow arthroplasty has been reported [8] with good results matching those for separate procedures. Finally, it must be remembered that the shoulder becomes a load-bearing joint following lower limb surgery when walking aids are employed and consideration of this must be given when planning the management of a polyarthritic patient.

Operative Considerations

The technique of unconstrained arthroplasty in the rheumatoid shoulder differs little from that in other pathologies. However, there are areas where special note and adaptations to the standard technique are necessary.

Patient Positioning

Rheumatoid patients are often thin and frail with skin and tissue quality to match. Great care must be taken to protect pressure areas during positioning with gentle handling and adequate padding of bony prominences.

Up to 80% of rheumatoid patients have radiological evidence of cervical spine involvement and 25% of rheumatoid admissions to hospital show signs of atlanto axial instability [9]. Subaxial problems are less frequently encountered. Dynamic flexion and extension lateral views are invaluable in the assessment of the rheumatoid neck with MRI assessment of use where doubt exists regarding the status of the cervical cord. General anesthesia or regional anesthesia using an interscalene block can be used. The advantage of regional anesthesia is that it avoids manipulating the cervical spine during intubation. Excellent analgesia and muscle relaxation can be achieved with an interscalene block.

We use the beach-chair position with the use of a neurosurgical head rest and an adjustable arm board (Figure 4.4). A folded towel medial to the medial border of the scapula stabilizes and facilitates access to the glenoid face (Figure 4.5). The patient must be positioned so that full extension of the shoulder can be achieved at the side of the table.

Approach

Many rheumatoid shoulders are markedly medialized and the deltoid muscle is nearly always thinned. We have found that using a more laterally placed incision commencing in front of the acromioclavicular joint and extending distally parallel to the chest wall results in less forceful retraction of deltoid and thinned skin (Figure 4.6). The deltopectoral interval is identified using the cephalic vein or associated fat stripe as a guide. We routinely tie off the thin walled cephalic vein proximally, where it penetrates the clavipectoral fascia and distally.

Deltoid is further protected by releasing the deltopectoral interval fully to the clavicle and elevating the muscle from the underlying

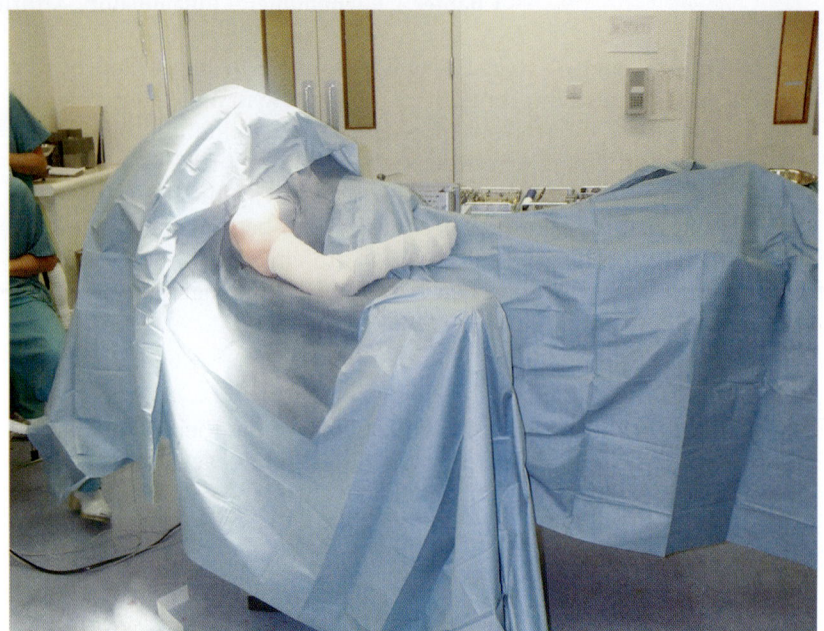

Figure 4.4. A patient positioned for surgery in the beach chair position. The patient must be positioned at the edge of the table to allow shoulder extension.

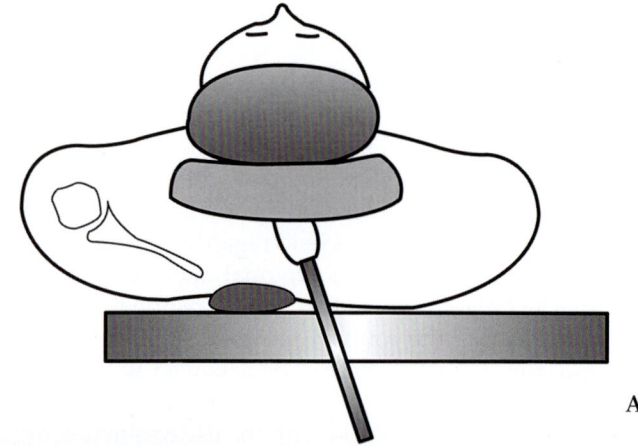

A

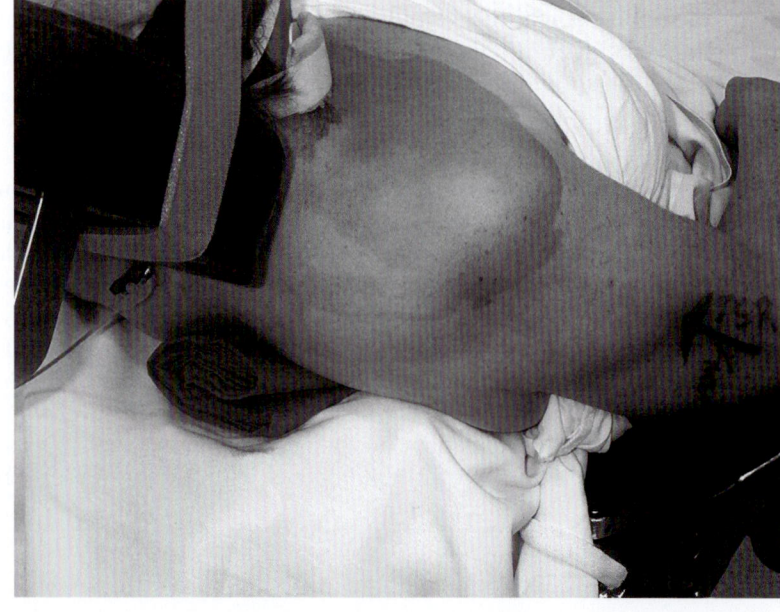

Figure 4.5. (A and B) A folded towel placed medial to the medial border of the scapula facilitates access to the glenoid face and stabilizes the scapula. **(A)** Correct positioning of the medial stabilizing towel.

B

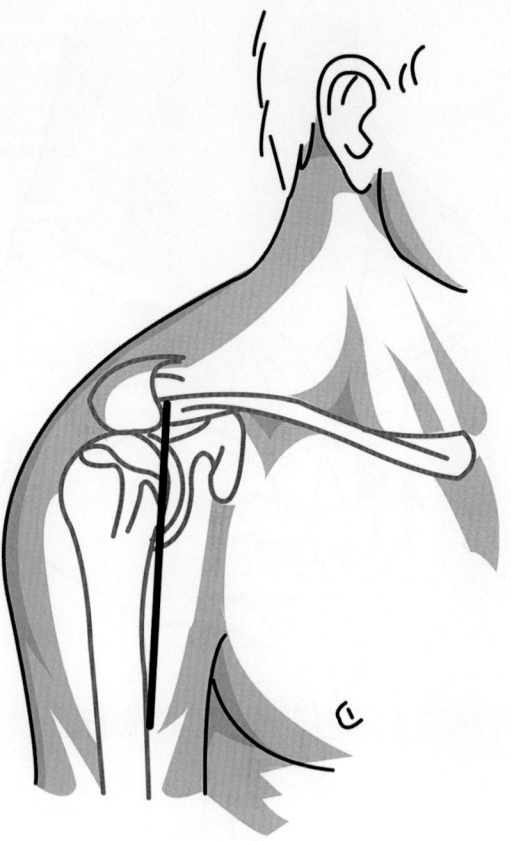

Figure 4.6. Skin incision extends from the acromioclavicular joint anteriorly distally parallel and 1 cm to 2 cm lateral to the chest wall. This incision is easily extended proximally to access the acromioclavicular joint.

clavipectoral fascia and humeral insertion using blunt finger dissection. A sensation of peeling a sticking plaster from the skin is felt distally as the deltoid is released. The finger is then advanced superiorly and posteriorly around humeral head before finally attempting penetration into the subacromial space (Figure 4.7). The subacromial space is frequently too narrow to admit a finger and here a blunt dissector to free the space is invaluable. Further exposure is frequently required and gained by sectioning of the upper centimeter of pectoralis major humeral insertion. Indeed, sectioning of the entire tendon may be necessary if the shoulder is particularly tight. This should be repaired, but may be difficult because of the poor quality of the rheumatoid tissues.

The rotator cuff is now assessed. In rheumatoid patients the supraspinatus is frequently thin and cuff tears are found in between 20% and 30% of shoulders [10–15]. Tears in the rotator cuff can be repaired about the prosthesis in standard fashion [16], but sometimes the thinned nature of the cuff precludes repair. Rozing and Brand [17] have reported on the difficulty of such repairs but have also indicated that, where they are possible, the result is superior to arthroplasty with a torn cuff. In the shoulders with a resorptive pattern, the cuff is usually

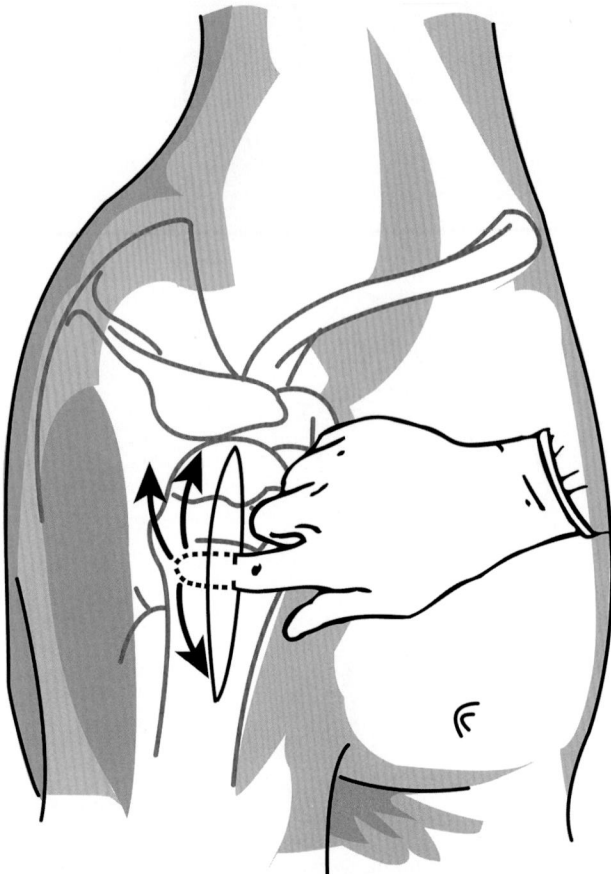

Figure 4.7. Elevation of deltoid from the humerus and clavipectoral fascia is initially performed distally to the muscle insertion, then superiorly both posterior and lateral to the humeral head before releasing into the subacromial space. It is important that all of the muscle is elevated.

thin and the joint much medialized. Although the tendon may be intact when first inspected, lateralizing the joint may well result in it losing its integrity. The quality of the tendon usually means that repair is not possible. In this situation the surgeon should be aware of the vulnerability of the cuff and be prepared to limit the releases and use a reduced offset prosthesis or avoid resurfacing the glenoid.

The coracoacromial ligament is usually intact and an attempt should be made to preserve it since it may act as a superior restraint when there is a deficient or absent rotator cuff.

Subscapularis is assessed in terms of available passive external rotation, and tendon thickness and integrity. Most rheumatoid patients coming to shoulder arthroplasty have grossly reduced external rotation or even fixed internal rotation deformities. Z lengthening of the subscapularis tendon is not appropriate in rheumatoid arthritis where the subscapularis tendon is too thin to permit its use. In most patients it is possible to section the tendon of subscapularis 5mm lateral to its humeral insertion and gain sufficient length by releasing the muscle and its tendon from the scapular neck and underside of the coracoid process. This subscapularis division is most easily accomplished by passing dissecting scissors beneath the tendon to emerge in the rotator interval proximally. The tendon is then incised directly onto the dissecting scissors after applying stay sutures to the medial margin of the tendon (Figure 4.8). The incision is carried superiorly into the rotator interval dividing the coracohumeral ligament. If on assessment the tendinous portion cannot be reached or the tendon is found to be too thin when the scissors are inserted access should be gained by osteotomizing the superficial portion of the lesser tuberosity. The anterior capsule is usually very thin and rarely produces the restriction seen in osteoarthritic shoulders. We would however excise it if it tethers the subscapularis tendon. On opening the capsule in line with the tendon any intra articular adhesions are released.

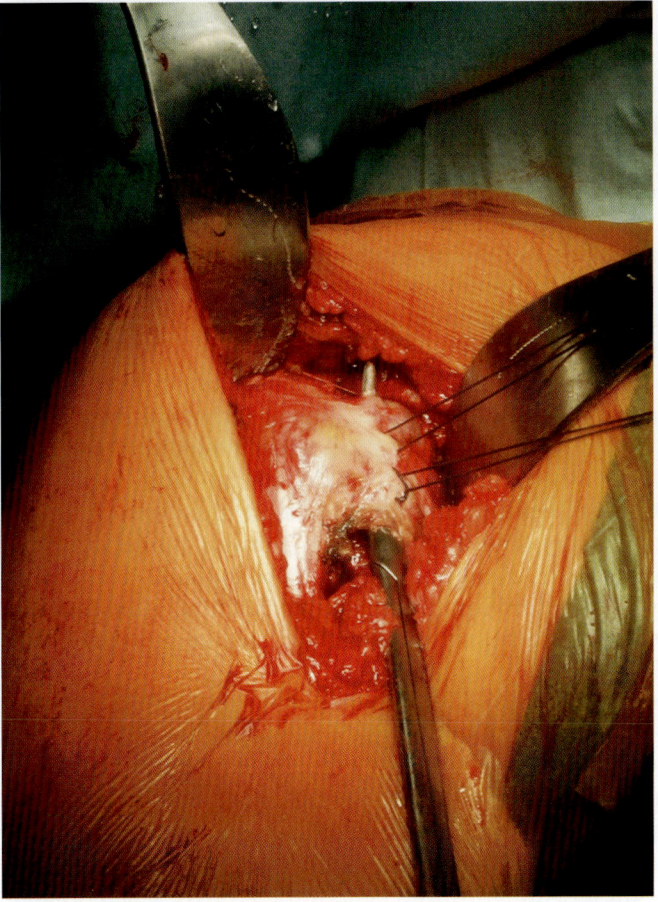

Figure 4.8. A dissecting scissor passed superiorly from the lower border of subscapularis to emerge at the rotator interval. Note that stay sutures have been applied medially prior to division of the tendon 5–10 mm from its insertion.

Since all of these shoulders will have medialized to some extent soft tissue releases will be required. To facilitate dislocation it is necessary to divide the inferior capsule. The axillary nerve is identified and protected. Slight external rotation is applied to the humerus and the inferior capsule is divided as far posteriorly as possible under direct vision. This dissection should be as close to the humeral head as possible, thus decreasing any chance of injury to the axillary nerve, which is usually medial. Further external rotation of the humerus should than allow easy anterior dislocation of the humeral head. If any resistance is encountered, external rotation is stopped and further capsular division undertaken. If there is still resistance total division of the tendon of pectoralis major is often helpful. Bone quality is reduced in these patients and iatrogenic fracture is a real risk with any maneuver requiring force.

At this stage the arm is extended at the side of the operating table and the humeral head dislocated and delivered gently into the wound using two retractors, one placed behind the humeral head beneath the acromion and the other behind the humeral head within the glenohumeral joint.

Humeral Preparation

Resection of the humeral head is performed with attention to the version and height of the bony cut using the cutting guide, which should be aligned with reference to the bicipital groove and the cuff insertion since bone deficiencies in the proximal humerus, and instability in the ipsilateral elbow frequently complicate head resection. By placing the point of the cutting guide toward the proximal part of the bicipital grove the version can be estimated. The insertion of the rotator cuff assists in determining the height of resection, the cut ideally emerging just proximal to the cuff insertion.

The bicipital groove acts as a reliable marker to identifying the initial reamer entry point in the humeral head (generally 5mm–10mm posterior to the groove). Rheumatoid bone is soft and porotic and the medullary cavity is generally capacious. This combination means that care with reamers and instrumentation of proximal humerus is paramount. Minimal force to enlarge the humeral medullary canal to the point that the reamer gently engages cortex is all that is required. A tight cortical fit, risking intraoperative fracture, is not essential since most rheumatoid humeral prostheses require cementing, as is discussed later.

Once the humerus is prepared appropriately, the trial prosthesis is inserted to match the cut surface, with the degree of version referenced against the alignment rods to give between 20 and 40 degrees of retroversion relative to the elbow. Instability of the elbow can obscure correct orientation of the component and alignment should be checked against the bicipital groove, correct orientation having the lateral fin of the prosthesis 5mm to 10mm behind the groove. When orientated correctly and seated properly the trial prosthesis is left in situ. This protects the proximal humerus during subsequent glenoid exposure and preparation.

Soft Tissue Releases/Glenoid Exposure

The posterior capsule is gently levered off the posterior glenoid rim with a blunt dissector. Formal posterior capsular releases are rarely required and may result in posterior laxity. The subscapularis muscle is now released through 360 degrees by elevating it from the anterior margin of glenoid, the scapular neck, and the undersurface of the coracoid process. There is a constant band extending from the underside of the coracoid process to the tendon and this must be released. This gains length and when complete gives a feeling of bounce or spring to the tendon when it is pulled on with the stay sutures.

The glenoid is exposed carefully with cobra retractors placed posterior to the glenoid protecting the proximal humerus and trial stem and anteriorly beneath the medially retracted subscapularis tendon on the neck of the scapula. If soft tissue release is adequate, exposure of the glenoid is good. If exposure of the glenoid is poor, it is likely that the soft tissue releases have been inadequate and further release of the inferior capsule and pectoralis major tendon will be necessary.

Glenoid Preparation

If present, the anterior osteophytic margin is excised, relatively lengthening the subscapularis further. If known to be large, the posterior osteophytes may be resected, but this is unusual in rheumatoid arthritis and resection is not usually performed.

The glenoid is usually eroded centrally with no excessive anterior or posterior erosion, and in some wet shoulders it may be completely preserved. The erosion usually progresses in a cephalad direction with the superior glenoid being eroded toward the base of the coracoid process but the inferior pole being preserved (Figure 4.9). If this position is accepted, any glenoid component also faces cephalad and this results in a reduced range of elevation and eccentric loading of the glenoid (Figure 4.10). It is our preference to remove the inferior pole using a burr and prepare the surface for resurfacing using the glenoid reamers whether implanting a glenoid component or not (Figure 4.11). This does further reduce glenoid bone stock, and, in theory, may weaken the glenoid, but the resulting arthroplasty is better balanced and we have had no problem with either glenoid fracture or early loosening. The central entry point for the glenoid reamer is identified and the line of reaming defined with the aid of a finger placed at the junction of the glenoid and scapula blade (Figure 4.12). This maneuver is particularly helpful in the presence of eccentric glenoid erosion.

The decision to resurface the glenoid or not is made intraoperatively unless there is inadequate bone stock as assessed by plane or CT radiography, or a massively deficient cuff. Many rheumatoid patients coming to shoulder arthroplasty are young but this is not a contraindication to glenoid resurfacing.

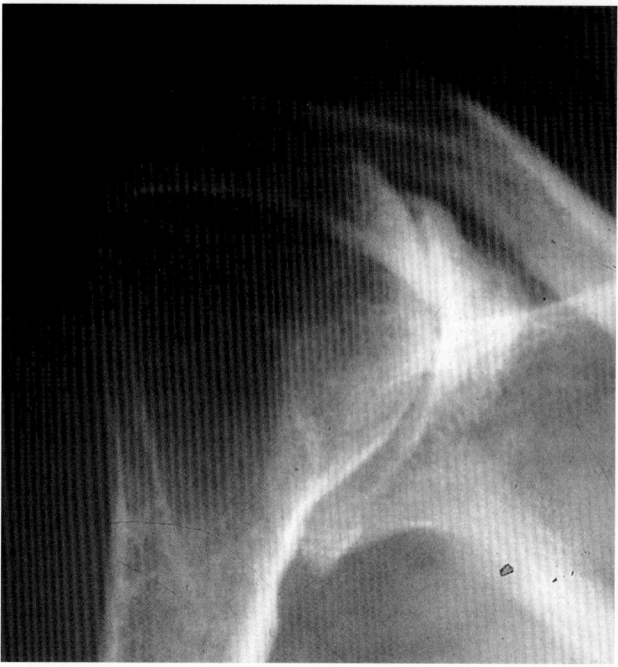

Figure 4.9. Characteristic cephalic erosion of the glenoid in a rheumatoid shoulder.

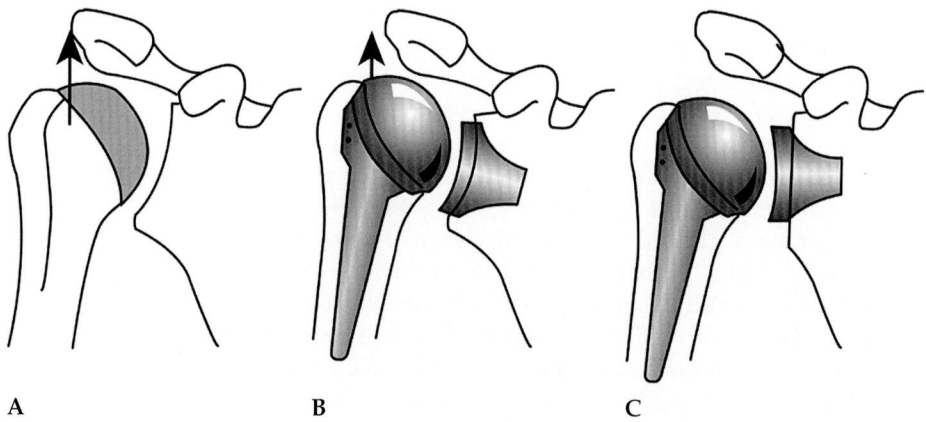

A   B   C

Figure 4.10. (A–C) In rheumatoid arthritis, the glenoid bone is frequently eroded in a cephalic direction as far as the base of the coracoid process while preserving the inferior pole **(A)**. Glenoid implantation without correction will result in superior subluxation **(B)**. Resection of the inferior pole of the glenoid is recommended to reorient the glenoid face **(C)**.

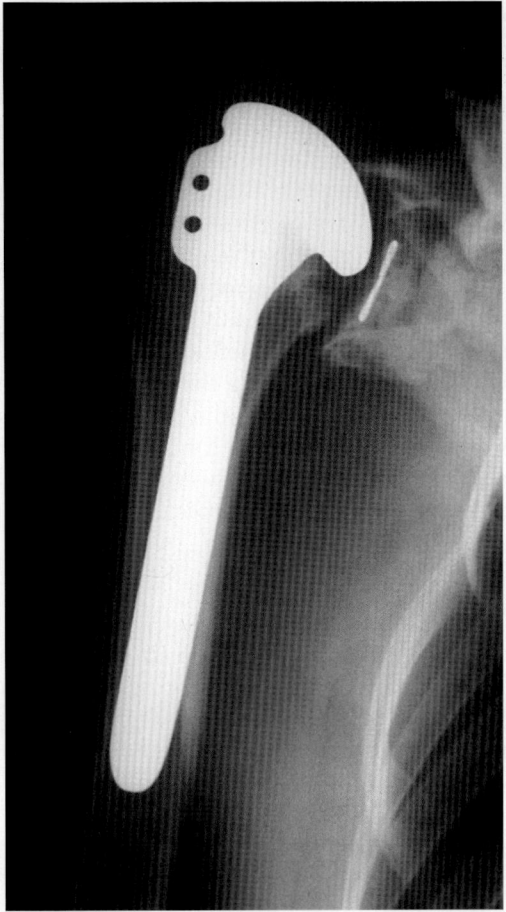

Figure 4.11. Failure to address cephalic erosion resulting in a superiorly angled component and subluxing humeral prosthesis.

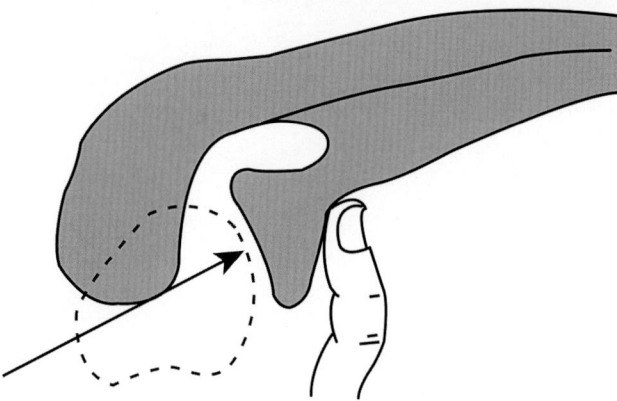

Figure 4.12. A fingertip placed at the junction of the glenoid and scapular blade allows correct alignment of instrumentation for the preparation of the glenoid face, especially where there is glenoid erosion.

Balancing the Shoulder

After all soft tissue releases have been performed and osteophytes removed, a trial humeral component with a head size equivalent to the narrowest head plus the width of the glenoid component is inserted (Figure 4.13). If with this component in situ and after simulated closure of subscapularis, 30 degrees of external rotation, 30% to 50% antero-posterior translation, and 90 degrees of internal rotation with the arm at 90 degrees of abduction are possible we proceed with glenoid resurfacing. If this degree of motion cannot be achieved, a glenoid component cannot be accommodated and only a humeral head component of a size that fulfills the previously mentioned criteria is inserted. This method ensures that after resurfacing the glenoid the shoulder will be balanced and accommodate at least the smallest humeral head component. However, our experience with humeral head replacement in the wet pattern of disease is such that we prefer total replacement and occasionally ream the glenoid more medially and accept less motion in order to do so.

Component Insertion

If a glenoid component is to be used, the sizing is determined by the reamer used and appropriate slot or peg holes are made in the already reamed glenoid face. Hand reaming of the glenoid is preferred as power reaming may destroy the soft glenoid bone. Care should be

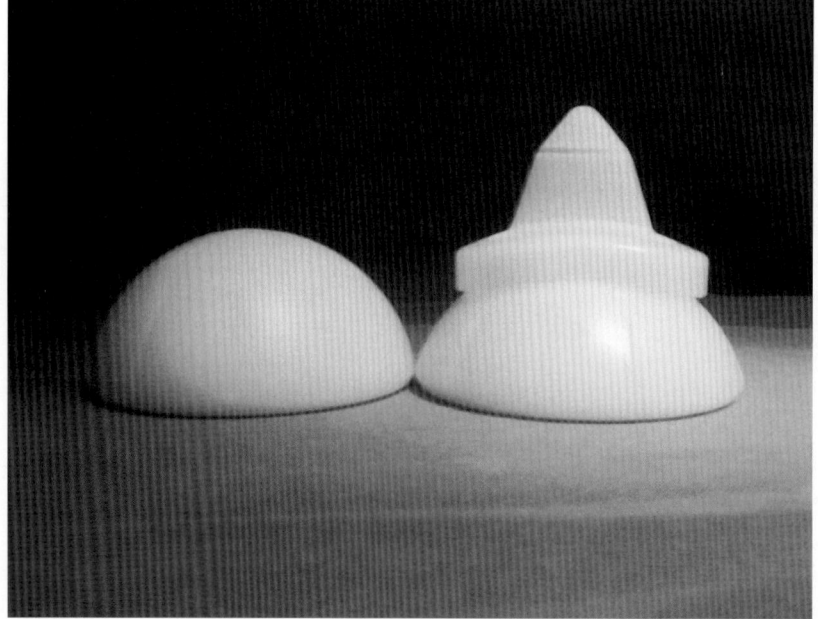

Figure 4.13. A large trial humeral head prosthesis with depth matching the combined depth of a smaller humeral head and glenoid component. If the large head is trialed and the shoulder can be balanced, then glenoid resurfacing with the smaller humeral head and glenoid will be possible.

taken to ensure that any inferior osteophytes have been removed and that the component is not seated too low. Glenoid fixation requires cement and several methods have been described. We prefer to compact the cancellous bone and use a stepwise insertion of doughy cement. Component insertion proceeds in the usual manner with pressure being maintained until the cement has cured.

Fixation of the humeral component in the rheumatoid patient is dependent on the bone quality and the prosthesis to be used. Porotic rheumatoid humeri tend to have capacious proximal medullary cavities. Press-fit components with slim proximal bodies do not gain adequate support and are prone to loosen. This has been confirmed both in our unit [14] and in a study from Denmark [13]. While cemented stems gave virtually no problems over 8 years, a significant proportion of noncemented stems subsided and loosened. More recently, Trail and Nuttall [18] have reported on the use of a broader proximal bodied prosthesis designed for noncemented use and have not seen any subsidence. Harris et al. [19] have demonstrated that if there is a good distal fix, a humeral prosthesis can be stabilized by proximal cementation alone. If the proximal humeral bone is deficient, we cement the humeral component with hand packed polymethylmethacrylate cement to fill the proximal flare of the humerus. Pressurization of the cement is not necessary in humeral implantation in the rheumatoid patient. Cement extrusion through thin osteoporotic bone confers no clinical benefit, damages already diseased bone further, and makes revision extremely difficult.

After the implantation of the glenoid component, it is necessary to recheck the soft tissue balancing so that the appropriate head size can be selected. The criteria outlined previously are used. If the proximal humerus remains uncovered by the standard head or soft tissue balancing is eccentric, consideration should be given to the use of an offset head.

Closure

After the shoulder is reduced the subscapularis is repaired according to the mode of opening. Attention has been drawn to the risk of failure of the subscapularis repair [20]. Our preferred method of closure has been direct suture of the tendon to its stump using long-term absorbable sutures (PDS Ethicon, Piscataway, NJ). If a good hold on the tendon or stump is not possible (an unusual situation), then transosseous sutures have to be added. Using the belly press test to assess subscapularis function in recent years has suggested that failure of the repair is a rare event in the rheumatoid patient. If an osteotomy of the lesser tuberosity was necessary to gain access, then reattachment to the humeral neck using suture anchors may gain length. In the presence of a cuff tear superiorly or a wide rotator interval, the subscapularis can be advanced superiorly to aid closure, augment depression of the humeral head, and assist future active elevation of the arm. We routinely use drains in rheumatoid shoulders, one deep to deltoid and one in the axillary recess. The deltopectoral interval is loosely approximated with interrupted absorbable sutures and the skin closed with subcuticular suture if the tissues permit, or surgical clips if not.

Special Operative Considerations

Acromioclavicular Arthritis

When there is painful disease of the acromioclavicular joint diagnosed clinically or by injection testing the excision of the outer end of the clavicle should be performed at the same time as glenohumeral arthroplasty, using the extensile incision described previously. The outer clavicle is approached from its superior aspect. Failure to recognize this problem compromises the result. Subacromial disease rarely requires attention since the exposure and the positioning of the arthroplasty decompress the space.

Massive Cuff Tear

Options for treatment of a rheumatoid shoulder with symptomatic glenohumeral arthritis and irreparable cuff tear include repair as previously discussed, cup arthroplasty in which an oversized resurfacing cup is applied over the tuberosities in a valgus orientation (Figure 4.14), a constrained arthroplasty, or arthrodesis.

Reversed geometry prostheses (Delta, DePuy, Warsaw, IN; Walker Bayley, Stanmore, Middlesex, UK) have gained in popularity in recent years and there have been two reports of their use in the rheumatoid shoulder [21, 22]. Unfortunately, these components rely on good

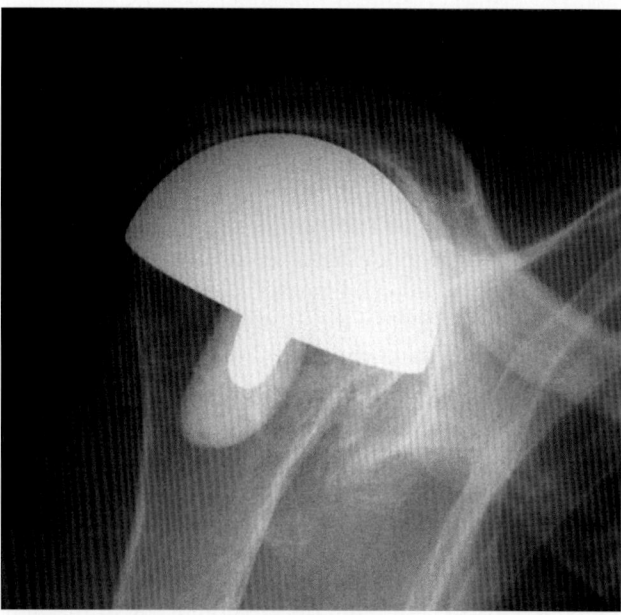

Figure 4.14. A Copeland cup arthroplasty placed in valgus orientation, resurfacing both the humeral head and greater tuberosity in rotator cuff arthropathy.

glenoid bone stock and uncemented screw fixation— precluding their use or increasing failure risks in many rheumatoid patients. In the eight Larsen V shoulders reported by Rittmeister and Kerschbaumer [21] and followed for 48 to 73 months, the Constant score improved from a mean of 17 to a mean of 63, but there were three glenoid loosenings, one of which was septic. The authors also drew attention to the fact that deltoid strength was crucial for function. Woodruff et al. [22] reported on the use of the Delta prosthesis in 17 rheumatoid patients, seven of whom were Larsen grade III, five grade IV, and only one grade V. All had massive tearing or "gross attenuation" of the cuff at surgery. Pain relief remained good at five years but glenoid radiolucencies were present in five of thirteen cases—with two glenoids radiologically loose. Stress shielding of the humerus proximally was universal. The high proportion of Larsen III shoulders in this series suggests that the glenoid bone stock was probably well preserved. The high rate of glenoid lucencies is therefore of serious concern.

If it is not possible to use a constrained prosthesis and the cuff deficiency is causing painful instability, then arthrodesis will have to be considered. Useful results have been achieved in rheumatoid patients when careful attention has been paid to the position selected and the preservation of elbow motion [23].

Intraoperative Fractures

Prevention is better than cure. Previously mentioned tips can avoid most of these problems—adequate soft tissue releases, resting a trial in the humeral cavity, care on dislocation and reduction and a respect for the diseased rheumatoid bone are all vital.

On occasion, however, fractures of the glenoid or humeral shaft occur. Importance here lies in the recognition of the event intraoperatively. On the glenoid side this most commonly consists of an anterior marginal fracture complicating glenoid insertion and is treated either conservatively or by resurfacing. On the humeral side most fractures occur at the midshaft level and require the use of a long stemmed prosthesis (Figure 4.15). No shoulder replacement should be embarked on without a long stemmed prosthesis available in the operating room.

Total Replacement or Humeral Head Replacement?

The potential advantages of glenoid replacement include a better fulcrum for improved strength and motion, increased stability, decreased friction, and elimination of the glenoid socket pain. Recent studies in the rheumatoid shoulder, however, have shown no significant difference between hemi and total shoulder arthroplasty (TSA) although some authors have found a subjective preference for total arthroplasty [24, 25, 26].

There are obviously some situations in which a glenoid component cannot be used such as when there is insufficient bone stock. Sojbjerg and colleagues [27] demonstrated that the use of a glenoid component when the bone stock was poor resulted in a high rate of loosening. If

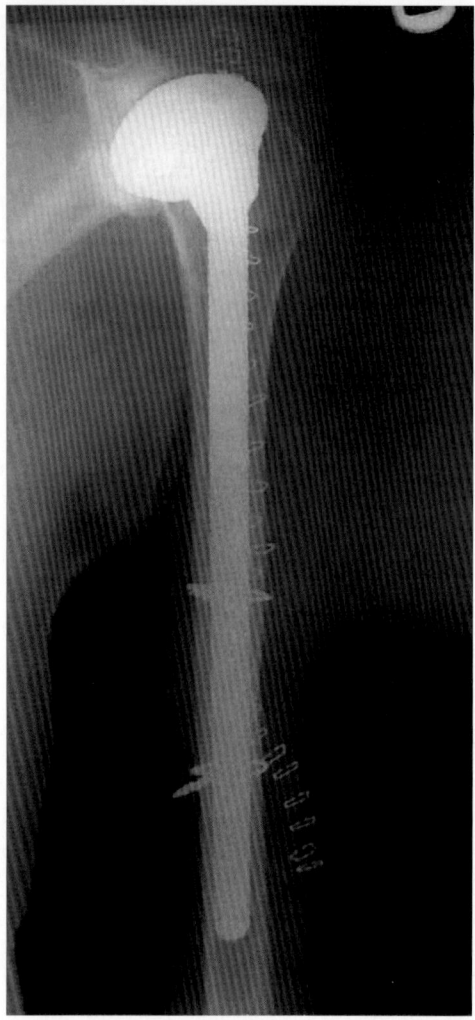

Figure 4.15. An intraoperative fracture treated with long stemmed prosthesis.

the rotator cuff is irreparably torn or very thin, there is a high likelihood that the humeral head will ride high and, in that situation, we prefer not to use a glenoid component.

We treat shoulder arthroplasty in the rheumatoid patient as a soft tissue procedure and base our choice of prosthetic components on the ability of the soft tissues to accommodate them. If our balancing criteria are met, then we proceed with total joint replacement; if not we insert only a humeral component with a head size that balances the shoulder. The slight exception to this rule is in the "wet" pattern of disease where we prefer total replacement. Our experience with this pattern of disease indicated that early and continuing glenoid erosion occurred in this group of patients when treated by hemiarthroplasty.

Postoperative Care

Unless there is the need to protect a fracture or a repaired rotator cuff, rehabilitation should commence on the first postoperative day. We follow the regime outlined by Neer commencing with passive motion of the shoulder but progressing to assisted active and then active movements as the patient is able. We have found that the patient is unwilling to externally rotate up to the range achieved at surgery in the early stages and therefore do not place any restrictions on this movement. However, we do not allow extension for the first three weeks to protect the repair of subscapularis tendon.

Isometric strengthening is introduced between four and six weeks and dynamic strengthening is carried out thereafter. Patients usually interact with their physiotherapist for about twelve weeks.

Hydrotherapy is particularly beneficial in these patients with multiple joint problems either in addition to or instead of the above regime.

Results

Results of shoulder arthroplasty in rheumatoid patients are generally inferior to those in osteoarthritis in terms of range of movement. This reflects the soft tissue and bone quality differences between the groups. Brenner et al. [28] have reported 73% survival at 11 years for all prostheses with 92% survival for the rheumatoid sub group. Torchia et al. [15] found the survival rate for all diagnostic groups was 88% at 15 years. Our experience suggests that demands placed on the arthroplasty are lower than in the osteoarthritic group of patients and that although function of the arthroplasty declines over time, revision is rarely necessary on clinical grounds.

Summary

Successful arthroplasty of the glenohumeral joint in the rheumatoid patient depends on an understanding of the disease process and pattern of the disease. An assessment of the entire patient and strict criteria for the diagnosis of the glenohumeral joint as source of the patient's symptoms is essential. The surgical technique necessitates meticulous care of the fragile soft and hard tissues with careful attention to soft tissue release, component orientation, and tissue balancing. If adhered to, the final result should be satisfying to both patient and the surgeon.

References

1. Petersson CJ. Painful shoulders in patients with rheumatoid arthritis. Scand J Rheumatol 1986;15:275–279.
2. Larsen A, Dale K, Eek M. Radiographic Evaluation of Rheumatoid arthritis and related conditions by standard reference films. Acta Radiol Diagn 1977;18:481–491.

3. Neer CS. Shoulder Reconstruction. Philadelphia: WB Saunders, 1990.

4. Kelly IG. Unconstrained shoulder arthroplasty in rheumatoid arthritis. Clin Orthop Related Res 1994;307(b):94–102.

5. Hirooka A, Wakitani S, Yoneda M, et al. Shoulder destruction in rheumatoid arthritis. Acta Orthop Scand 1996;67:258–263.

6. Kelly IG. The source of shoulder pain in rheumatoid arthritis: usefulness of local anesthetic injections. J Shoulder Elbow Surg 1994;3:62–65.

7. Grennan DM, Gray J, Louden J, et al. Methotrexate and early post operative complications in patients with rheumatoid arthritis undergoing elective orthopaedic surgery. Ann Rheum Dis 2001;60(3):214–217.

8. Kocialkowski A, Wallace WA. One stage arthroplasty of the ipsilateral shoulder and elbow. J Bone Joint Surg 1990;72B:520.

9. Agarwal AK, Peppelman WC, Kraus DR, et al. The cervical spine in rheumatoid arthritis. Br Med J 1993;306:79–80.

10. Neer CS, Watson KC, Stanton FJ. Recent experience in total shoulder arthroplasty. J Bone Joint Surg 1982;64A:319–337.

11. Cofield RH. Total shoulder arthroplasty with the Neer prosthesis. J Bone Joint Surg 1984;66-A:899–906.

12. Kelly IG, Foster RS, Fisher WD. Neer total shoulder replacement in rheumatoid arthritis. J Bone Joint Surg 1987;69B:723–736.

13. Sneppen O, Fruensgaard S, Johannsen HV, et al. Total Shoulder replacement in rheumatoid arthritis: proximal migration and loosening. J Shoulder Elbow Surg 1996;5:47–52.

14. Stewart MP, Kelly IG. Total Shoulder replacement in rheumatoid arthritis: a seven to thirteen year follow up of 37 joints. J Bone Joint Surg 1997; 79B:68–72.

15. Torchia ME, Cofield RH, Settergren CR. Total shoulder arthroplasty with the Neer prosthesis: long term results. J Shoulder Elbow Surg 1997;6:495–505.

16. Pollock RG, Efrain DD, McIlveen SJ, Flatow EL, Bigliani LU. Prosthetic replacement in rotator cuff deficient shoulders. J Shoulder Elbow Surg 1992;1:173–186.

17. Rozing PM, Brand R. Rotator cuff repair during shoulder arthroplasty in rheumatoid arthritis. J Arthroplasty 1998;13(3):311–319.

18. Trail IA, Nuttall D. The results of shoulder arthroplasty in patients with rheumatoid arthritis. J Bone Joint Surg 2002;84B:1121–1125.

19. Harris TE, Jobe CM, Dai QG. J Shoulder Elbow Surg 2000;9(3):205–210.

20. Miller SL, Hazrati Y, Klepps S, et al. Loss of subscapularis function after total shoulder replacement: a seldom recognized problem. J Shoulder Elbow Surg 2003;12:29–34.

21. Rittmeister M, Kerschbaumer F. Grammont reverse total shoulder arthroplasty in patients with rheumatoid arthritis and nonreconstructable rotator cuff lesions. J Shoulder Elbow Surg 2001;10(1):17–22.

22. Woodruff MJ, Cohen AP, Bradley JG. Arthroplasty of the shoulder in rheumatoid arthritis with rotator cuff dysfunction. Intern Orthop (SICOT) 2003;27:7–10.

23. Rybka V, Raunio P, Vainio K. Arthrodesis of the shoulder in rheumatoid arthritis: a review of 41 cases. J Bone Joint Surg 1979;61B:155–158.

24. Rodosky MW, Bigliani LU. Indications for glenoid resurfacing in shoulder arthroplasty. J Shoulder Elbow Surg 1996;5:231–247.

25. Gschwend N, Bischof A. Clinical experiences in arthroplasty according to Neer. J Orthop Rheumatol 1991;4:135–143.

26. Boyd AD, Thomas WH, Scott RD, et al. Total shoulder arthroplasty versus hemiarthroplasty. Indications for glenoid resurfacing. J Arthroplasty 1990; 5:329–336.

27. Sojbjerg JO, Frich LH, Johannsen HV, Sneppen O. Late results of total shoulder replacement in patients with rheumatoid arthritis. Clin Orthop Related Res 1999;366:39–45.
28. Brenner BC, Ferlic DC, Clayton ML, et al. Survivorship of total shoulder arthroplasty. J Bone Joint Surg 1989;71A:1289–1296.

Chapter 5

Arthroplasty for Proximal Humerus Fractures, Nonunions, and Malunions

Edward W. Lee and Evan L. Flatow

Treatment of complex fractures and fracture-dislocations of the proximal humerus in both the acute and late settings represent some of the most difficult injuries to assess and treat in the shoulder girdle. While the vast majority of proximal humerus fractures (more than 85%) are nondisplaced and amenable to nonoperative treatment, the remaining minority may involve multiple fragments or *parts*, comminution, and articular surface damage and represent a significant therapeutic challenge.

Based on Codman's anatomical description of fractures about the proximal humerus [1], Neer [2] published a comprehensive four-part classification scheme of these complex injuries in 1970. Wide use of this system has allowed for more uniformity in evaluation and has directed treatment in this area for the last three decades.

In conjunction with adequate evaluation of the proximal humeral anatomy, whether it is an acute fracture or the sequelae of an old injury, the therapeutic course should be guided by the surgical goal of anatomic restoration of the proximal humerus and patient-determined factors, such as age, function, and quality of remaining bone. With respect to acute fractures, all two-part, most three-part, and some four-part fractures are well treated by closed reduction or open reduction and internal fixation techniques. When soft bone, impaired head vascularity, or articular damage make fixation difficult or ill-advised, prosthetic arthroplasty is a reasonable option.

Use of a humeral head prosthesis for proximal humerus fractures was first reported in the 1950s. Multiple designs were emerging [3–7], but Neer's metal prosthesis became the most commonly used. In 1953, Neer [7] reported the first use of his prosthetic humeral head in a complex fracture-dislocation of the proximal humerus. In 1955 and 1970, he reported his series of 27 and 43 patients, respectively, with fracture-dislocations treated with prosthetic replacement [7, 8].

Advances in design since Neer's first-generation monoblock prosthesis and his subsequent redesign in 1973 have included the use of modular head and stem components. Restoration of soft tissue ten-

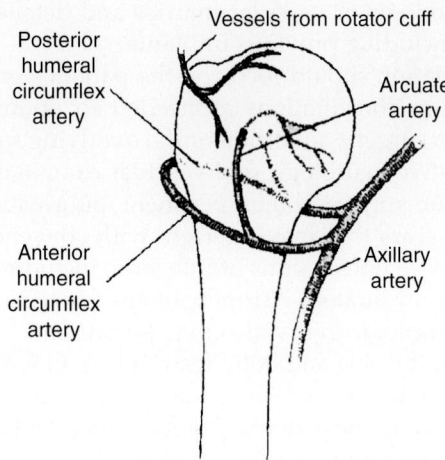

Figure 5.1. Blood supply to the proximal humerus. (By permission of TF Schlegel, RJ Hawkins, J Am Acad Orthop Surg 2:54–66, 1994.)

sioning may be more reliable with a wider variety of head sizes and offset. In addition, should conversion to a total shoulder become necessary, removable heads allow for better visualization of the glenoid while permitting preservation of a well-fixed stem [9, 10].

Blood Supply

Laing [11] was the first to describe the arcuate artery, a continuation of the ascending branch of the anterior humeral circumflex artery, which is itself the major blood supply to the humeral head. It usually enters the bone in the area of the intertubercular groove and gives branches to the greater and lesser tuberosities. A smaller contribution to the blood supply is provided by the posterior humeral circumflex arteries and tendinous-osseous anastomoses from the rotator cuff. Gerber et al. [12] found that vascularization of the head was only possible through the ascending branch of the anterior humeral circumflex; injury to this structure would likely compromise its main blood supply leading to avascular necrosis (Figure 5.1).

Patient Evaluation

As in management of any fracture, a thorough history and physical examination is essential before initiating any treatment regimen. In addition to an account of the injury and its mechanism, information such as hand dominance, preinjury functional level, medical history, cognitive deficits, and available social supports should be sought to direct the method of treatment and assess the patient's ability to protect the tuberosity repair and participate in postoperative physical therapy. In cases of failed treatment, additional history becomes relevant such as associated neurologic or vascular injuries and detailed accounts of initial treatment including previous implants.

Physical examination should focus on the patient's general medical condition, obtaining consultations as needed to optimize comorbid conditions prior to surgery, condition of the overlying soft tissues, and a careful preoperative neurologic and vascular examination.

In cases of prior surgery, other pertinent information should be documented. Old scars that may interfere with conventional surgical approaches should be noted; signs of infection, including erythema or drainage, must be evaluated. Atrophy of the shoulder musculature from disuse or neurologic injury also may be present.

Assessment of soft tissue and bony restraints to motion, particularly passive, is important in preoperative planning. Forward flexion, lateral elevation, and internal and external rotation may be limited by contractures and bony impingement from malunited fragments; soft tissue releases and osteotomies may need to be performed at the time of surgery to address these problems.

Strength and integrity of the rotator cuff should also be carefully evaluated. Weakness in external rotation may be anticipated with greater tuberosity malunions as the functional length of the supraspinatus, infraspinatus, and teres minor are shortened. Integrity of the subscapularis and lesser tuberosity can be evaluated by the Gerber lift-off [13] and belly-press tests.

Instability can be evaluated with conventional provocative maneuvers. A greater tuberosity malunited posteriorly can lever the humeral head over the glenoid and simulate anterior instability [14]. Addressing the problem intraoperatively can be done with soft tissue procedures or adjustment of humeral version.

Radiographic Evaluation

Definitive diagnosis and preoperative planning begin with adequate plain radiographs. The standard trauma series, anteroposterior and lateral in the scapular plane and an axillary view, allow evaluation of the proximal humerus in three perpendicular planes. The addition of supplemental views can be useful to estimate displacement of specific segments. Phemister [15] recommended rotational anteroposterior views to visualize fractures of the greater tuberosity obscured by the humeral head; Morris et al. [16] found that anteroposterior views clearly showed superior displacement of greater tuberosity fractures but were misleading in assessment of posterior retraction. A good quality axillary (standard or Velpeau) is generally sufficient to evaluate posterior retraction of the greater tuberosity and overlap of the fragment with the articular surface [17].

Other radiologic diagnostic tests may provide additional information. Computed tomography (CT) is a helpful adjunct in identifying the bony anatomy in complex acute fractures, nonunions, and malunions. CT has been shown to more accurately judge greater tuberosity displacement than plain films [16]. CT is also valuable in assessing the amount of articular involvement with head-splitting or impression fractures, chronic fracture-dislocations, and associated glenoid rim fractures.

Magnetic resonance imaging (MRI) is not routinely obtained in the setting of proximal humerus fractures but does provide information about both the bone and soft tissues. MRI can help judge integrity of rotator cuff and its relationship to the tuberosities; furthermore, early stages of avascular necrosis can be detected sooner than on standard radiographs.

Indications for Humeral Head Replacement

The use of arthroplasty in the management of proximal humerus fractures has evolved from the results of closed and open treatments of these injuries. In general, prosthetic replacement of the proximal humerus is reserved for those patients with poor bone stock and fracture patterns that preclude stable internal fixation or viability of the humeral head.

Nonunions and malunions of the proximal humerus after failed non-operative or operative therapy present another difficult management problem. Patients with minimal symptoms or those who have low functional demands may be treated nonoperatively. Many patients, however, have pain and severe functional impairment; in these cases, indications for arthroplasty include osteoporosis precluding internal fixation, severe head cavitation, avascular necrosis, or post-traumatic glenohumeral arthritis [18].

Indications for Arthroplasty: Three- and Four-Part Fractures and Fracture Dislocations

Neer obtained 63% satisfactory results with internal fixation of three-part fractures and 100% failure of fixation of four-part fractures; however, 96% of four-part injuries treated with hemiarthroplasty had satisfactory or excellent results [8].

While preservation of the humeral head remains the preferred method of treating most three-part fractures, select cases may be more amenable to humeral head replacement. In situations in which significant injury to the articular segment or its blood supply was apparent or when osteoporosis would result in unstable internal fixation, primary hemiarthroplasty is indicated to allow for earlier mobilization of the shoulder.

Traditional treatment of displaced four-part fractures has come under scrutiny by several studies. These injuries, with or without associated dislocations, have been associated with the development of avascular necrosis in as many as 90% of cases [8]. This is especially true for *classic* 4-part fracture-dislocations, in which the head is dislocated and has lost all soft tissue attachments (Figure 5.2). This led Neer to recommend prosthetic arthroplasty in four-part displacements. Paavolainen et al. [19] concurred with Neer's findings and found open reduction and internal fixation unsuccessful in four-part fractures.

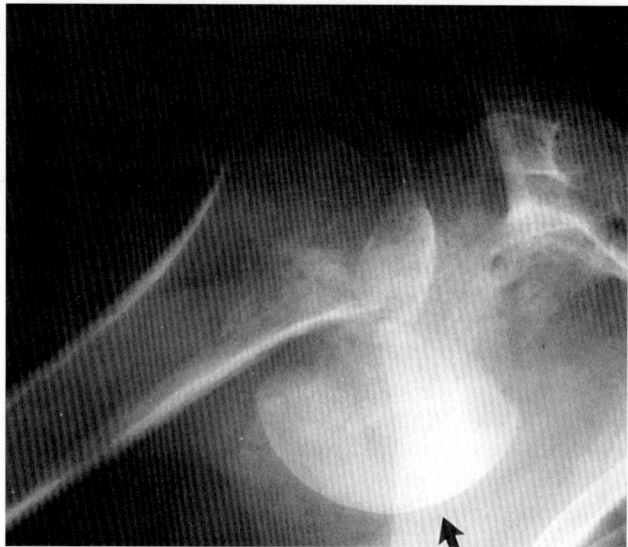

Figure 5.2. Anteroposterior radiograph of a *classic* 4-part proximal humerus fracture-dislocation with the head fragment displaced into the axilla.

A number of studies, however, have revisited the use of internal fixation for severe proximal humerus fractures with encouraging results. In their study of 19 patients, Lee and Hansen [20] reported no cases of posttraumatic avascular necrosis in four-part proximal humerus fractures with an average follow-up of two years.

Esser [21] treated 26 patients (average age, 55 years) with three- or four-part fractures with a modified cloverleaf plate with no cases of avascular necrosis at average follow-up of six years. He concluded that open reduction and internal fixation should be the initial treatment of displaced three and four-part fractures with primary hemiarthroplasty reserved for elderly patients with poor bone quality.

Darder et al. [22] described tension band and K-wire fixation of displaced four-part fractures in 33 patients at an average of seven years postoperatively. Satisfactory or excellent results were obtained in 64% according to Neer's criteria, but again, emphasis was on the younger (average age, 59 years), active, healthy patient.

In a study by Gerber et al. [23] the authors found satisfactory clinical results in patients with osteonecrosis in the setting of anatomic healing of the tuberosities. In those patients in whom anatomic or near-anatomic healing occurred, outcomes were comparable to those treated with hemiarthroplasty for complex proximal humerus fractures. They concluded that a fracture at risk for avascular necrosis must be reduced anatomically if a joint-preserving procedure is performed.

Siebler and Kuner [24] and later Szyszkowitz et al. [25] suggested that internal fixation of three- and four-part fractures could produce good outcomes. The latter found 70% excellent or satisfactory outcomes in three-part fractures and 22% in four-part fractures (compared with Neer's 0%). The authors noted that even with failure of internal fixation, hemiarthroplasty could be used as a late salvage procedure.

In a subset of patients, Jakob et al. [26] reported a pattern termed the "four-part valgus impacted fractures" in which open reduction and internal fixation may be indicated. In these injuries, the head is impacted on the shaft and the tuberosities are split but in close proximity to the head and shaft. The head is not dislocated or displaced laterally, and some contact with the glenoid is maintained (Figure 5.3). While not a true four-part fracture according to the Neer classification, it must be discerned from its severely displaced counterpart. The authors reported 74% satisfactory results and avascular necrosis in only 26% with elevation of the head and fixation with multiple pins. The findings of Resch et al. [27] further suggested that these injuries could be adequately treated with limited dissection and internal fixation.

Despite these studies, the results of internal fixation of four-part displacements are generally poor [19, 25, 28–32]. With the possible exception of the young, active patient with the head in continuity with the glenoid and some soft tissues attachments, the treatment of choice for most displaced four-part fractures and fracture-dislocations is immediate prosthetic replacement.

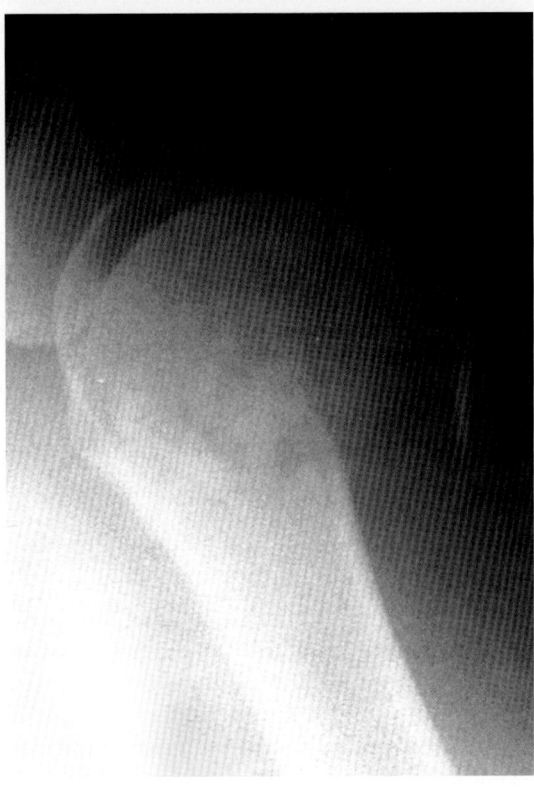

Figure 5.3. Anteroposterior radiograph of a valgus-impacted proximal humerus fracture.

Consensus on definitive treatment of two-part anatomic neck fractures is difficult given its rarity (only 0.54% [33] proximal humerus fractures) and a paucity of reports in the literature [34–37]. If fixation of the head fragment to the proximal humerus cannot be secured or the fragment is devoid of soft tissue attachments, then excision followed by humeral head replacement may be considered.

Articular Surface Fractures: Impression, Head-Splitting

The role of arthroplasty in the management of articular impression fractures is dictated by the size of the defect and the time from injury. In cases of acute posterior dislocations (within 2–3 weeks) with less than 20% involvement of the anterior articular surface, closed reduction followed by immobilization in external rotation is usually sufficient [38]. Defects between 20% and 45% present less than 6 months may be treated with the McLaughlin procedure or its modification as reported by Hawkins et al. [38]. For articular defects greater than 45%, or with a dislocation older than 6 months old, prosthetic replacement is the preferred method of treatment. Involvement of the glenoid, whether from fracture or secondary wear from an incongruent joint, may require total shoulder arthroplasty (TSA).

Head-splitting fractures also usually require hemiarthroplasty (Figure 5.4). Although technically demanding with a high likelihood of failure, open reduction and internal fixation may be considered in the case of a young patient with minimal comminution and adequate bone stock.

Proximal Humerus Malunion/Nonunion

The indications to proceed with prosthetic arthroplasty in cases of nonunion and malunion are based on the patient's quality of life, adequacy of residual bone stock, and condition of the glenohumeral joint. As noted previously, significant functional disability and pain must be present. Poor bone quality, residual intraarticular step-off, osteonecrosis of the head, or secondary degenerative joint disease precludes the use of corrective osteotomies or internal fixation to salvage malunited or nonunited segments; humeral head replacement should be considered in these situations (Figure 5.5).

Surgical Approach/Technique

Acute Fracture

The patient is placed in the modified beach-chair position under a regional (i.e., interscalene block) and/or general anesthesia. The deltopectoral approach is used in performing shoulder arthroplasty, providing exposure of both the proximal humerus and, if necessary, the glenoid. The skin incision is started just inferior to the clavicle, extending across the coracoid process, and extending laterally to the deltoid insertion. The deltoid origin and insertion are preserved with this approach. The deltopectoral interval is identified by the cephalic vein,

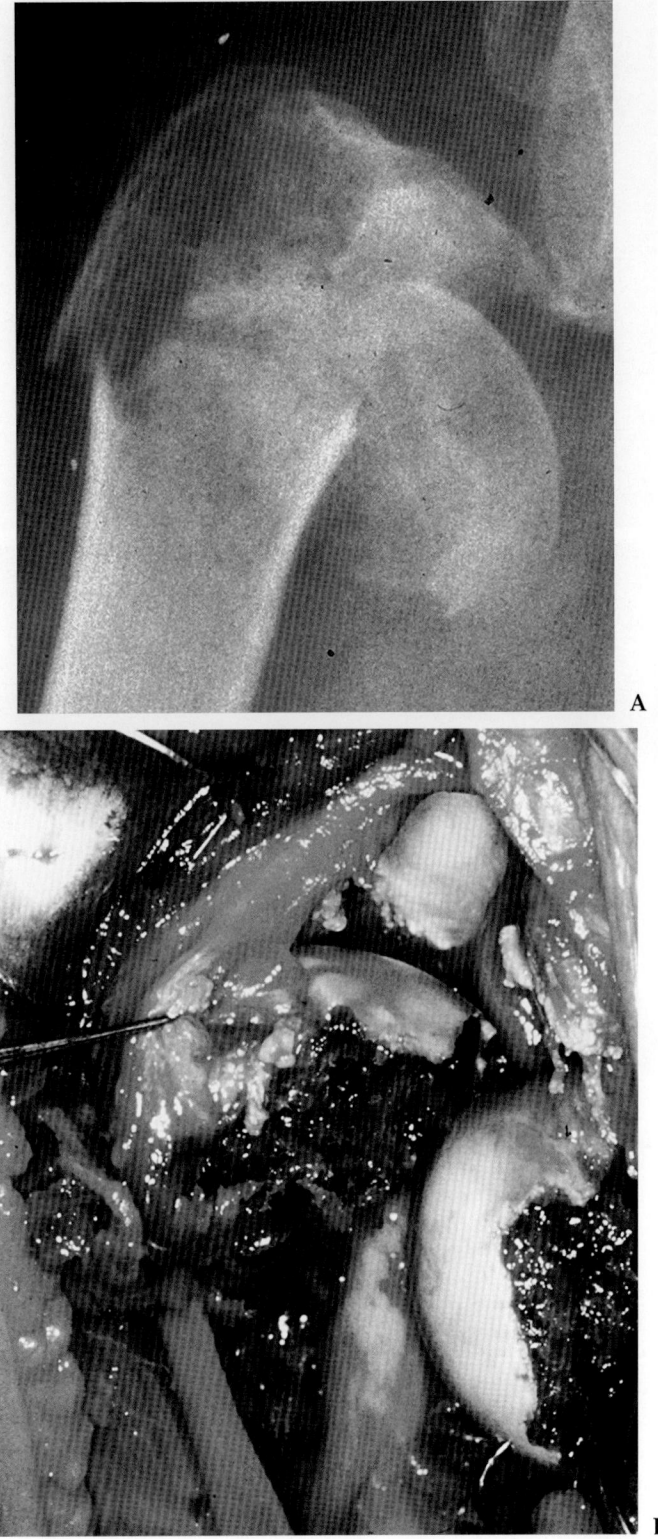

Figure 5.4. (A) Anteroposterior view of a head-splitting fracture. **(B)** Intraoperative picture demonstrating 2 major head fragments.

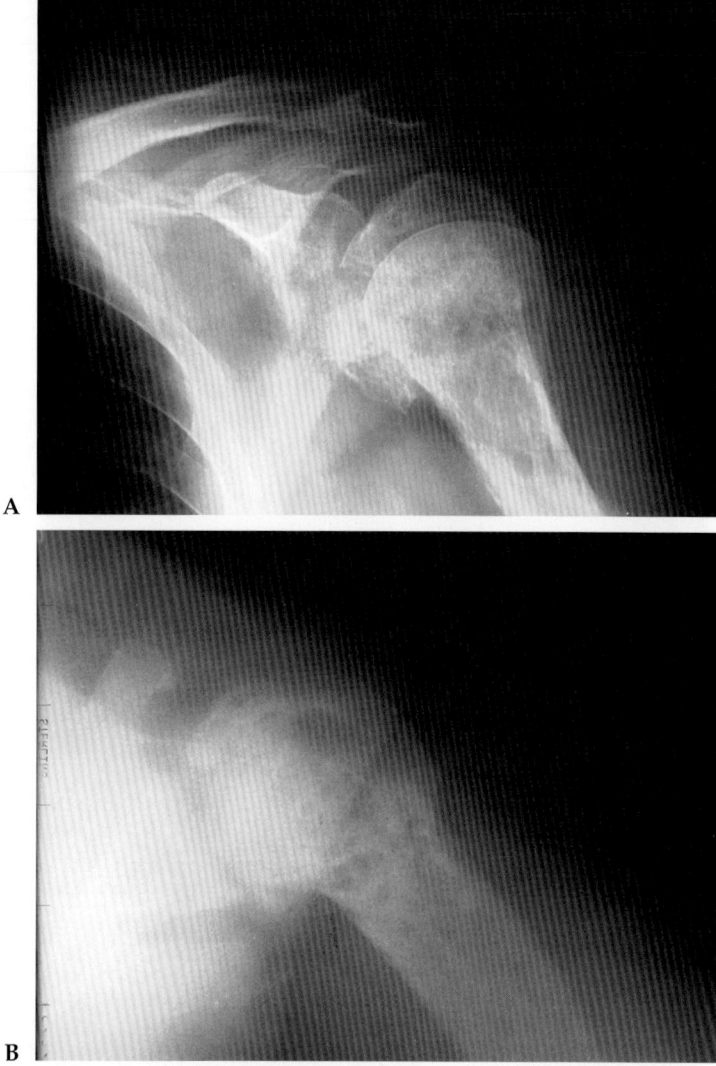

Figure 5.5. (A) Anteroposterior and (B) axillary radiographs of a four-part proximal humerus malunion.

which can be retracted either medially or laterally. If more exposure is needed, the upper 1 cm to 2 cm of the pectoralis major tendon can be released. The leading edge of the coracoacromial ligament is excised to facilitate exposure. This does not affect the structural stability or the ligament or its role as a superior restraint to the humeral head.

The condition of the biceps tendon should be evaluated. If it is intact with no evidence of fraying or tendinopathy, the biceps may be preserved. Otherwise, the intraarticular portion of the tendon should be transected followed by a tenodesis to adjacent soft tissue or the pectoralis major tendon at the conclusion of the procedure. Some surgeons prefer to routinely sacrifice the biceps during prosthetic reconstruction to remove it as a possible source of postoperative pain or stiffness.

Identification of the tuberosity fragments requires careful dissection. Intact soft tissue attachments and nondisplaced fracture lines should be preserved when possible. In some cases in which the tuberosities remain connected to each other and the rotator interval remains intact, the entire unit may be lifted superiorly to expose the head segment. If the tuberosities are separated, the lesser tuberosity is retracted medially and the greater tuberosity laterally. Usually, the biceps is with the lesser tuberosity, and the fracture line is 5mm to 6mm lateral to the bicipital groove. Heavy nonabsorbable sutures can be placed for traction around the bone-tendon junction of the fragments. During mobilization of the lesser tuberosity and the associated subscapularis, caution must be taken to protect the axillary nerve at the inferior border of the tendon. Use of the *tug-test* [39] can assist in localization and protection of the nerve.

Great care should be taken when extracting the head fragment in anterior fracture-dislocations. In this situation, the head lies in close proximity to the axillary artery and brachial plexus. This relationship becomes particularly important in delayed reconstructions when scarring and adhesions place these structures at risk during dissection and removal of the head. Once freed, the fragment may be used as a template for the trial head as well as a source of cancellous graft placed beneath the tuberosities (Figure 5.6).

Restoring functional tension to the deltoid and rotator cuff is dependent on recreating humeral length with the prosthesis. Placing the stem too low leads to inferior subluxation of the prosthesis and inability to elevate the extremity. Placing the implant too high subjects the rotator cuff and tuberosity repair to excessive tension and potential early failure. Judging the proper height for the prosthesis is a crucial step. Historically, surgeons have used many methods to help with this determination, including using a jig that measures humeral length referenced from the elbow (Tornier, Montbonnot, France), placing the tuberosities below the collar of the prosthesis, allowing slight overlap with the metaphysis, setting the stem at a height which allows the head to be translated about 50% of its diameter both inferiorly and posteriorly, and using a radiograph of the contralateral shoulder as a template (Figure 5.7). In our experience, the most reliable method for judging prosthetic height is a technique we term the *jig-saw puzzle* approach: The fracture fragments are re-assembled to determine the proximal humeral anatomy, which is then precisely reconstructed with the prosthetic implant (Figures 5.8 and 5.9). There is usually a calcar gap of about 5mm to 7mm that must be recreated.

Stability of the glenohumeral joint and the tuberosity repair is also dependent on recreating appropriate version with the prosthesis. Furthermore, excessive retroversion places the greater tuberosity repair under tension when the arm is brought into internal rotation against the body [40]. Thus, in a fracture, retroversion is set at about 20 degrees to counteract this problem. This may be measured against the forearm axis, remembering that 5 to 10 degrees is added by the epicondylar axis

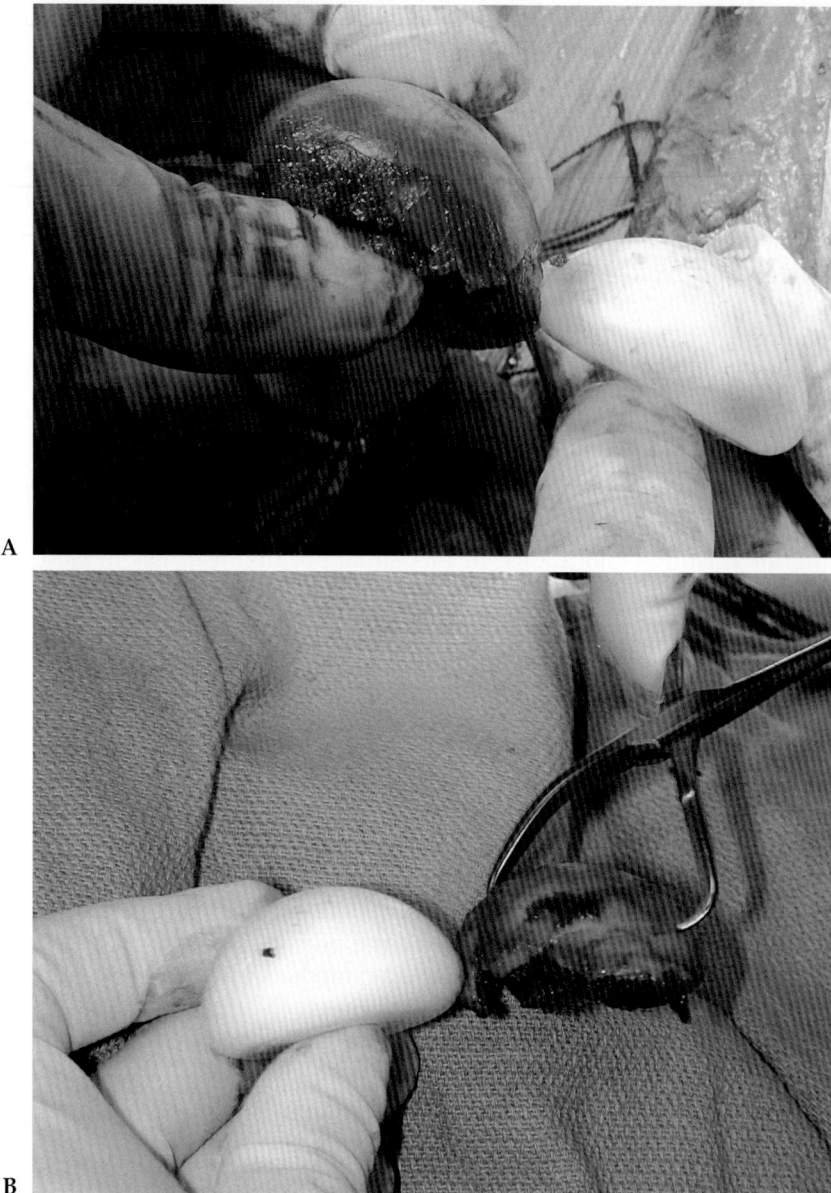

Figure 5.6. (A and B) Humeral head size is estimated after extracting the head fragment and measuring against the prosthesis with templates or using radiographs of the contralateral shoulder if available.

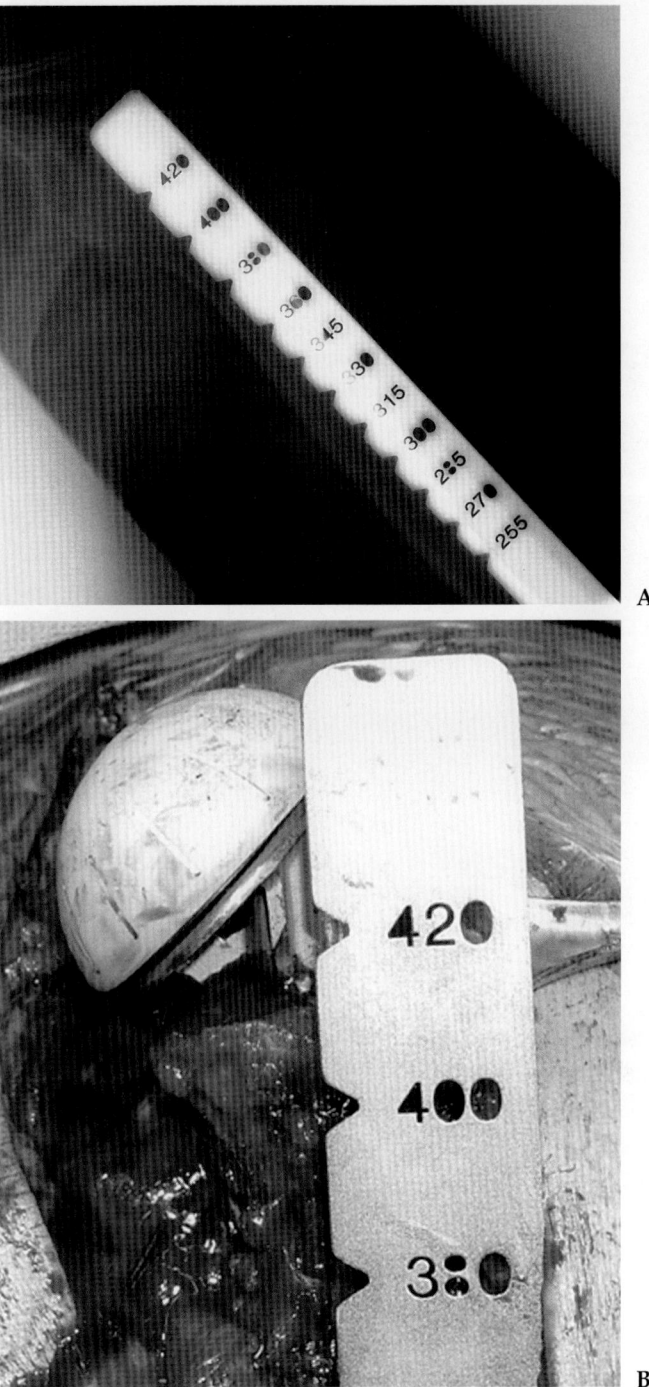

Figure 5.7. **(A)** Measuring humeral height from radiograph of the contralateral proximal humerus. **(B)** Recreating height as measured from the plain film.

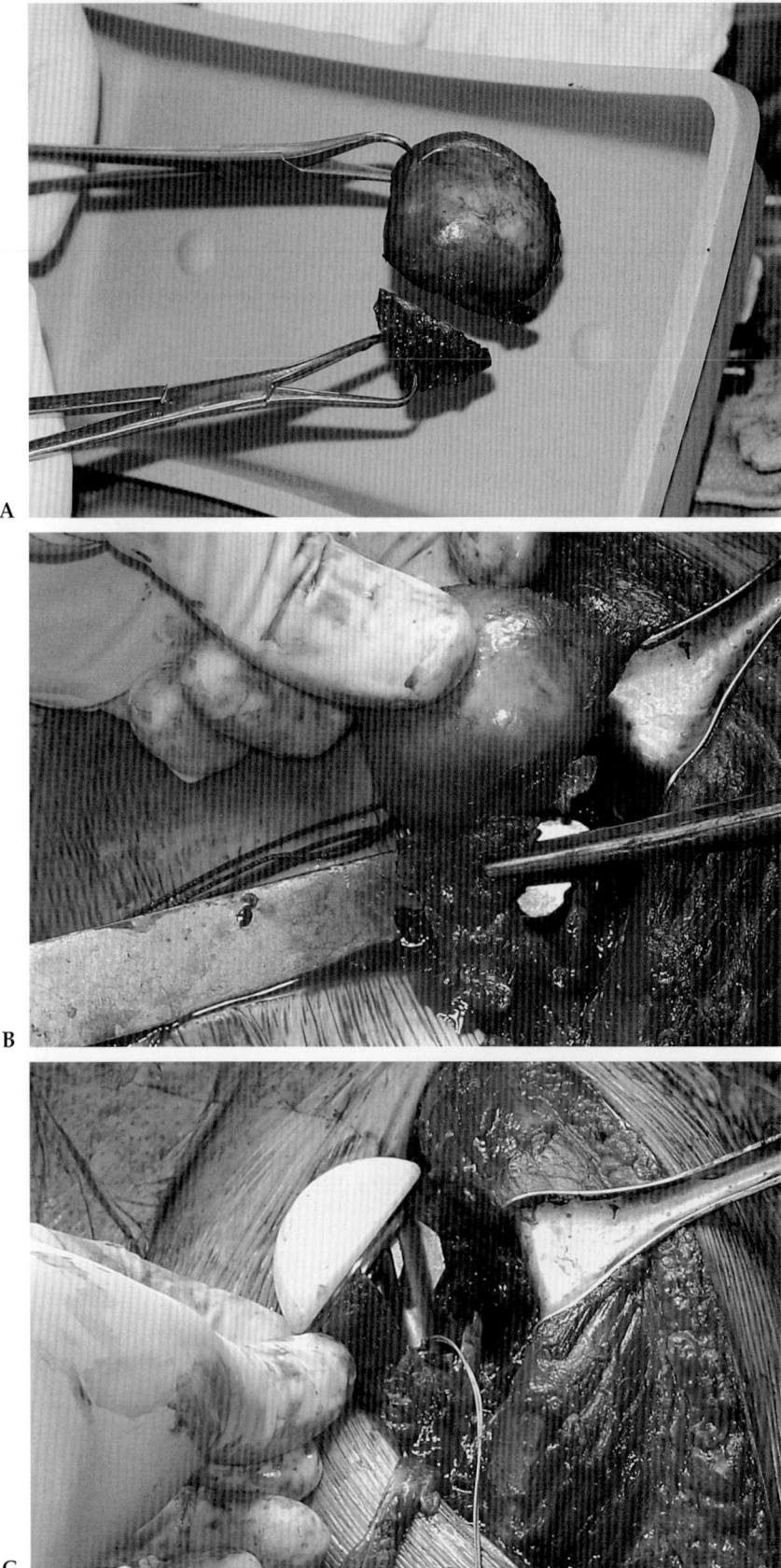

Figure 5.8. **(A)** Reassembly of head and medial calcar fragments. **(B)** Recreating humeral head height with medial calcar fragment. **(C)** Restoration of height with trial prosthesis.

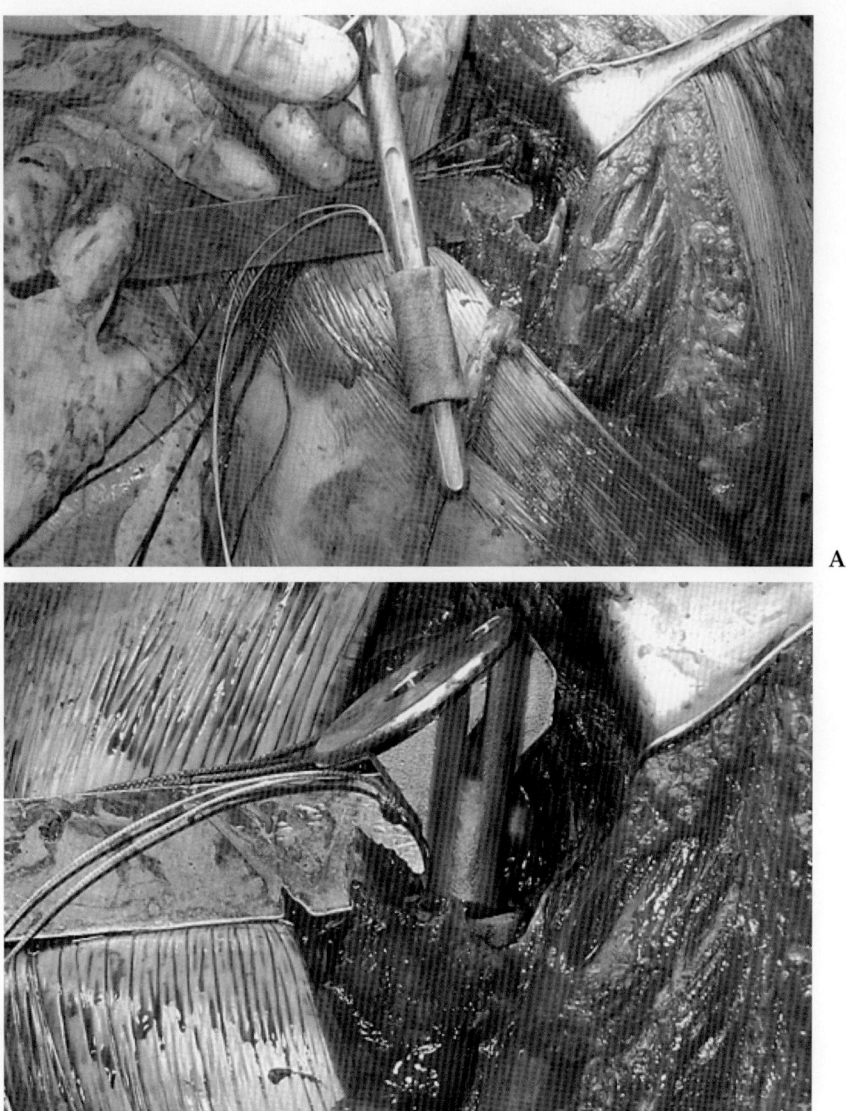

A

B

Figure 5.9. (A and B) Use of foam spacers (Zimmer, Warsaw, IN) to provisionally hold trial stem in place.

(thus, 20–30 degrees with respect to the forearm) (Figures 5.10 and 5.11).

As noted previously, a wider selection of head configurations with modular systems further facilitates restoration of proper tension to the surrounding musculotendinous structures as well as making revision or conversion to a total shoulder arthroplasty easier. The use of an offset head can relieve tension on the rotator cuff when a patient's anatomy results in an eccentrically placed stem. In cases in which revision of the head or resurfacing of the glenoid become necessary in the

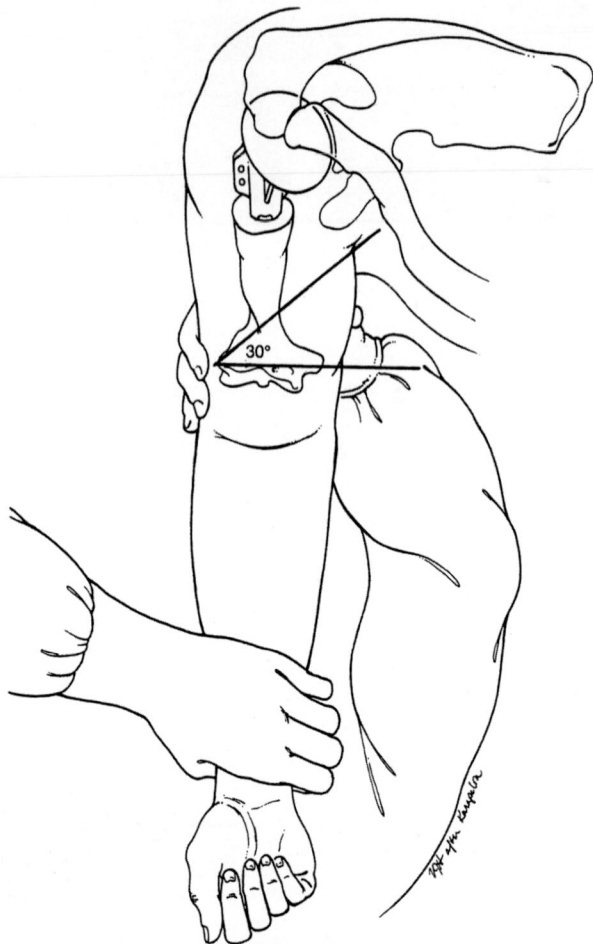

Figure 5.10. Illustration depicting appropriate amount of retroversion (aim for approximately 20 to 30 degrees to avoid tension on the greater tuberosity repair with the arm internally rotated in the sling). The distal epicondylar axis is utilized as a reference for head position. (By permission of LJ Bigliani, in Post M, Bigliani LU, Flatow EL, et al., editors. The Shoulder: Operative Technique. New York: Lippincott Williams & Wilkins, 1998;3–71.)

future, removal of the modular head from the taper would avoid extraction of a potentially well-fixed stem.

The use of polymethylmethacrylate with final implantation of the humeral stem is routinely required in the setting of fracture and is one factor associated with favorable postoperative results [41–43]. Cement increases stability, allows the component to seat at the proper height, and prevents rotation within the humeral canal.

The goal of fixation of the tuberosities is to ensure bony union with the humeral shaft and to permit early postoperative mobilization. This is accomplished through securing the tuberosities to each other and to the humeral shaft with heavy braided nonabsorbable sutures (e.g., No. 5 Ethibond [Ethicon/Johnson & Johnson, Somerville, NJ] and No. 2

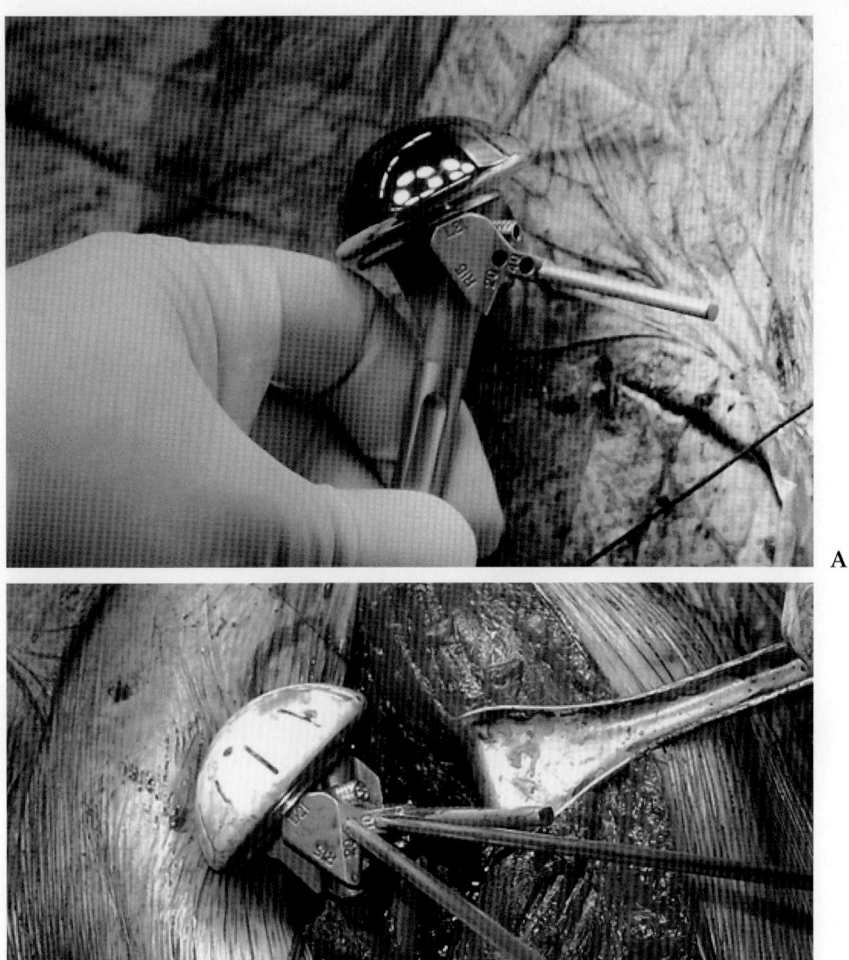

A

B

Figure 5.11. (A and B) Detachable fin clamps with retroversion guide pins (Zimmer, Warsaw, IN) assist in reestablishing proper humeral height and rotation.

FiberWire [Arthrex, Naples, FL]). Two sutures should be placed from the greater to the lesser tuberosity either through the fin of the prosthesis or around the medial aspect of the implant stem. More recently, we have used 1.3-mm titanium cables, which come on a large needle, as this has greatly increased implant security. Two sutures can then also be passed through two drill holes in the humerus lateral and one medial to the bicipital groove prior to cementation, providing vertical fixation of the lesser and greater tuberosities, respectively. A figure-of-eight tension band suture in and out of the infraspinatus tendon at its insertion and similarly with respect to the subscapularis is also used to reduce reliance on the soft, osteoporotic bone (Figure 5.12). Cancellous bone graft from the head is placed beneath the tuberosities to aid in healing (Figure 5.13).

Once the tuberosity repair is complete, the shoulder should be taken through a gentle range of motion to assess fixation and determine the

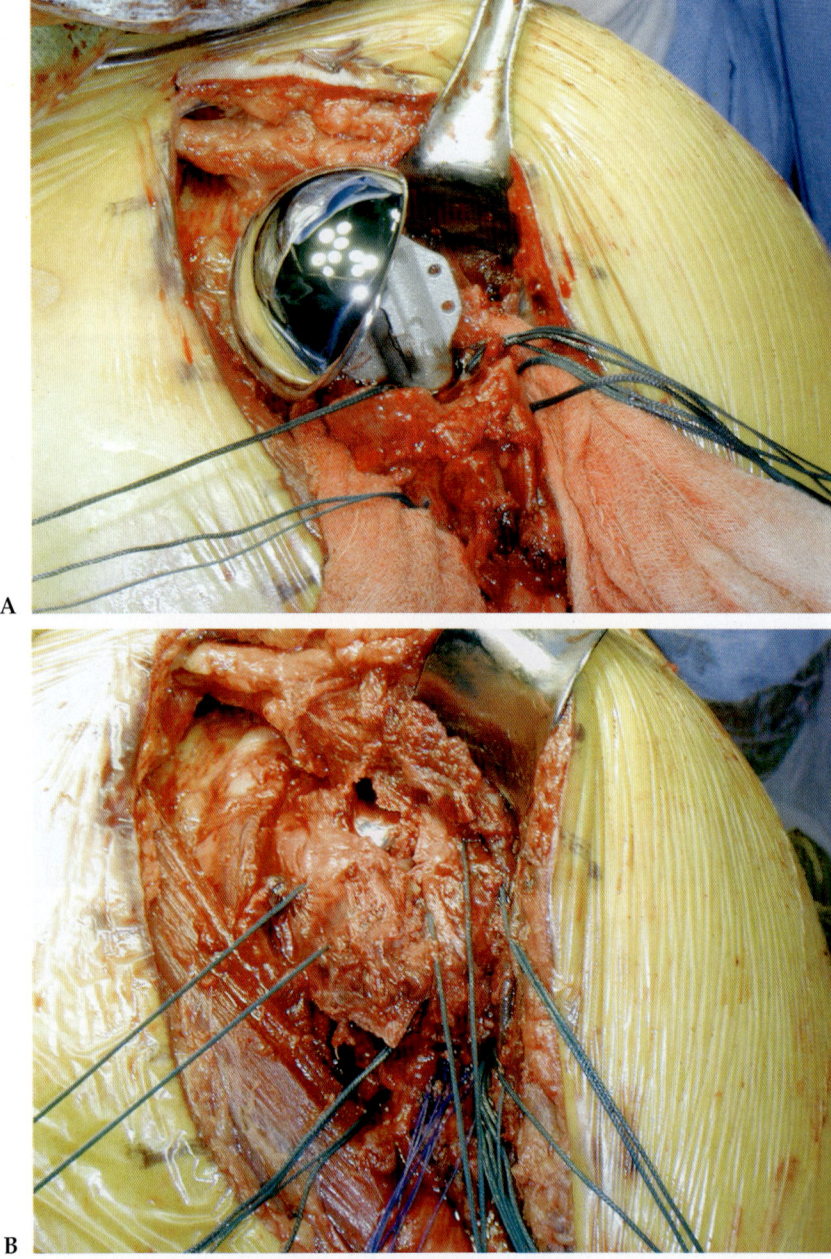

A

B

Figure 5.12. Tuberosity fixation. **(A)** Heavy nonabsorbable sutures medial and lateral to the bicipital groove that were placed prior to insertion of the final prosthesis. **(B)** Tuberosities positioned beneath the articular surface.

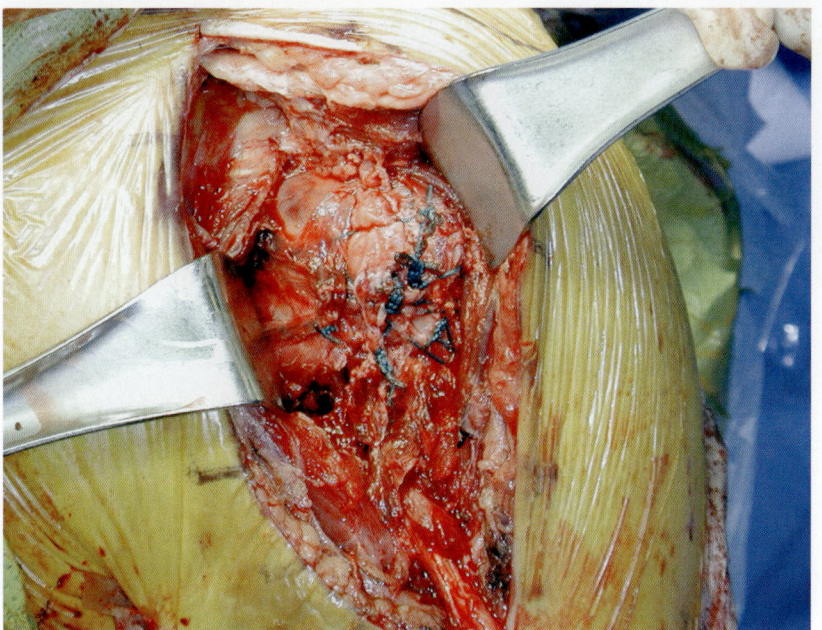

C

Figure 5.12. (*Continued*) **(C)** Tuberosities secured into position followed by closure of the rotator interval.

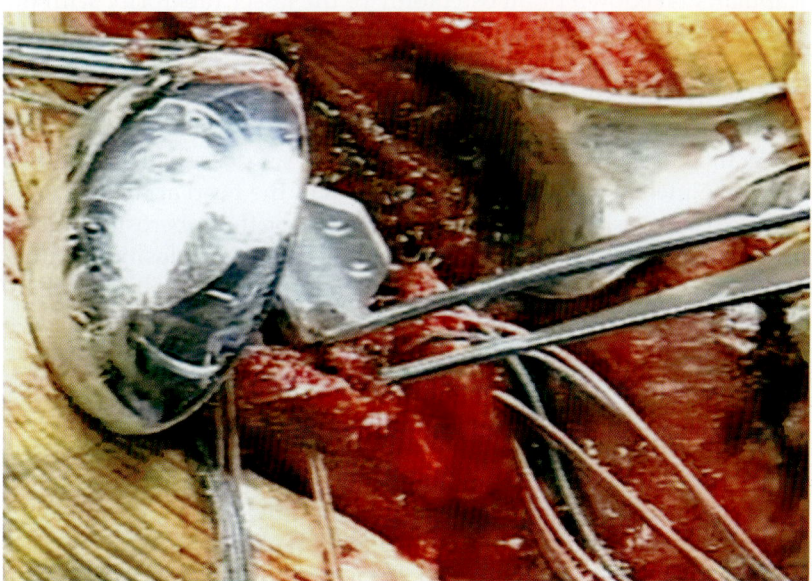

Figure 5.13. Cancellous bone graft retrieved from the humeral head is placed beneath the tuberosities.

limits of postoperative rehabilitation. After suction drains are placed under the deltoid, the deltopectoral interval is reapproximated followed by a layered closure of the subcutaneous tissues.

Considerations in Proximal Humerus Nonunion/Malunion

The few published series on the surgical treatment of proximal humerus nonunions report bone grafting and internal fixation yield poor results [18, 44–47], with better outcomes using modified Enders rods and a tension band construct [18] or blade plate fixation [48]. The use of these techniques is, again, limited by the presence of adequate bone stock and the absence of joint involvement.

When the proximal fragment is deemed unsuitable for internal fixation, a humeral head replacement is indicated (Figure 5.14). The use of the extended deltopectoral approach is usually sufficient in most acute and chronic fracture cases. However, complex pathology in the setting of some chronic fractures may require the more extensile anteromedial approach, which incorporates the deltopectoral exposure with release of the clavicular and anterior acromial origins of the deltoid [32]. After mobilization of the deltoid and release of subacromial and subdeltoid adhesions, the tuberosities can be identified using the biceps tendon as a landmark. In the case of a surgical neck nonunion, the medial calcar may have resorbed providing access to the head fragment through the nonunion site and the rotator interval. If this is not possible, a subscapularis takedown or an osteotomy of the lesser tuberosity with the associated subscapularis attachment is carefully performed.

The head can be excised using an osteotome or oscillating saw, leaving the tuberosities. Stem height is assessed by recreating the contour of the medial cortex (Figure 5.15). Version can be determined using the distal humeral epicondylar axis, as described previously. When the medial calcar is absent, removal of the head at the anatomic neck leaves a c-shaped fragment consisting of the tuberosities and a medial gap. In this case, a large corticocancellous graft fashioned from the head fragment is placed medially beneath the prosthesis (Figure 5.16). If the medial cortex is intact, osteotomy of the head results in a ring-shaped remnant containing the tuberosities and the medial calcar. The stem of the prosthesis can be skewered through this segment and across the nonunion site followed by placement of cancellous graft.

A successful outcome in arthroplasty for malunited fractures of the proximal humerus requires strict attention to the soft tissue component of the deformity in addition to the more obvious bony pathology. Careful lysis of subdeltoid and subacromial adhesions helps increase shoulder abduction and forward flexion. Capsular contractures are usually present and should be released. In malunions, it is usually preferable to adjust the humeral implant to the tuberosity rather than perform a corrective osteotomy. The impact of cutting and repositioning the tuberosities should not be underestimated, with several authors linking this procedure with a compromised outcome [49–52]. With severe malunions, however, tuberosity osteotomy may be required [53]. In most cases, an osteotomy is not necessary [54]. Acromioplasty may

Figure 5.14. **(A)** Anteroposterior and **(B)** axillary views demonstrating a nonunion at the surgical neck with cavitation of the head. Intraoperatively, the subscapularis and lesser tuberosity were found separate from the head and greater tuberosity fragment. **(C)** Anteroposterior view after hemiarthroplasty and tuberosity reconstruction. A titanium cable was used to reinforce the tuberosity fixation.

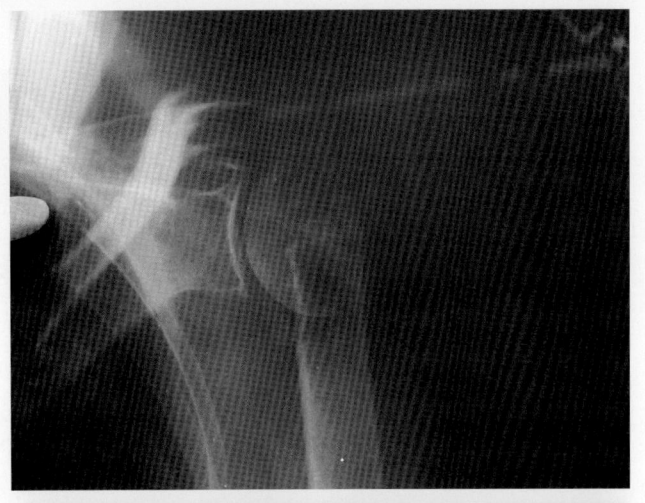

A

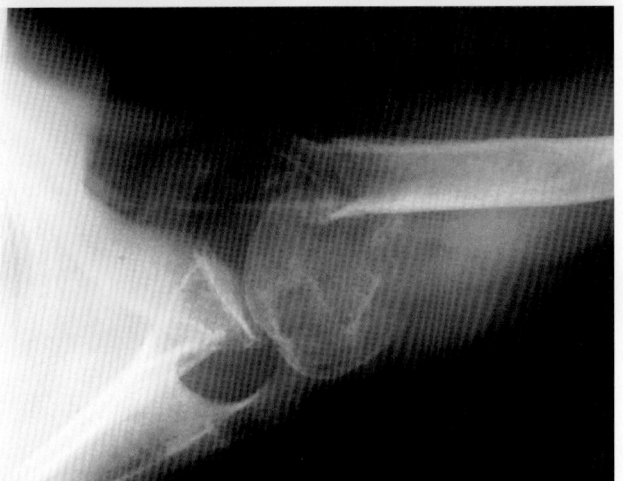

B

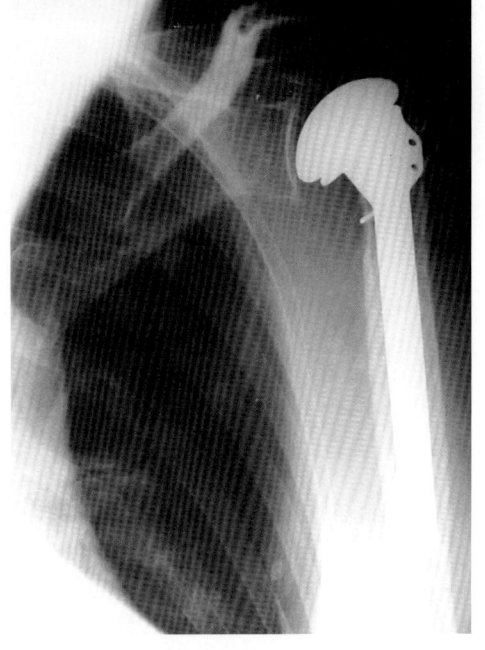

C

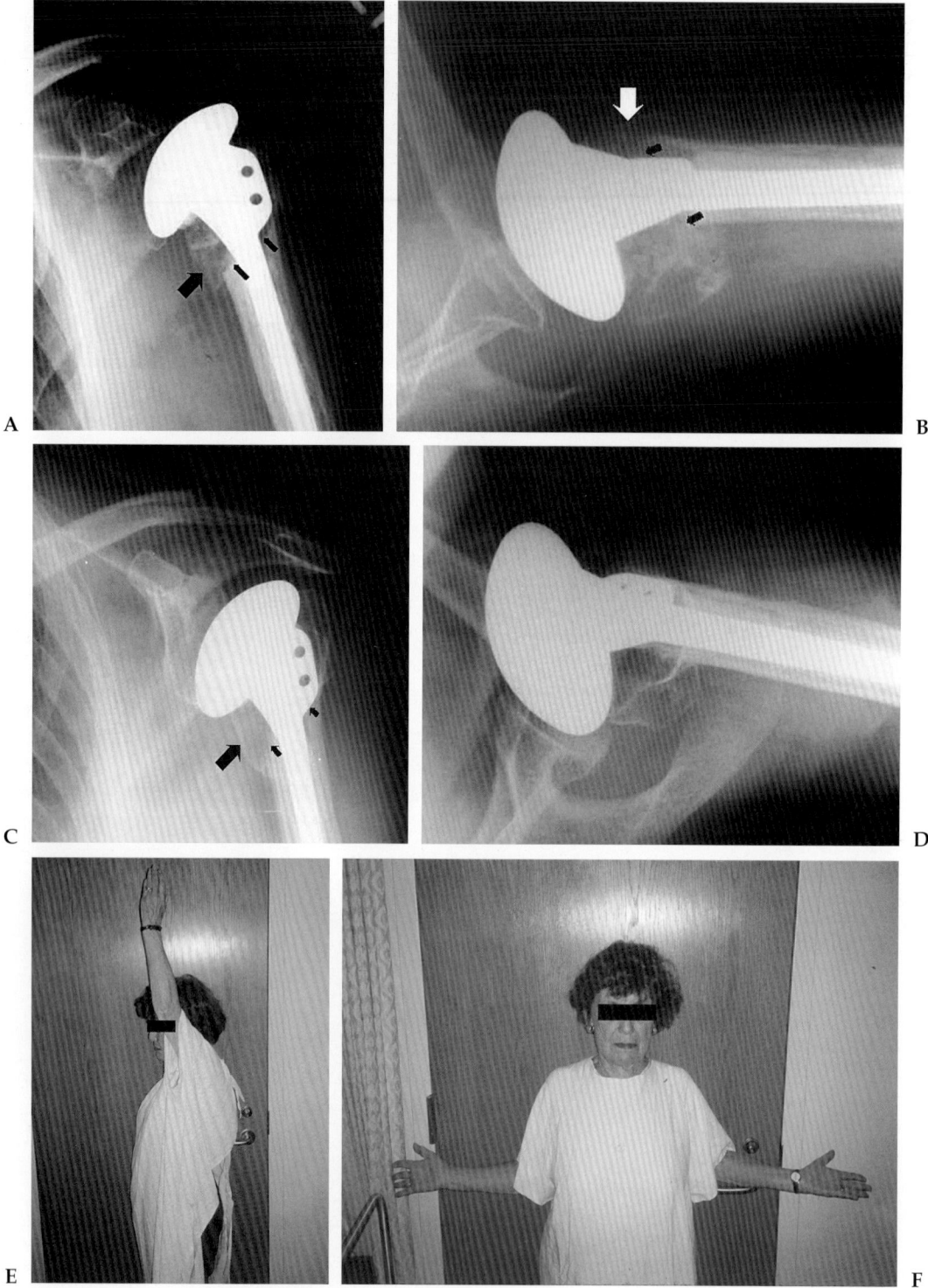

Figure 5.15. **(A)** Anteroposterior and **(B)** axillary views demonstrating restoration of humeral contour. The surgical neck nonunion site (*small arrows*) and the bone graft (*large arrows*) are easily visualized at 6 weeks postop, while at 2 years postop, the **(C)** anteroposterior and **(D)** axillary views show healing with obliteration of the nonunion site. Clinical photographs taken 4 years postoperatively. Patient has regained full elevation **(E)** and external rotation **(F)**.

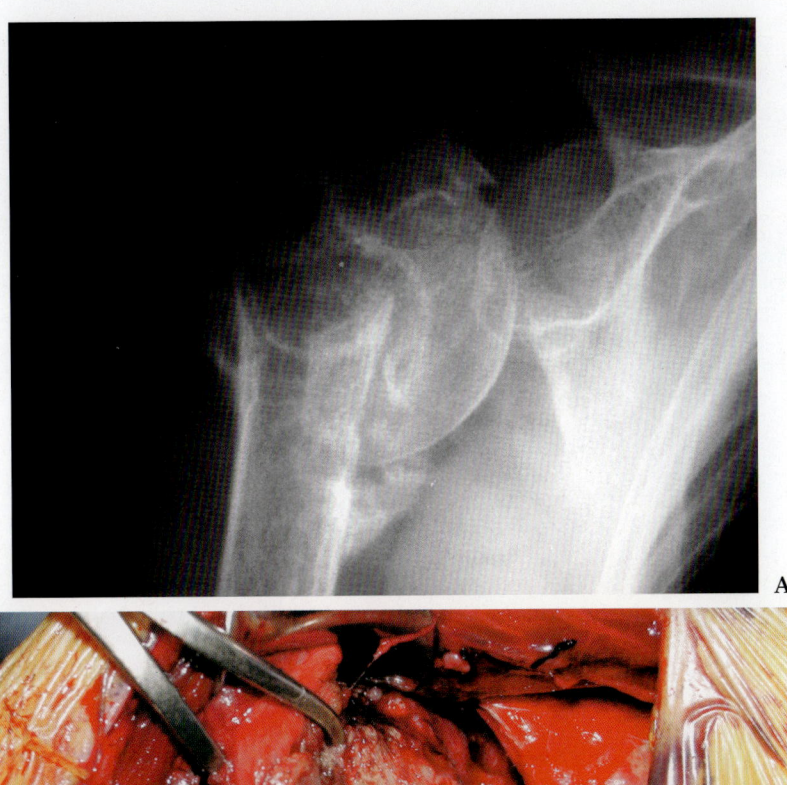

A

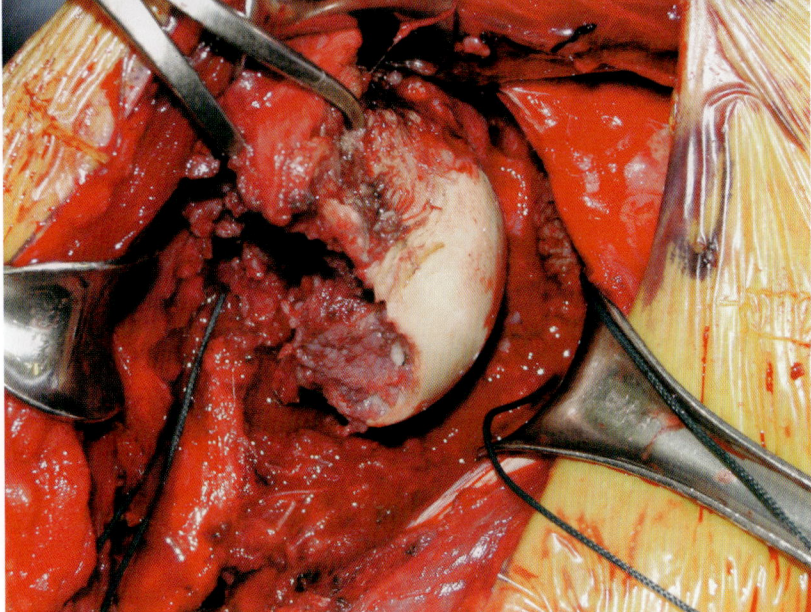

B

Figure 5.16. (A) Anteroposterior radiograph demonstrating surgical neck nonunion with calcar resorption. **(B)** Intraoperative picture showing cavitation of the head fragment.

(Continued)

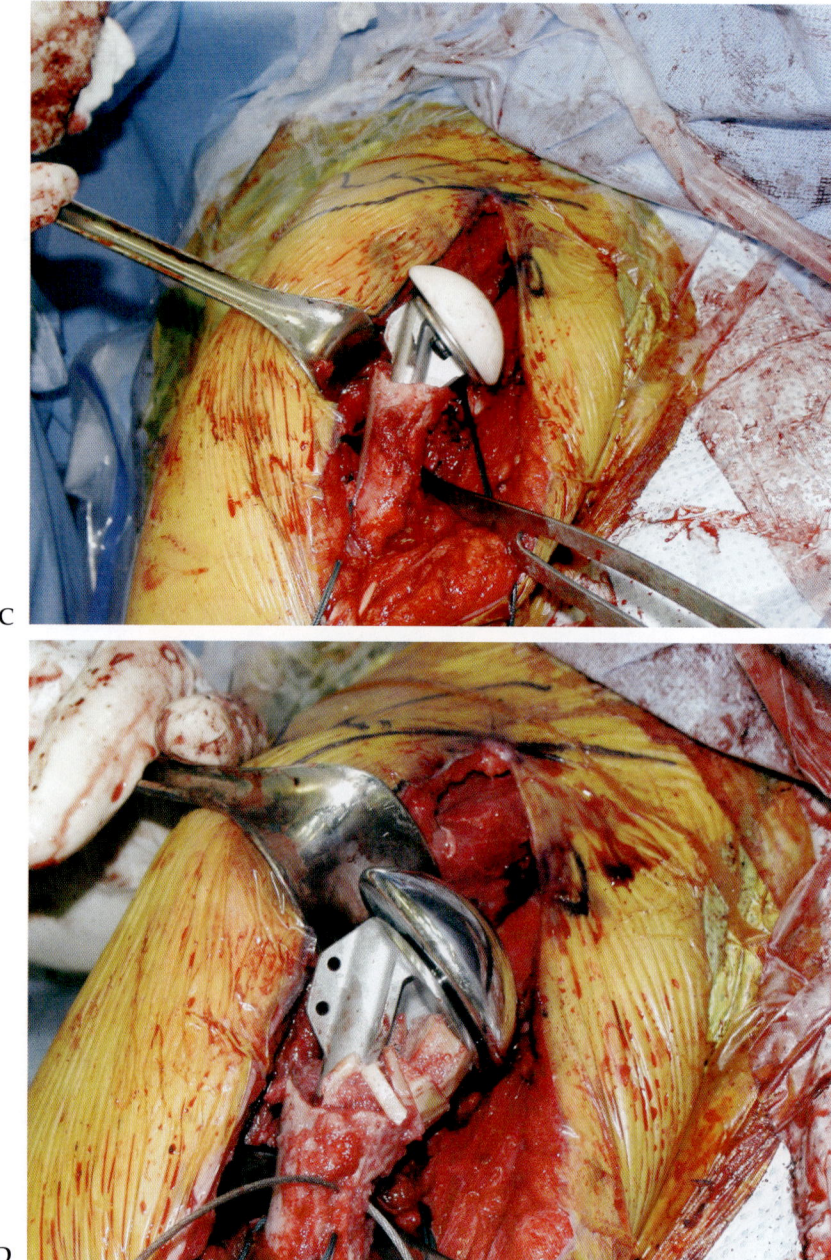

C

D

Figure 5.16. (*Continued*) **(C)** Trial prosthesis is assessed for proper height and version. Note bone loss in calcar region. **(D)** Bone graft placed along medial cortex after cementation of the humeral component.

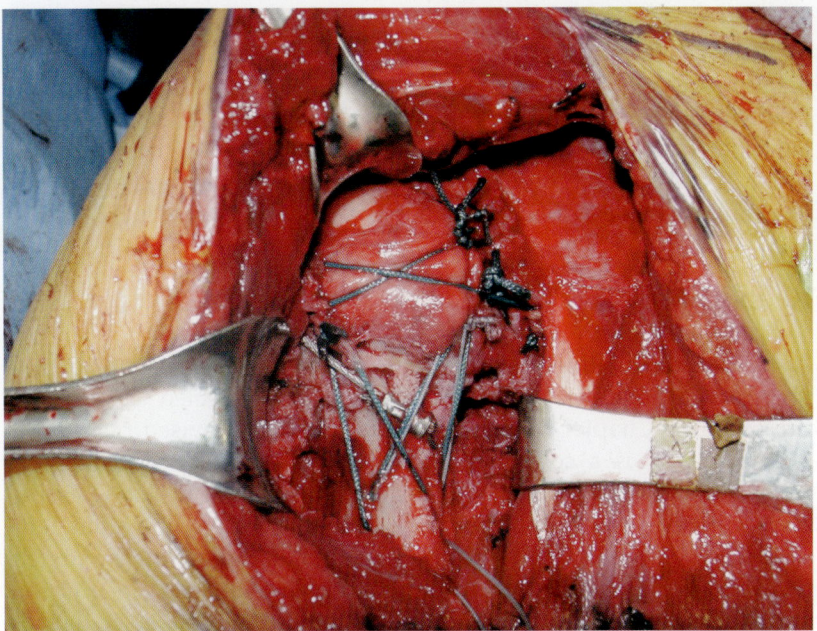

E

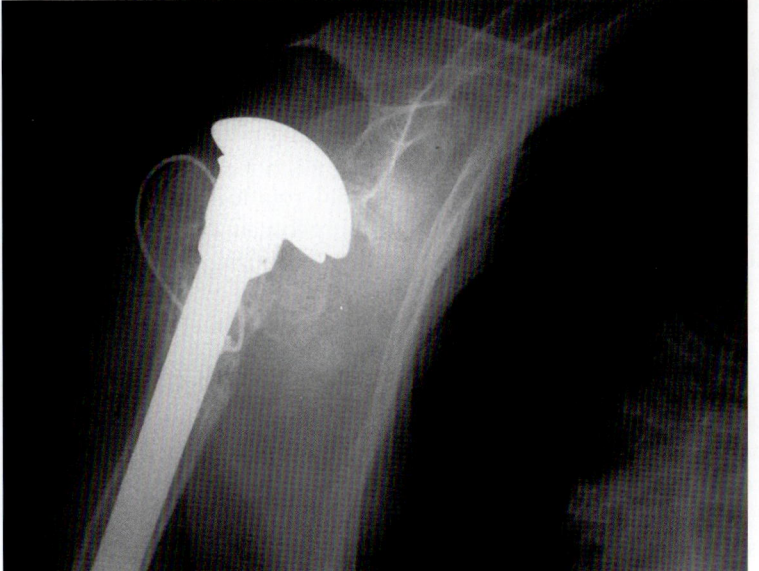

F

Figure 5.16. (*Continued*) **(E)** The tuberosities are secured with a cable; figure-of-eight suture fixation of the tuberosities further reinforces placement of the graft. **(F)** Postoperative anteroposterior radiograph.

be used as needed to improve clearance of a mildly malpositioned tuberosity. Malunion of the lesser tuberosity may lead to posterior subluxation of the head or cause impingement against the coracoid in internal rotation [55]. An attempt should be made to maintain bulk of the tuberosities while excising as little bone as possible. The greater and lesser tuberosity osteotomies are typically biplanar and uniplanar, respectively, as described by Tanner and Cofield (Figure 5.17) [32].

Rehabilitation

A structured rehabilitation program is essential to regain function after proximal humerus fracture reconstruction. The detailed exercises are presented in Chapter 8. The three-phase system devised by Hughes and Neer [56] is a commonly employed protocol. Phase I involves passive-assistive motion in the early postoperative period. Phase II starts with evidence of tuberosity healing and employs active and light-resistive exercises. Finally, phase III is aimed at a more intense stretching and strengthening program to maximize and maintain function. Each program is individualized and based on the quality of the soft tissues, bone quality, security of tuberosity fixation, intraoperative range of motion, and the patient's ability to comprehend and participate in the prescribed regimen. Exercises are performed three to four times daily for 20 to 30 minutes.

Phase I exercises can be started on the first postoperative day. Gentle gravity-assisted pendulum exercises, passive elevation in the plane of the scapula as well as supine external rotation with a stick within defined limits are permitted with surgeon and therapist guidance. Elbow, wrist, and hand motion are also encouraged.

Phase II is initiated with evidence of tuberosity healing at approximately 6 to 8 weeks after surgery. Assisted elevation with a pulley system and supine followed by erect isometric strengthening exercises are performed. Stretches to improve forward elevation, extension, abduction, external and internal rotation are done in addition to encouraging gradual use of the extremity in activities of daily living to promote strength and endurance.

At approximately 3 months from surgery, phase III exercises are instituted. Progressive resistive exercises with TheraBands and light weights are incorporated into the daily routine along with more aggressive stretching. Patients should be informed that maximal return of function will take up to 12 to 18 months in conjunction with diligence to the prescribed postoperative routine.

Results

The results of primary prosthetic replacement for proximal humerus fractures in the literature have been somewhat mixed. Pain relief has been a reliable outcome with most series reporting adequate symptom resolution in the majority of patients; however, functional return

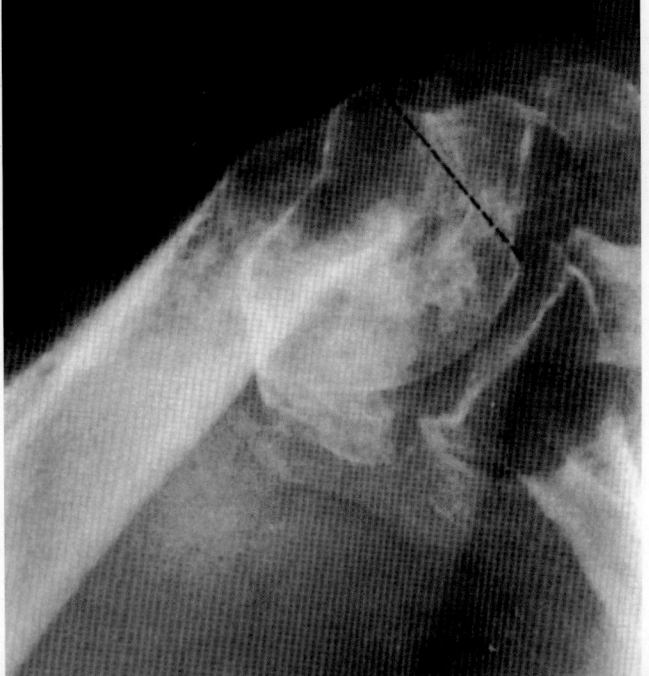

A

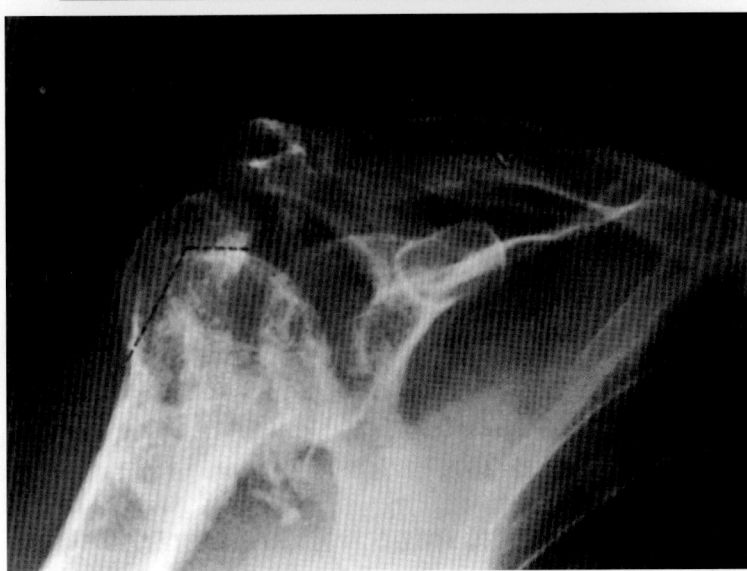

B

Figure 5.17. Tuberosity osteotomy. **(A)** Axillary view with dotted lines indicating uniplanar osteotomy of the lesser tuberosity. **(B)** Anteroposterior view with dotted line indicating biplanar osteotomy of the greater tuberosity. (From Tanner MW, Cofield RH [32], by permission of Clin Orthop.)

has been more variable [42, 43, 57–60]. The less than dramatic gains in strength and motion postoperatively could be attributed to a number of factors including patient age, fracture type, adequacy of rotator cuff or tuberosity reconstruction, restoration of version and soft tissue tensioning, and compliance with the vigorous rehabilitation program.

The debate over the merits of acute prosthetic replacement versus delayed treatment after either failed nonoperative treatment or failed internal fixation has been gradually borne out in the literature. At issue is the assumption that unsuccessful humeral head-preserving procedures can be effectively salvaged with late hemiarthroplasty. A number of authors, however, have found inferior results and higher complication rates compared with primary arthroplasty.

Tanner and Cofield [32] studied 43 patients with a fracture or fracture-dislocation of the proximal humerus treated with prosthetic arthroplasty. The patients were divided into those treated acutely with primary arthroplasty and those treated for chronic postfracture problems. The complications encountered in the acutely treated group were related to tuberosity healing and rotator cuff failure. Complications were more frequent in the chronic post-injury group and were generally related to surgical difficulty, scarring, and distortion of anatomy. Pain relief was satisfactory in both groups but function was dependent on security of the tuberosity repair, protection post-surgery, and long-term physiotherapy. The authors concluded that when possible, surgery should be performed early to avoid the complications and limits in postoperative recovery with chronic fractures.

We reported our [61] experience with prosthetic replacement of 4-part and head-splitting proximal humerus fractures. Sixty-five cases were followed for an average of 3 years. Complications were infrequent with tuberosity detachment (6%) the most commonly encountered problem. Ninety-seven percent of patients were pain free with average active elevation of 124 degrees, although functional outcome was less reliable than pain relief. The authors noted that results were highly dependent on the patient's compliance with the postoperative rehabilitation regimen.

In another report of 23 patients evaluating arthroplasty after failed initial treatment of three- and four-part fractures, Norris et al. [47] found late humeral head replacement was a satisfactory reconstructive option. However, they also emphasized the technical difficulty and inferior results compared to acute shoulder arthroplasty.

A retrospective review by Beredjiklian et al. [62] examined 22 of 39 patients with a proximal humeral malunion involving glenohumeral joint incongruity managed with prosthetic replacement. 74% had a satisfactory result, with the authors underscoring the importance of correcting both the osseous and soft tissue abnormalities at the time of surgery.

The effect of tuberosity osteotomy on outcome has been highlighted by a number of authors. Neer [49] suggested slight malpositioning of the humeral component to avoid tuberosity osteotomy. Dines et al. [50] studied late posttraumatic reconstructions with prosthetic arthroplasty and found better results with patients younger than 70 and those who did not require tuberosity osteotomy. Boileau et al. [51] similarly found greater tuberosity osteotomy as the most likely reason for poor results after late prosthetic replacement. More recently, in two separate studies examining shoulder arthroplasty for nonunions and malunions, Antuña et al. [52, 63] found that patients who underwent operative treatment and those who underwent tuberosity osteotomy or had problems with tuberosity healing were at risk of having a poorer result. In cases of nonunion, preservation of the tuberosities with calcar grafting can potentially avert these complications.

Miller et al. reported their experience with 9 patients with surgical neck nonunions complicated by severe humeral head destruction and inadequate bone stock. All patients underwent humeral head replacement with calcar grafting. Graft resorption was noted in 2 patients, however, all tuberosities healed with most patients achieving a dramatic improvement in range-of-motion and pain [64]. Trabecular metal components (Zimmer, Warsaw, IN) are currently evolving and show promise in the treatment of nonunions through bone ingrowth at the implant-bone interface.

Conclusion

Treatment of proximal humerus fractures poses one of the most difficult management problems for the orthopedic surgeon. Shoulder arthroplasty remains the preferred treatment for more complex fracture patterns in lower demand, elderly patients with osteoporotic bone and significant compromise of the articular surface or its blood supply. Although associated with inferior results and higher complication rates, late reconstruction for proximal humerus fractures is a viable option for patients with significant functional impairment and pain associated with poor bone stock and glenohumeral joint damage.

References

1. Codman EA. Rupture of the supraspinatus tendon and other lesions in or about the subacromial bursa. In The Shoulder, EA Codman, Editor. New York: G. Miller, 1934;331–334.
2. Neer CS II. Displaced proximal humerus fractures. Part I. Classification and evaluation. J Bone Joint Surg 1970;52A:1077–1089.
3. De Anquin CL, De Anquin A. Prosthetic replacement in the treatment of serious fractures of the proximal humerus. In Shoulder Surgery, I Bayley, Kessel L, Editors. New York: Springer-Verlag, 1965.
4. Edelman G. Immediate therapy of complex fractures of the upper end of the humerus by means of acrylic prosthesis. Presse Med 1951;59:1777–1778.
5. Fellander M. Fracture-dislocations of the shoulder joint. Acta Chir Scand 1954;107:138–145.
6. Lasher WW. Fracture of the head of the humerus. JAMA 1925;84:356–358.
7. Neer CS, Brown TH, McLaughlin HL. Fracture of the neck of the humerus with dislocation of the head fragment. Am J Surg 1953;85:252–258.
8. Neer CS. Indications for replacement of the proximal humeral articulation. Am J Surg 1955;89:901–907.
9. Moeckel BH, Dines DM, Warren RF, et al. Modular hemiarthroplasty for fractures of the proximal part of the humerus. J Bone Joint Surg 1992; 74A:884–889.
10. Shaffer BS, Giordano CP, Zuckerman JD. Revision of a loose glenoid component facilitated by a modular humeral component. A technical note. J Arthroplasty 1990;5(Suppl):S579–S581.

11. Laing PG. The arterial supply of the adult humerus. J Bone Joint Surg 1956; 38A:1105–1116.

12. Gerber C, Schneeberger A, Vinh JS. The arterial vascularization of the humeral head: an anatomic study. J Bone Joint Surg 1993;2:S30.

13. Gerber C, Krushell RJ. Isolated rupture of the tendon of the subscapularis muscle. Clinical features in 16 cases. J Bone Joint Surg Br 1991; 73(3):389–394.

14. Craig EV. Open reduction and internal fixation of greater tuberosity fractures, malunions, and nonunions. In Master techniques in orthopaedic surgery, the shoulder, EV Craig, Editor. New York: Raven Press, 1995; 289–307.

15. Phemister DB. Fractures of the greater tuberosity of the humerus. With an operative procedure for fixation. Ann Surg 1912;56:440–449

16. Morris ME, Kilkoyne RF, Shuman W, et al. Humeral tuberosity fractures. Evaluation by CT scan and management of malunion. Orthop Trans 1987; 11:242.

17. Flatow EL, Cuomo F, Maday MG, Miller SR, McIlveen SJ, Bigliani LU. Open reduction and internal fixation of two-part displaced fractures of the greater tuberosity of the proximal part of the humerus. J Bone Joint Surg 1991;73(8);1213–1218.

18. Duralde XA, Flatow EL, Pollock RG, Nicholson GP, Self EB, Bigliani LU. Operative treatment of nonunions of the surgical neck of the humerus. J Shoulder Elbow Surg 1996;5:169–180

19. Paavolainen P, Björkenheim JM, Slätis P, et al. Operative treatment of sever proximal humeral fractures. Acta Orthop Scand 1983;54:374–379.

20. Lee CK, Hansen HR. Post-traumatic avascular necrosis of the humeral head in displaced proximal humeral fractures. J Trauma 1981;21:788–791.

21. Esser RD. Treatment of three- and four-part fractures of the proximal humerus with a modified cloverleaf plate. J Orthop Trauma 1994;8: 15–22.

22. Darder A, Sanchis V, Gastaldi E, et al. Four-part displaced proximal humeral fractures: operative treatment using Kirschner wires and a tension band. J Orthop Trauma 1993;7:497–505.

23. Gerber C, Hersche O, Berberat C. The clinical relevance of posttraumatic avascular necrosis of the humeral head. J Shoulder Elbow Surg 1998;7: 586–590.

24. Siebler G, Kuner EH. Luxationsfracturen des proximalen humerus. Ergebnisse nach operativer Behandlung. Eine AO studie uber 167 falle. Hefte zur Unfallheilkunde 1987;186:171–178.

25. Szyszkowitz R, Seggi W, Schleifer P, et al. Proximal humeral fractures. Management techniques and expected results. Clin Orthop 1993;292:13–25.

26. Jakob P, Miniaci A, Anson PS, et al. Four-part valgus impacted fractures of the proximal humerus. J Bone Joint Surg 1991;73B:295–298.

27. Resch H, Beck E, Bayley I. Reconstruction of the valgus-impacted humeral head fracture. J Shoulder Elbow Surg 1995;4:73–80.

28. Kristiansen B, Christensen SW. Plate fixation of proximal humeral fractures. Acta Orthop Scand 1986;57:320–323.

29. Mills HJ, Horne G. Fractures of the proximal humerus in adults. J Trauma 1985;25:801–805.

30. Stableforth PG. Four-part fractures of the neck of the humerus. J Bone Joint Surg 1984;66B:104–108.

31. Sturzenegger M, Fornaro E, Jakob RP. Results of surgical treatment of multifragmented fractures of the humeral head. Arch Orthop Trauma Surg 1982;100:249–259.

32. Tanner MW, Cofield RH. Prosthetic arthroplasty for fractures and fracture-dislocations of the proximal humerus. Clin Orthop 1983;179:116–128.
33. Neer CS. Fractures about the shoulder. In Fractures in adults, CA Rockwood, Green DB, Editors. Philadelphia: Lippincott, 1984;675–721.
34. Checchia SL, Santos PD, Miyazaki AN. Surgical treatment of acute and chronic posterior fracture-dislocation of the shoulder. J Shoulder Elbow Surg 1998;7(1):53–65.
35. Norris TR. Fractures of the proximal humerus and dislocations of the shoulder. In Skeletal Trauma, BD Browner, Jupiter JB, Levine AM, Trafton PG, Editors. Philadelphia: WB Saunders, 1992;1201–1290.
36. Galanakis IA, Kontakis GM, Steriopoulos KA. Posterior dislocation of the shoulder associated with fracture of the humeral anatomic neck. J Trauma 1997;42(6):1176–1178.
37. Ogawa K, Yoshida A, Inokuchi W. Posterior shoulder dislocation associated with fracture of the humeral anatomic neck. J Trauma 1999;46(2):318–323.
38. Hawkins RJ, Neer CS II, Pianta RM, et al. Locked posterior dislocation of the shoulder. J Bone Joint Surg 1987;69:9–18.
39. Flatow EL, Bigliani LU. Tips of the trade. Locating and protecting the axillary nerve in shoulder surgery: the tug test. Orthop Rev 1992;21(4): 503–505.
40. LeHeuc JC, Boileau P, Sinnerton R, et al. Tuberosity osteosynthesis. In Shoulder Arthroplasty, G Walch, Boileau P, Editors. Berlin: Springer-Verlag, 1999;323–329.
41. Green A, Barnard WL, Limbird RS. Humeral head replacement for acute, four-part proximal humerus fractures. J Shoulder Elbow Surg 1993;2: 249–254.
42. Hawkins RJ, Switlyk P. Acute prosthetic replacement for severe fractures of the proximal humerus. Clin Orthop 1993;289:156–160.
43. Compito CA, Self EB, Bigliani LU. Arthroplasty and acute shoulder trauma: reasons for success and failure. Clin Orthop 1994;307:27–36.
44. Healy WL, Jupiter JP, Kristiansen TK, et al. Nonunion of the proximal humerus. A review of 25 cases. J Orthop Trauma 1990;4:424–431.
45. Nayak N, Schickendantz MS, Regan WD, et al. Operative treatment of nonunion of surgical neck fractures of the humerus. Clin Orthop 1995;313: 200–205.
46. Scheck M. Surgical treatment of nonunions of the surgical neck of the humerus. Clin Orthop 1982;167:255–259.
47. Norris TR, Green A, McGuigan FX. Late prosthetic shoulder arthroplasty for displaced proximal humerus fractures. J Shoulder Elbow Surg 1995; 4:271–280.
48. Ring D, McKee MD, Perey B. The use of a blade plate and autogenous cancellous bone graft in the treatment of ununited fractures of the proximal humerus. J Shoulder Elbow Surg 2001;10:501–507.
49. Neer CS II. Glenohumeral arthroplasty. In Shoulder reconstruction. Philadelphia: WB Saunders, 1990;143–269.
50. Dines DM, Warren RF, Altchek DW, et al. Posttraumatic changes of the proximal humerus: malunion, nonunion, and osteonecrosis-treatment with modular hemiarthroplasty or total shoulder arthroplasty. J Shoulder Elbow Surg 1993;2:11–21.
51. Boileau P, Trojani C, Walch G, et al. Shoulder arthroplasty for the treatment of the sequelae of fractures of the proximal humerus. J Shoulder Elbow Surg 2001;10(4):299–308.
52. Antuña SA, Sperling JW, Sanchez-Sotelo J, et al. Shoulder arthroplasty for proximal humeral malunions: long-term results. J Shoulder Elbow Surg 2002;11:122–129.

53. Siegel JA, Dines DM. Proximal humerus malunions. Orthop Clin North Am 2000;31:35–50.
54. Beredjiklian PK, Iannotti JP. Treatment of proximal humerus fracture malunion with prosthetic arthroplasty. Instr Course Lect 1998;47:135–140.
55. Siegel JA, Dines DM. Techniques in managing proximal humeral malunions: J Shoulder Elbow Surg 2003;12:69–78.
56. Hughes M, Neer CS. Glenohumeral joint replacement and postoperative rehabilitation. Phys Ther 1975;55:850–858
57. Goldman RT, Koval KJ, Cuomo F, et al. Functional outcome after humeral head replacement for acute three- and four-part proximal humerus fractures. J Shoulder Elbow Surg 1995;4:81–86.
58. Kay SP, Amstutz HC. Shoulder hemiarthroplasty at UCLA. Clin Orthop 1988;228:42–48.
59. Wretenberg P, Ekelund A. Acute hemiarthroplasty after proximal humerus fracture in old patients. A retrospective evaluation of 18 patients followed for 2 years. Acta Orthop Scand 1997;68:121–123.
60. Bodey WN, Yeoman PM. Prosthetic arthroplasty of the shoulder. Acta Orthop Scand 1983;54:900–903.
61. Fischer RA, Nicholson GP, McIlveen SJ, et al. Primary Humeral Head Replacement for Severely Displaced Fractures of the Proximal Humerus. Presented at the American Academy of Orthopaedic Surgeons Annual Meeting, Washington, D.C., February 1992.
62. Beredjiklian PK, Iannotti JP, Norris TR, et al. Operative management of malunion of a fracture of the proximal humerus. J Bone Joint Surg 1998;80:1484–1497.
63. Antuña SA, Sperling JW, Sanchez-Sotelo J, et al. Shoulder arthroplasty for proximal humeral nonunions. J Shoulder Elbow Surg 2002;11:114–121.
64. Miller S, Klepps S, Lin J, et al. Effectiveness of Replacement Arthroplasty with Calcar Grafting for the Treatment of Surgical Neck Nonunions of the Humerus. Presented at the American Academy of Orthopaedic Surgeons Annual Meeting, New Orleans, Louisiana, February 2003.

Chapter 6

Revision Shoulder Arthroplasty and Related Tendon Transfers

Ilya Voloshin, Kevin J. Setter, and Louis U. Bigliani

In 1994, approximately 10,000 shoulder replacements were performed in the United States [1]. With new and emerging technology, expanding operative indications, and an increasing elderly population, this number will continue to rise. Increasing application of shoulder arthroplasty in a younger patient population relative to knee and hip arthroplasty [2] will also contribute to this expected increase. As the number of primary procedures grows, an expanding need for revision surgery after shoulder arthroplasty will likely follow.

Currently, information concerning the diagnosis and treatment of failed shoulder arthroplasty is limited. Revision shoulder arthroplasty is performed infrequently, and few centers have extensive experience with such procedures. The literature suggests revision rates of 5% to 10% following shoulder arthroplasty [3], although the subsequent outcomes remain poorly defined. Neer et al. suggested that revision shoulder arthroplasty is the most difficult of joint arthroplasty procedures [4, 5]. Complicating factors include bone deficiency, increased risk of fracture, muscle atrophy, and contracted and scarred soft tissues. The goals of revision surgery are similar to those for primary procedures. They include restoration of normal anatomy and preservation of bone stock with necessary soft tissue balancing to maximize pain relief and optimize function. Myriad potential problems after failed shoulder arthroplasty frequently complicate achievement of these goals. Although the outcomes after revision surgery are generally considered inferior to those after primary arthroplasty, a comprehensive and detailed approach can lead to successful results. This chapter outlines a systematic approach to failed shoulder arthroplasty, with an overview of the most common problems encountered in revision surgery and detailed surgical techniques to address them.

Evaluation of Failed Shoulder Arthroplasty

A careful history is of course critical in evaluating the failed shoulder arthroplasty. An early and essential consideration is whether the patient enjoyed a pain-free interval after the primary procedure. This has important clinical implications. The presence of an initial pain-free interval suggests causative factors unrelated to the primary procedure. Alternatively, the absence of a pain-free interval may imply failure to identify and address concomitant contributing diagnoses, as well as technical errors or intraoperative complications related to the initial surgery.

A review of all past records is equally important, especially if the patient was originally treated elsewhere. Operative reports are particularly valuable, providing information such as tissue quality and particular implants used in the primary procedure. Such records facilitate preoperative planning, ensuring that the appropriate instrumentation for implant extraction, components for modular replacement, custom prosthesis, and necessary bone or soft tissue grafts are available for the revision surgery.

A comprehensive physical examination should be performed, including a meticulous assessment of range of motion, muscle strength, and stability. Excessive stiffness may be indicative of oversized or malpositioned components or soft tissue contracture. Instability may also suggest component malposition, as well as soft tissue inadequacy. Weakness and muscle atrophy may indicate mechanical problems such as a rotator cuff tear, or neurological deficits. When indicated, electrodiagnostic studies can help differentiate between these.

Preoperative diagnostic imaging should include true AP images of the scapula in neutral, internal and external rotation, as well as an axillary lateral and an outlet view. If questions exist regarding the size of the glenoid vault or retroversion of the glenoid, a CT scan is obtained. As artifact from the prosthesis may limit MRI interpretation, an arthrogram is recommended to evaluate suspected rotator cuff tears and component loosening.

Another diagnostic and therapeutic modality for failed shoulder arthroplasty is shoulder arthroscopy. Evaluation of the glenoid, rotator cuff musculature, and capsular structures can be performed with the arthroscope. Subacromial decompression, acromioclavicular joint resection, synovectomy, and contracture release can also be performed arthroscopically as indicated.

Surgical Approach

The challenges encountered in surgical approaches for revision surgery are numerous and warrant special attention. One of the most complicated challenges is soft tissue contracture, which may distort the normal anatomy and place neurovascular structures at risk. Customary landmarks such as the coracoid and acromion may not be as reliable to help guide in the development of safe tissue planes. Specifically, soft tissue contracture during an anterior approach may alter the locations of the musculocutaneous and axillary nerves. It is important to start laterally to avoid damage to those neurovascular structures typically located medial and inferior to the coracoid.

An extended deltopectoral skin incision is used, incorporating the previous skin incision if possible. A new skin incision is made if required. The vascularity of the subcutaneous tissue around the shoulder is excellent, and skin necrosis has been a rare problem in our practice. The deltopectoral interval should be approached from a lateral direction. Previous injury to the cephalic vein and obliteration of fascial planes from scarring can make this task challenging. Blunt dissection and electrocautery are used to separate the clavicular portion of the pectoralis major and the deltoid muscles (Figure 6.1). When there is extensive scarring, it is easier to start the dissection distally over the humeral shaft near deltoid insertion. Rotating the humerus may also be helpful to identify the interval between the muscles. Once the deltopectoral interval has been developed, the coracoacromial ligament is excised to facilitate superior exposure. Next it is crucial to release and recreate the subdeltoid and subacromial spaces. This step cannot be overemphasized—it will aid in glenoid exposure as well as help increase postoperative range of motion. Often it is easier to delineate the subacromial space once the clavipectoral fascia has been incised. This space is contiguous with the subdeltoid space. The subdeltoid and subacromial spaces are released in a blunt fashion using an elevator

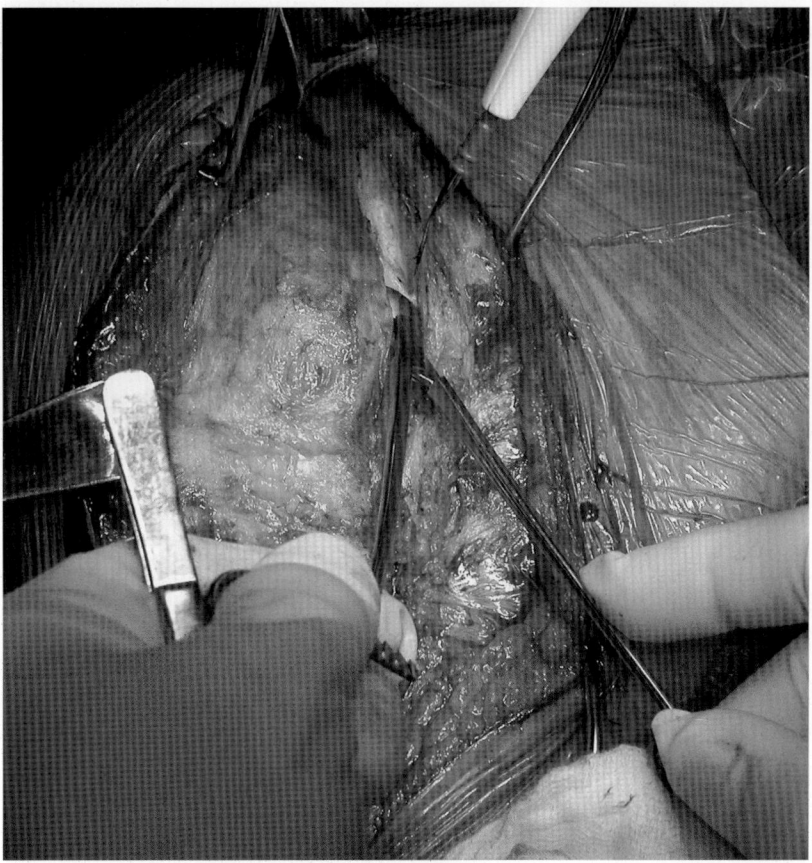

Figure 6.1. Scarred deltopectoral interval.

(Figure 6.2). One has to exercise caution in the inferior aspect of the subdeltoid bursa to prevent injury to branches of the axillary nerve emerging from the quadrangular space. The elevator should *hug* the proximal humerus to avoid injury to those branches of the nerve that travel on the surface of the subdeltoid fascia. Recreation of normal muscular excursion and gliding planes is important for adequate exposure and postoperative range of motion. The pectoralis major muscle is retracted medially. Releases between the strap and the pectoralis major muscles may be necessary for adequate exposure. At this point, a scarred bursa over the subscapularis and clavipectoral fascia is frequently encountered. It is necessary to develop a plane between the strap muscles and the subscapularis and again, this task is often complicated by extensive scar. The interval can initially be identified using electrocautery, but further release medially should be performed in a blunt fashion using a soft tissue elevator (Figure 6.3). Adequate release is essential for medial retraction of the strap muscles to establish adequate exposure, as well as contributing to necessary subscapularis release for adequate muscular excursion. Extreme care should be exercised inferiorly in this plane to avoid injury to the axillary nerve coursing around the inferior border of the subscapularis on its way to the quadrangular space.

At this point, the condition and integrity of the subscapularis insertion is assessed. Specific techniques addressing subscapularis deficiency are covered in the section Instability After Total Shoulder Arthroplasty later in this chapter. In the majority of patients undergoing revision arthroplasty, the subscapularis muscle is adherent to the

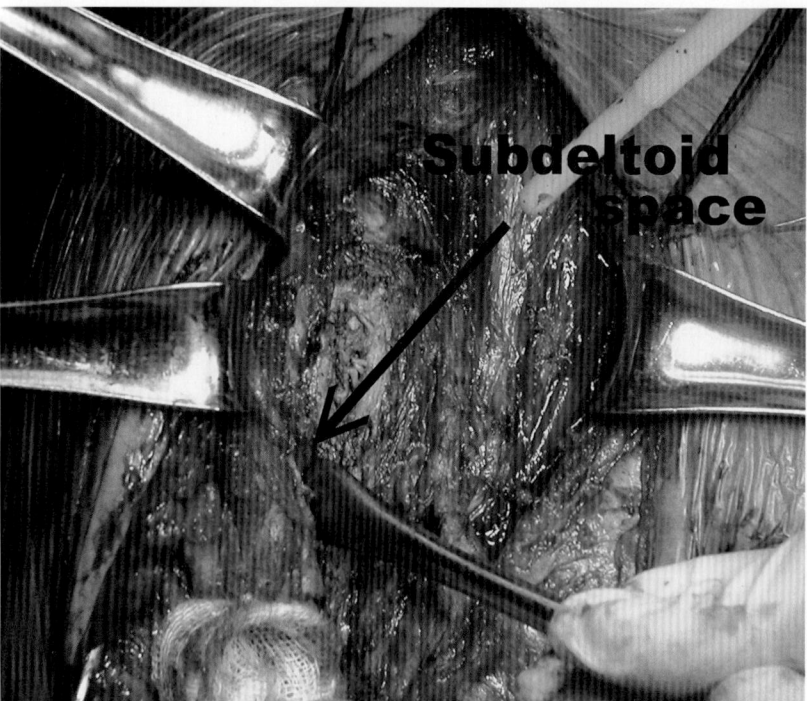

Figure 6.2. Release of subdeltoid space.

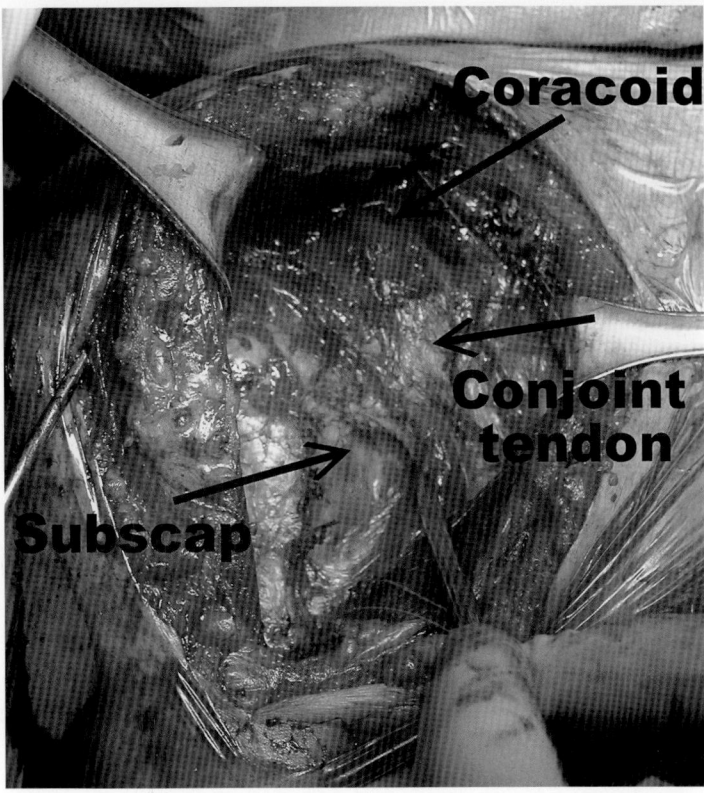

Figure 6.3. Adhesions between conjoint tendon and subscapularis.

surrounding tissues and contracted. This limits external rotation and the joint volume available for certain reconstructive options such as larger humeral head sizes and prosthetic glenoid insertion. Especially in the revision setting, it is important to maximize the length of the available subscapularis for later repair. It is often necessary to release the coracohumeral ligament to improve the excursion of the superior aspect of the subscapularis. The tendon is released directly off the lesser tuberosity in conjunction with the joint capsule (Figure 6.4). Inferiorly, the release is extended onto the shaft of the humerus. As long as the dissection is performed subperiosteally, the axillary nerve should be out of harm's way. Care should be taken not to detach the latissimus dorsi tendon. Once that tendon is encountered, the capsular release is extended posteriorly, above the latissimus dorsi tendon and along the medial neck of the humerus. Scar tissue around humeral head and neck has to be cleared to externally rotate the arm for exposure. The head of the modular prosthesis can be removed for better exposure (Figure 6.5). It is important to externally rotate and adduct the humerus during the inferior capsular release to protect the axillary nerve. The plane of dissection moves away from the nerve with the external rotation of the arm. The inferior capsular release must be performed beyond the 6 o'clock position, and often to the 8 o'clock position for a right shoulder, to obtain adequate exposure and successfully deliver the proximal humerus into the operative field. Further work on the

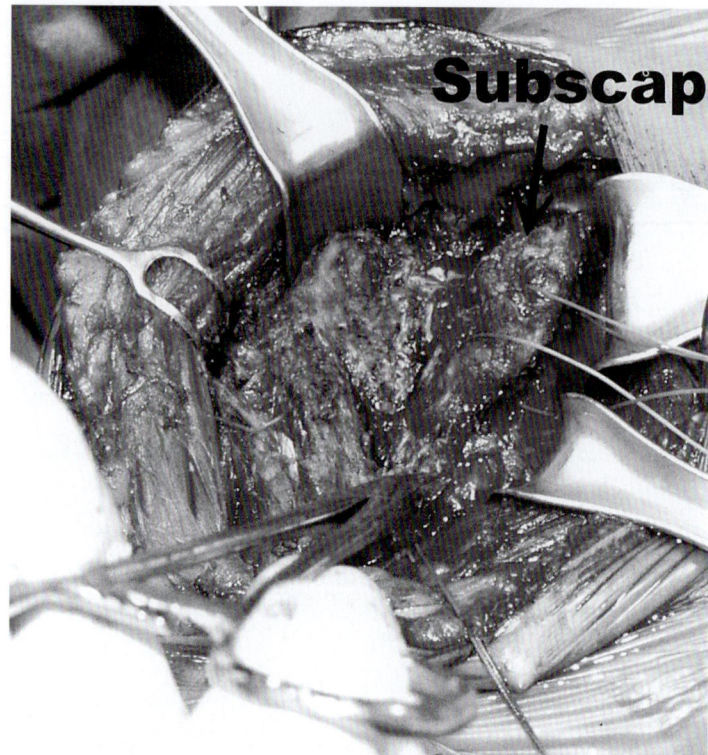

Figure 6.4. Subscapularis detachment off the humerus.

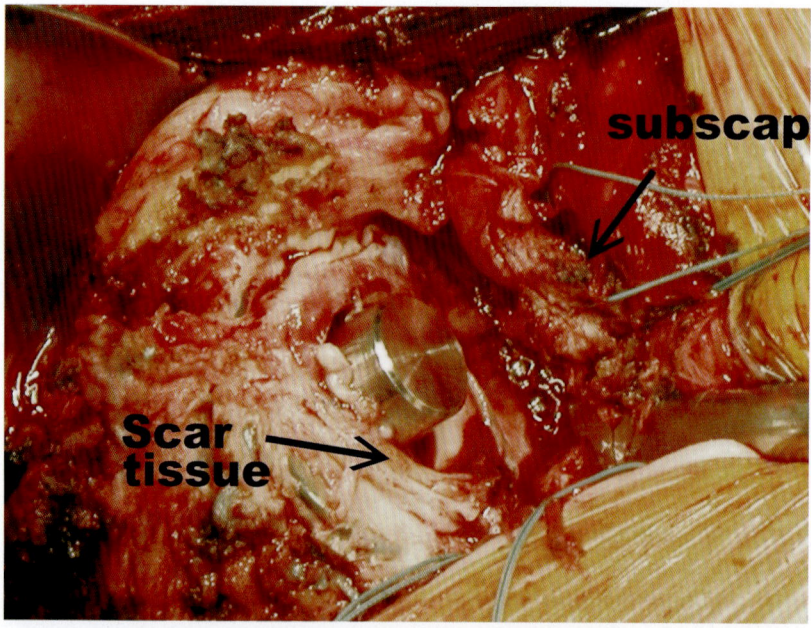

Figure 6.5. Extensive scarring around the humeral neck and prostheses.

proximal humerus depends on specific potential problems particular to the case.

After adequate exposure of the proximal humerus is obtained, further exposure is required to gain adequate access to the glenoid. Modular components allow the surgeon to leave the humeral stem undisturbed. At this point attention is returned to the subscapularis to complete the circumferential release of this muscle. This step is crucial for exposure and restoration of external rotation and soft tissue balance. The interval between the subscapularis and the anterior capsule is developed at the level of the glenoid. In the revision setting this interval is often obliterated and needs to be recreated for adequate release of the undersurface of the muscle. This is usually started with electrocautery at the glenoid, and then continued medially using blunt dissection to prevent potential denervation of the muscle (Figure 6.6). The coracohumeral ligament may require further release if the initial release was not satisfactory. Next, the anterior capsule is excised following its separation from the subscapularis. The lateral portion of the capsule confluent with the tendon can be left attached for preservation of more

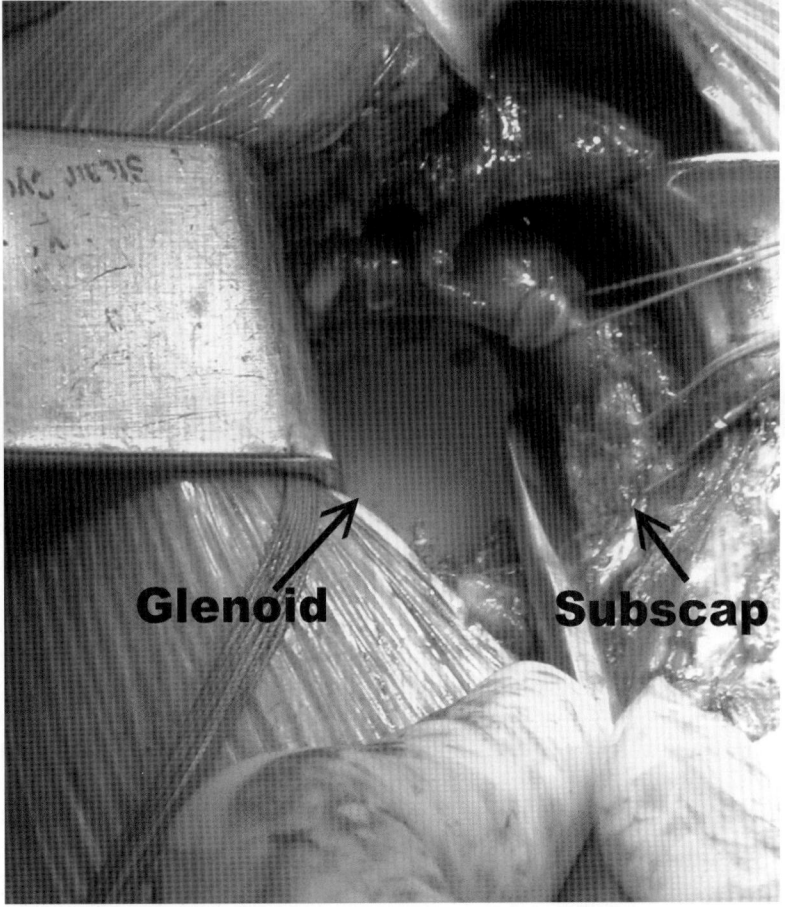

Figure 6.6. Release of subscapularis from the capsule at the level of the glenoid.

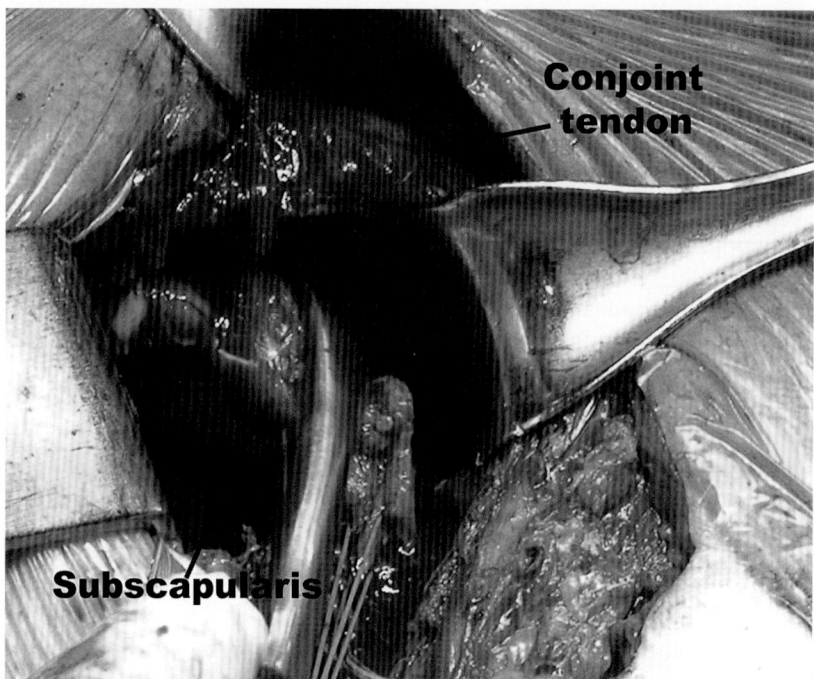

Figure 6.7. Circumferential subscapularis release addressing multiple potential sites of adhesions. It is important to repeat previously performed steps to ensure adequate release.

stout tissue for repair. The subscapularis release can be extended further medially in a blunt fashion all around the muscle until adequate excursion and length are achieved (Figure 6.7). At this point, further capsular release can be performed with electrocautery superiorly around the glenoid and inferiorly as needed to achieve adequate exposure. If the exposure remains limited, the contracted long head of the biceps tendon, if present, can be released with subsequent tenodesis at the biceps groove. Further work on the glenoid depends on specific issues that need to be addressed during revision surgery.

Obtaining adequate exposure can be a great challenge in revision arthroplasty due to contracted soft tissue. It is important to perform necessary releases of the subdeltoid and subacromial spaces as well as circumferential subscapularis release. The releases should be performed predominantly with blunt dissection to avoid injury to the neurovascular structures. The surgeon needs to be patient and use gentle retraction of tissues to avoid potential intraoperative fractures of osteopenic bone. Great care should be exercised to preserve the attachment of the anterior deltoid. Dysfunction of the anterior deltoid postoperatively is a disastrous complication without any viable options for correction. In rare situations, if exposure is still limited after all soft tissue releases, the deltoid can be detached to facilitate exposure. The anterior deltoid is removed from the anterior clavicle and acromion, leaving a stout periosteal sleeve of tissue for subsequent repair (Figure 6.8A and 6.8B). The deltoid is then split at the raphe between the

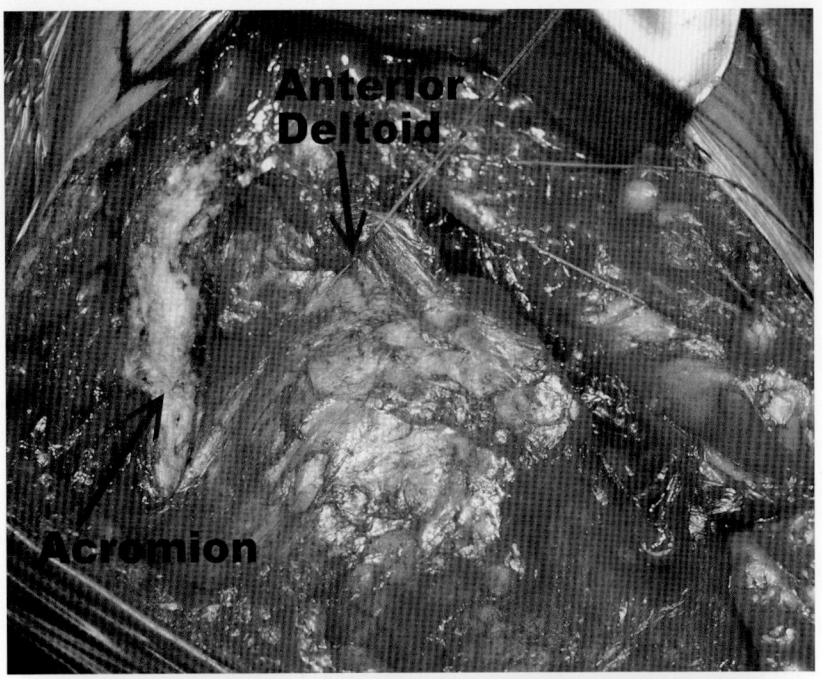

A

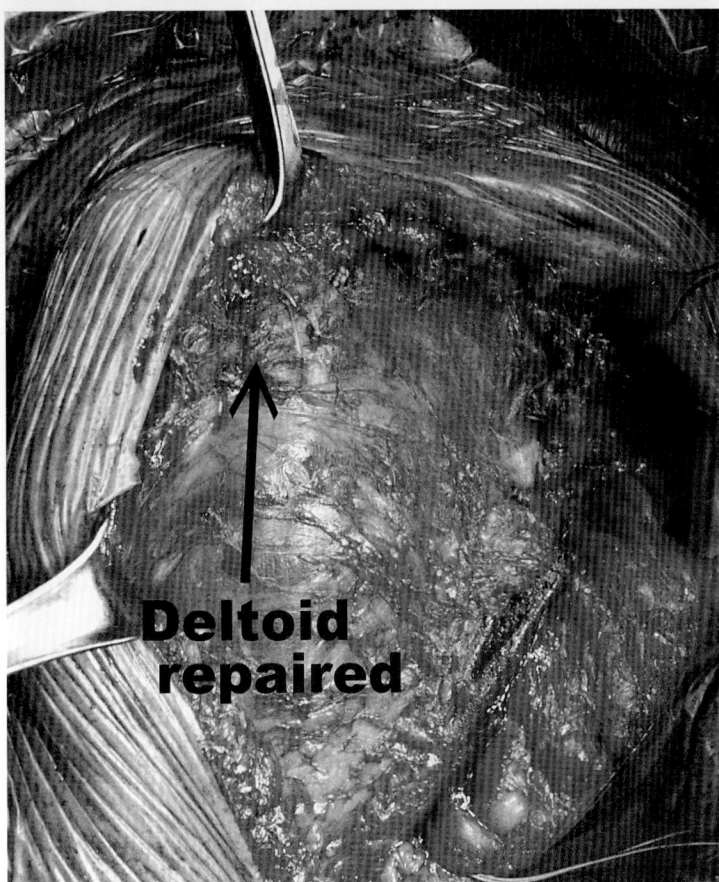

B

Figure 6.8. **(A)** Detachment of the anterior deltoid leaving stout tissue on the acromion for subsequent repair. **(B)** Subsequent repair of the anterior deltoid.

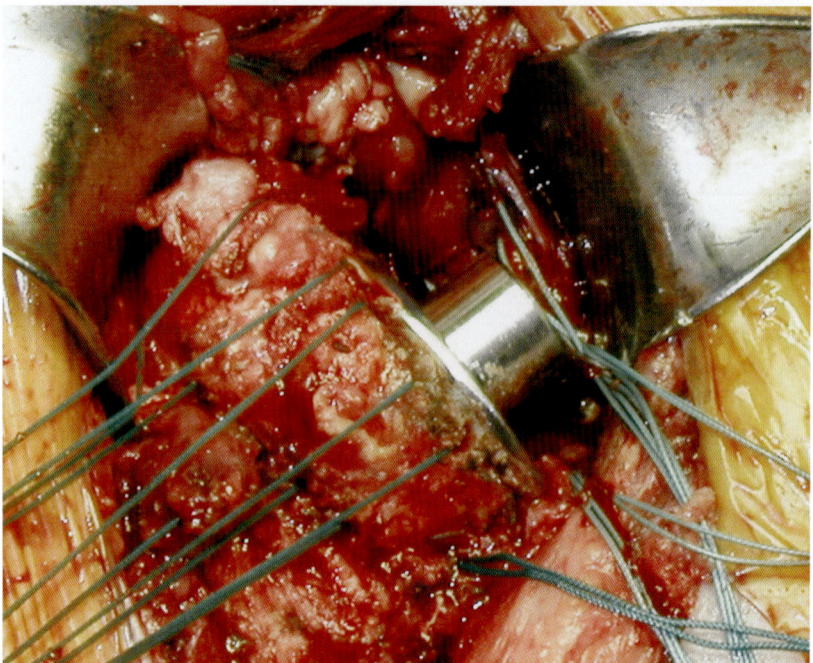

Figure 6.9. Placement of transosseous sutures for subscapularis repair.

anterior and middle deltoid longitudinally. This split is extended no more than 4 cm lateral to the acromion to avoid injury to the axillary nerve. This takedown provides superior exposure, and with internal rotation of the humerus the posterior rotator cuff can be easily exposed. Meticulous repair of the deltoid is essential. If the soft tissue repair is deemed inadequate, the deltoid should be repaired through drill holes in the clavicle and acromion. Postoperative rehabilitation must focus on protection of this repair, which may compromise the functional result of surgery. We have performed this approach several times in difficult revisions and have not compromised deltoid function postoperatively. We do not recommend detaching the deltoid insertion distally.

The subscapularis muscle repair is crucial in revision surgery. The insertion of the subscapularis can be medialized by repairing it to the osteotomized humeral neck with heavy transosseous sutures, allowing further gain in functional length (Figure 6.9). In general, each centimeter gain in length of the anterior tissues increases external rotation by 20 degrees.

Most pathology in revision surgery can be addressed through the deltopectoral approach. However, in some situations, such as locked posterior instability, a combined anterior and posterior approach may be necessary. If a combined anterior and posterior approach is necessary, the patient is placed in the beach chair position to allow access to the anterior and posterior aspects of the shoulder. The table can be *airplaned* to either side to facilitate exposure. For the posterior approach, an oblique skin incision is made. The deltoid is split along the direction of its fibers, beginning at the posterior lateral corner of the acromion and extended for no more than 5 cm. The deltoid is detached from the lateral acromion for 1 cm to 2 cm and from the scapular spine for 3 cm to 4 cm. The infraspinatus tendon is then distinguished from the supraspinatus superiorly and from the teres minor inferiorly. Two anatomic considerations can be used to help delineate the infraspinatus from the teres minor. As the infraspinatus is a bipennate muscle, when three groups of muscle fibers can be seen, the upper two represent the infraspinatus. Second, the infraspinatus inserts on the greater tuberosity on a broad facet, whereas teres minor inserts on a distinct smaller facet, which is typically palpable. Once clearly defined, the infraspinatus can be separated from the underlying posterior capsule. Laterally, the tendon and capsule are confluent and it can prove challenging to separate the two. It is often helpful to identify the plane medially where the muscle bellies separate more easily. The tendon is incised approximately 1 cm from the tuberosity. The posterior capsule can then be incised 1 cm from its lateral insertion on the humerus. Posterior pathology, whether a locked posteriorly dislocated prosthesis or a patulous posterior capsule causing posterior instability, can then be addressed.

Bone Deficiency

While revision arthroplasty of the shoulder can present multiple technical challenges, one of the most difficult and unfortunately most common issues is bone deficiency of the glenoid or proximal humerus. The etiology of bone deficiency can be from multiple factors, acting individually or in combination with one another. Abnormal or eccentric wear, instability, infection, malaligned components, and intraoperative bone loss during component removal can all produce bone deficiency. In addition to addressing existing bone deficiency, the etiology of the problem must be determined and corrected to prevent the recurrence after revision surgery.

Component Removal

Before addressing the technical options to deal with bone deficiency, it is important to review the appropriate techniques for component removal. Potential problems of component malposition, loosening, and mechanical failure may necessitate component extraction. The removal of the humeral and glenoid components usually requires special equipment and a great deal of patience. System-specific extractors as well as universal extraction tools are essential. Flexible osteotomes can be quite helpful to detach the prosthetic surfaces at the bone/cement interface. One has to be very careful and patient to prevent intraoperative fracture and the removal of excessive amounts of bone. Different types of extraction devices are available. They usually hook under the collar and are attached to a slap hammer (Figure 6.10). Also, a heavy chisel is helpful to create a vertical force under the collar. The best extractors are those that are in line with the humeral shaft. Cement removal may be difficult as the humeral cortex may be thin and susceptible to fracture. In difficult cases, we have used ultrasonic wave devices to melt the cement and facilitate its removal.

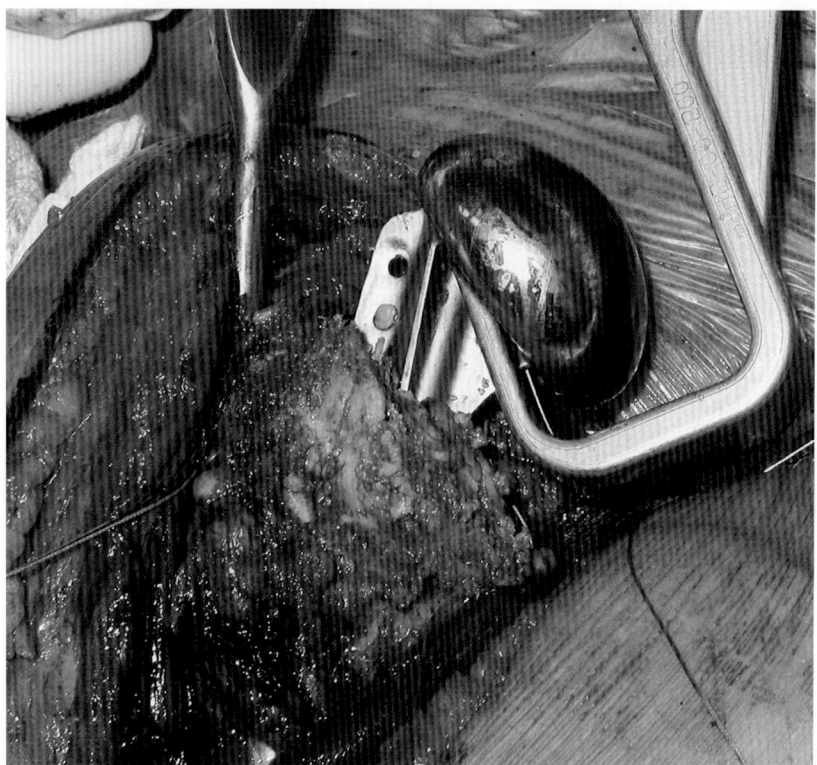

Figure 6.10. Humeral component removal.

An anterior humeral osteotomy can be performed to gain exposure to the entire length of the humeral stem. An extended incision is required in this technique to gain exposure distally to the shaft of the humerus. The deltopectoral approach is extended distally. Medially, care needs to be exercised to prevent injury to the musculocutaneous nerve. An anterior L-shaped window of the proximal humerus is created, extending down distally and ending several centimeters proximal to the tip of the prosthesis. This is performed using a combination of the sagittal saw and osteotomes. The horizontal limb of the osteotomy enables a window of cortex to be hinged open, creating excellent access to the cement mantle and the entire humeral prosthesis. Care is exercised proximally to prevent a fracture of the tuberosities. Using flexible osteotomes, the prosthesis/cement/bone interface is disrupted for unobstructed removal of the humeral component. The remainder of the cement can be removed using special rasps. The anterior bone window is closed and secured in place with cerclage wires. This fixation is quite stable and restores the integrity of the humeral shaft for placement of a new component. Care must be taken to prevent injury to the radial nerve by remaining subperiosteal while placing the cerclage wires.

Removal of the glenoid component is usually performed in the setting of loosening and/or mechanical failure. Loosening of the glenoid is the most common cause of failure leading to revision after total shoulder arthroplasty [3] (Figure 6.11). Symptomatic loosening of

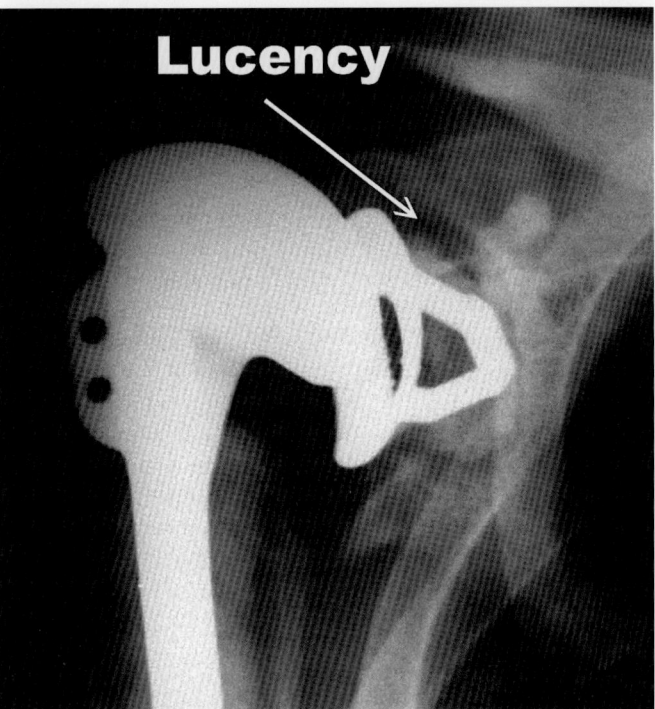

Figure 6.11. AP radiograph demonstrating loosening all around glenoid component.

the glenoid is treated by removal of the component. Again patience and accurate technique are extremely important to prevent unnecessary bone loss. Flexible osteotomes and a rongeur are useful in glenoid extraction. It is sometimes necessary to cut the keel or pegs of the polyethylene glenoid component for successful extraction. O'Driscoll and associates have reported good results in small series of patents treated with arthroscopic removal of loosened polyethylene glenoids [6]. This technique has limited applications since the additional pathology usually present in failed shoulder arthroplasty cannot be addressed. Also, bone grafting of the glenoid cavity cannot be performed.

Proximal Humeral Bone Deficiency

The most common scenarios contributing to proximal humeral bone deficiency include excessive bone loss during component removal, malunion, nonunion, and infection. Several treatment options can deal with this bone deficiency including resection arthroplasty, arthrodesis, osteotomy, and restoration of the proximal humerus with autograft, allograft, a custom prosthesis, or an allograft-prosthetic composite. The main goals of proximal humerus reconstruction are to achieve secure fixation of the humeral component, restore the humeral height, and securely repair the rotator cuff and deltoid muscles to the anatomically positioned tuberosities. Determining the appropriate humeral height can be a challenging task. This is a common problem in the setting of hemiarthroplasty for fracture and can contribute to failure of this procedure. Greater tuberosity malunion and nonunion can also be challenging in terms of proximal humerus bony reconstruction. Tuberosity malunion may cause painful subacromial impingement. If the superior displacement of the greater tuberosity is mild, anterior acromioplasty may provide adequate decompression of subacromial space. Severe displacement may necessitate tuberosity osteotomy and repair. Tuberosity nonunion can lead to loss of motion and weakness, as well as superior migration from compromised rotator cuff function. Achieving bony union is often a challenge.

The humeral component needs to be cemented into the canal in appropriate version with the humeral head centered in the glenoid after gentle traction on the arm is applied (Figure 6.12). The traction is important to restore the physiologic myofascial tension around the shoulder. If the tuberosities are detached, repair of the tuberosities with heavy nonabsorbable sutures is performed and autogenous bone graft is placed to augment healing. Wire or cable fixation can also be added to provide additional stability of the tuberosities. When bone deficiency is extensive as often is the case after component removal, the tuberosi-

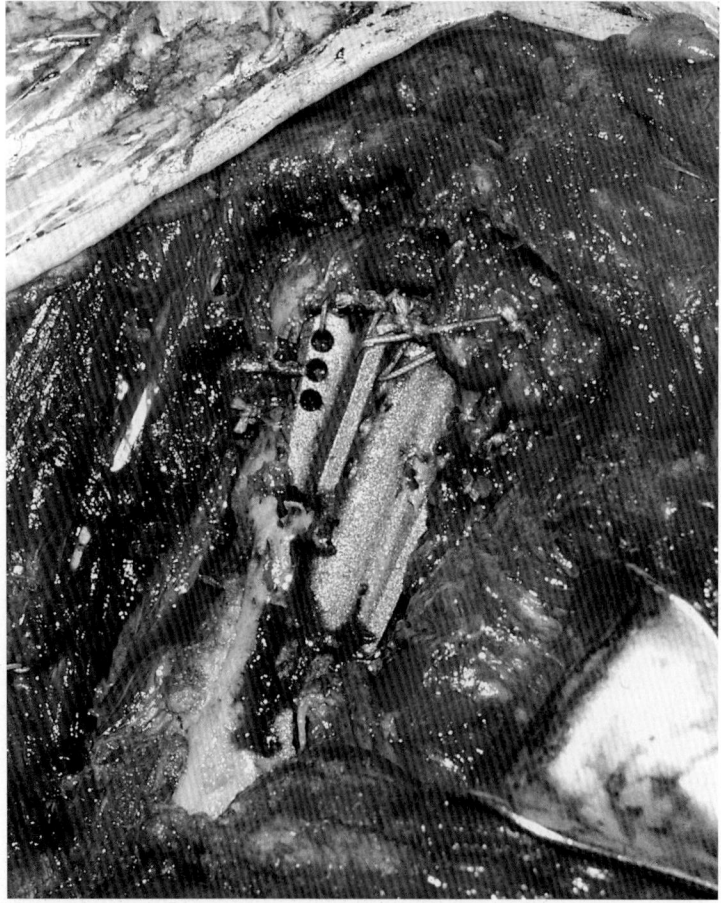

Figure 6.12. Humeral stem placed at appropriate height despite substantial proximal bone loss.

ties cannot be approximated to the shaft of bone. In these cases, cortical strut allograft in combination with autograft can be used. Cerclage
wires are used to achieve fixation of the strut allograft to the shaft of
the humerus distally and to the prosthesis proximally. Again caution
should be exercised to prevent injury to the axillary and radial nerves
during wire placement.

Recent evidence has suggested that uncemented humeral prostheses
may have a higher rate of loosening at intermediate-term follow-up
than prostheses implanted with modern cementing techniques [7, 8, 9,
10]. This evidence coupled with frequent compromise of bone stock in
the revision setting suggests that uncemented humeral prostheses are
rarely indicated in revision surgery.

Trabecular metal implants represent an emerging technology that
has great potential in the setting of revision surgery. Our initial experience with these has been extremely satisfying in terms of achieving
tuberosity fixation in cases of nonunion. Trabecular metal (TM) prostheses allow for bone and even soft tissue ingrowth, achieving firm
attachment around the proximal part of the humeral stem (Figure 6.13).

Osteoarticular allografts and allograft-prosthetic composites are primarily indicated in the setting of tumor surgery, and discussion of their
use is beyond the scope of this text.

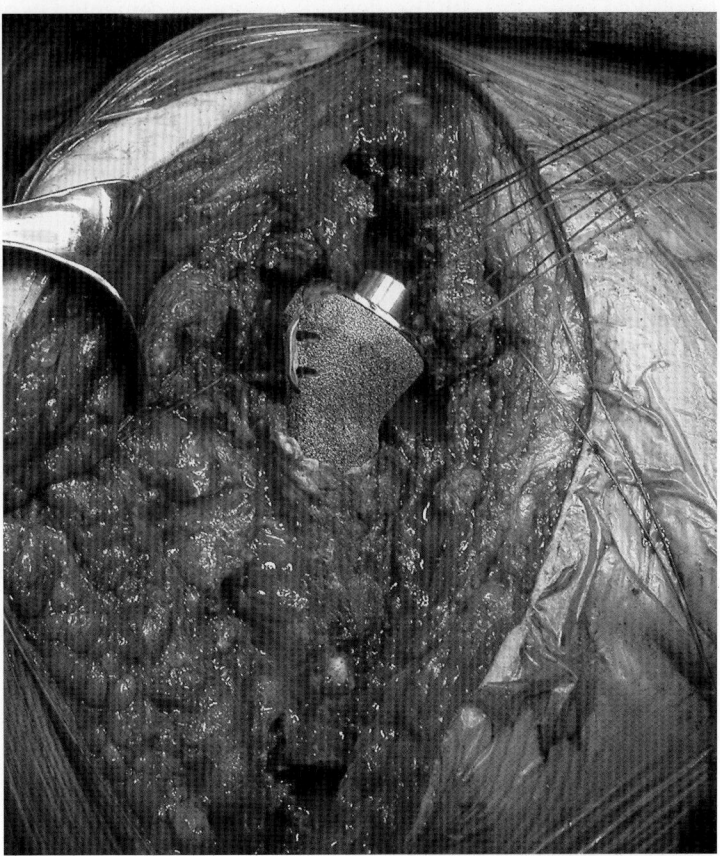

Figure 6.13. Placement of trabecular metal humeral stem in a case with extensive proximal bone deficiency and nonunion of the greater tuberosity.

Glenoid Bone Deficiency

The most important issue to resolve in the setting of glenoid deficiency is whether implantation of a new glenoid component remains technically feasible. Glenoid implantation if often desirable, as the literature suggests that total shoulder arthroplasty provides better pain relief than hemiarthroplasty alone [11, 12, 13]. The integrity and repairability of the rotator cuff, the availability of sufficient bone stock, and the presence of adequate joint volume affect the feasibility of glenoid implantation. Massive rotator cuff deficiency precludes the use of a glenoid component to avoid the creation of a *rocking horse* glenoid [14]. Insufficient bone stock to achieve secure fixation of the glenoid component also prohibits implantation. Extensive contracture of the musculature around the shoulder can cause dramatic reduction of joint volume despite all of the necessary releases previously described. In this situation, overstuffing the joint with a glenoid component renders postoperative range of motion unacceptable. In these clinical scenarios, a surgeon has several options depending on the specific pathology present. Antuna et al. have described patterns of glenoid bone loss as being central, peripheral, or combined [15]. With in each category, the bone loss can be further categorized as mild, moderate, or severe. In cases of mild to moderate central bone deficiency, particulate allograft can be packed centrally with the glenoid component cemented in place. In cases of severe central deficiency, a two-stage procedure with glenoid implantation at a later time may be necessary. In cases of eccentric wear and abnormal version, the native glenoid can be reamed to restore appropriate version. This technique is covered elsewhere in this text. Eccentric posterior wear is often present in failed hemiarthroplasty (Figure 6.14). In these cases, eccentric reaming and component place-

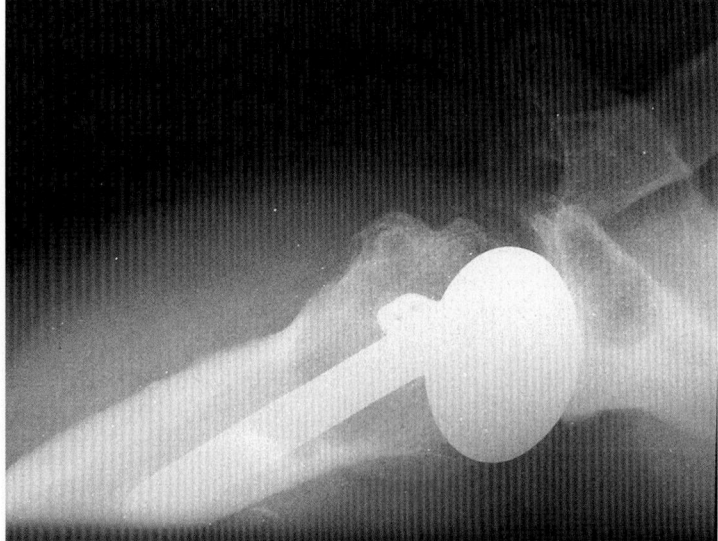

Figure 6.14. Axillary radiograph of a painful hemiarthroplasty demonstrating posterior glenoid wear.

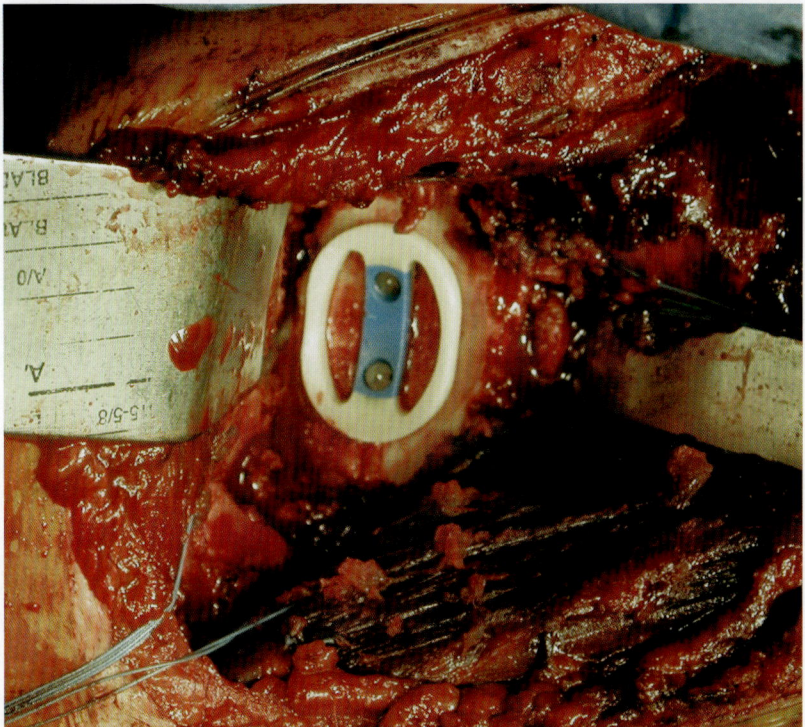

Figure 6.15. Open-faced glenoid provisional with 46-mm outer diameter and 52-mm inner (articular) diameter.

ment can be accomplished easier when glenoid components with two different radii of curvature are available for use. The shoulder system used in our institution has the versatility to go up or down one size on the articulating surface compared with the nonarticular surface. This versatility allows placement of a glenoid component with 40-mm curverture on the nonarticular side and a 46-mm curverture on the articular side, or 46-mm curverture on the nonarticular side and 52-mm curverture on the articular side (Figure 6.15). This feature of the glenoid component is extremely useful when glenoid bone stock is limited and the size of the humeral head is large. Coracoid transfer can be used to address anterior uncontained glenoid deficiency (i.e., the Latarjet procedure) [16, 17]. An osteotome or sagittal saw is used to perform an osteotomy of the coracoid distal to the coracoclavicular ligaments. Care is exercised not to damage neurovascular structures medial to the coracoid. The coracoid is shaped to fit the anterior glenoid defect and secured in place with two 3.5-mm cortical screws. Another option is iliac crest bone graft to reconstruct anterior or posterior glenoid. For patients with insufficient bone stock to support the glenoid, removal of the glenoid without reimplantation is necessary. A soft tissue resurfacing of the glenoid rather than simple removal of the glenoid prothesis may decrease the incidence of postoperative pain [18]. Achilles allograft, fascia lata, or meniscal allograft each represent potential options for soft tissue resurfacing. At our institution, meniscal allograft has been used for resurfacing of the glenoid in selected young patients. A lateral meniscus allograft is shaped to fit the glenoid surface. Bio-absorbable suture anchors are placed into the glenoid face and the allograft tissue is secured to the glenoid and surrounding tissue. Limited information is available to date regarding the results of this technique, although early follow-up has been encouraging.

Glenoid implantation in the setting of bone deficiency is a challenging task. Preoperative CT or MRI is important in determining the amount of bone available for implantation. In most cases it is possible and desirable to adjust the version of the glenoid by reaming of the high side. Typically, a sufficient vault remains for implantation of the glenoid component. In cases of massive deficiency, a structural bone graft to augment the worn side of the glenoid can be used to restore appropriate version [5]. A posterior approach or percutaneous technique can be used to achieve fixation of structural bone graft for posterior glenoid deficiency. After secure fixation of the graft, reaming is performed to achieve a concentric glenoid in appropriate version.

Recently, trabecular metal components have also been used in glenoid implantation (Figure 6.16A). This technology offers exciting theoretical advantages over cementation techniques and conventional press-fit components. A trabecular metal glenoid implant can be useful in achieving good fixation in compromised bone in the revision setting, and our early limited clinical experience with this has been encouraging (Figure 6.16B).

Instability After Total Shoulder Arthroplasty

Instability after total shoulder arthroplasty can be classified on the basis of the direction of instability as superior, inferior, posterior, or anterior. Instability can vary from mild subluxation to severe dislocation. The chronicity of instability is an important factor in determining its etiology. Early instability may be related to component malposition or failure of the subscapularis repair. Superior instability occurs most commonly due to rotator cuff insufficiency and an incompetent coracoacromial arch. Inferior instability occurs most commonly due to inappropriate height of the humeral component. This typically mandates component removal and reinsertion with restoration of the appropriate height. Anterior and posterior instability are among the most common complications after total shoulder arthroplasty and often necessitate prosthetic repositioning and soft tissue rebalancing. Tendon transfers may be necessary if the rotator cuff tendons are deficient.

Frequent contributing factors to both anterior and posterior instability include malalignment of the glenoid and/or humeral components, soft tissue contracture or imbalance, and a rotator cuff tear, especially subscapularis failure in case of anterior instability [2, 19]. The results of revision surgery in the setting of instability are inferior to those of primary arthroplasty, accentuating the importance of correct component placement and meticulous subscapularis repair during the primary procedure. Malposition of the glenoid and/or humeral

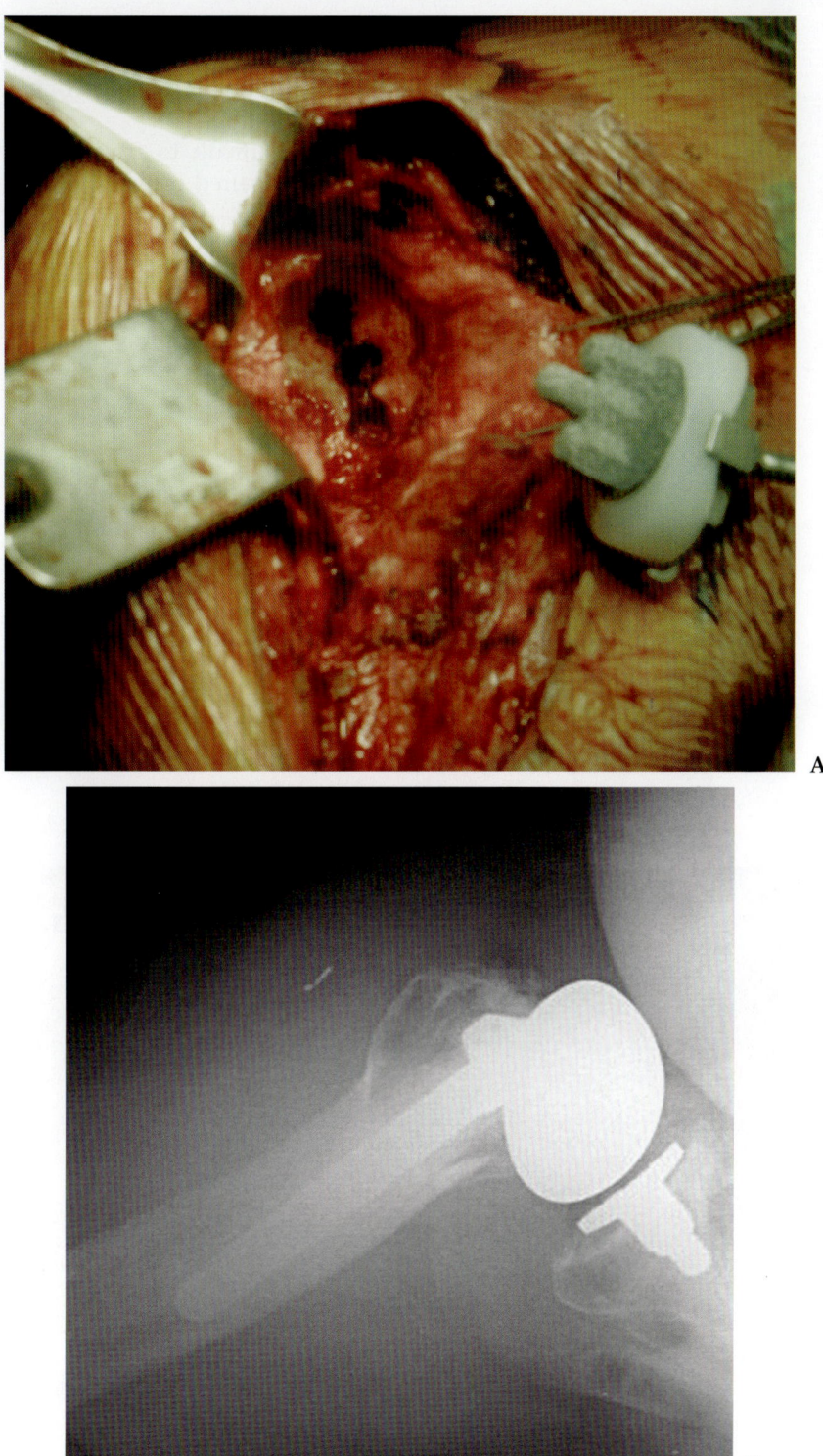

Figure 6.16. (A) Revision case for symptomatic glenoid loosening. Trabecular metal component was used in compromised bone. Excellent initial fixation was achieved. **(B)** Postoperative axillary view demonstrating trabecular metal component.

components is the most common cause. Such components must be removed using techniques described previously, any bone deficiency must be addressed, and well-fixed and appropriately aligned components must be placed.

Subscapularis insufficiency is especially difficult to treat (Figure 6.17A and 6.17B). The subscapularis can be repaired primarily if ade-

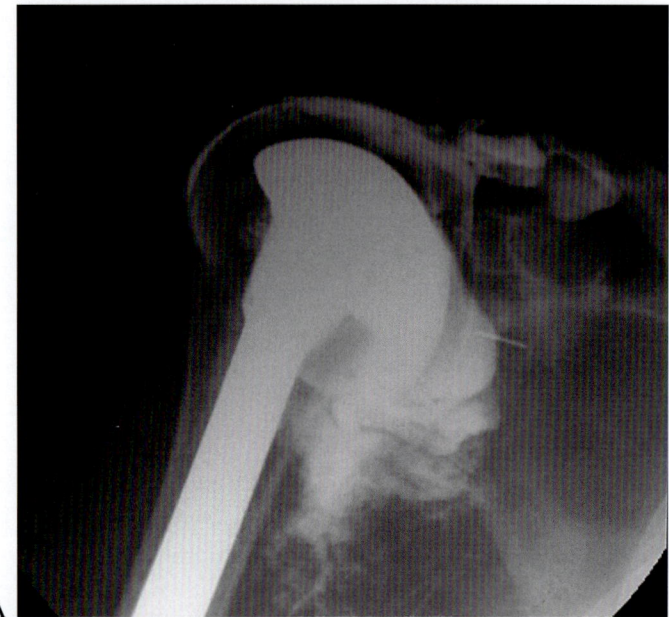

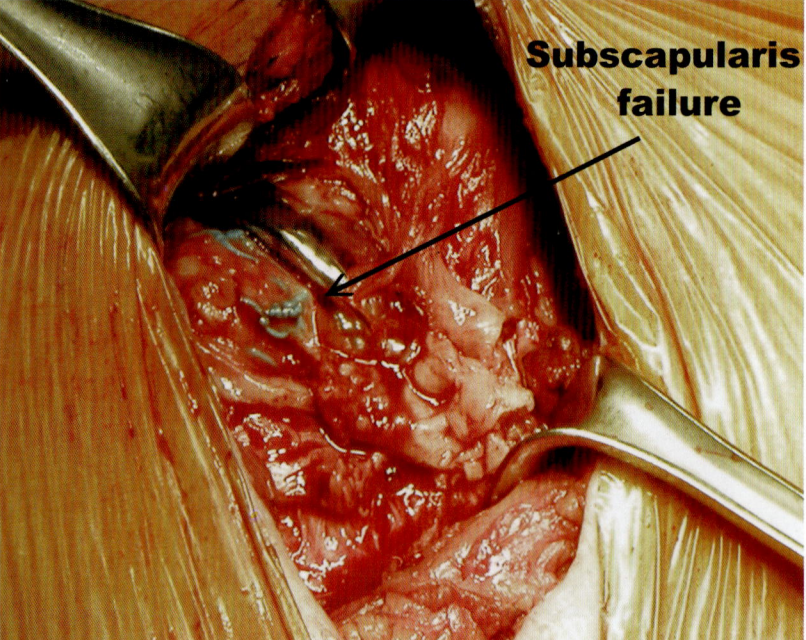

Figure 6.17. **(A)** Arthrogram demonstrating leakage of contrast indicating subscapularis tear. **(B)** Subscapularis failure identified during surgery. Adequate tissue of the tendon was found to allow direct repair.

quate tissue is present. Subscapularis releases previously described can be used to achieve adequate length and excursion to allow for primary subscapularis repair (see Figures 6.6 and 6.7). Often, inadequate tissue is available for stable, low-tension repair. In these cases various tendon transfers are used to substitute for the deficient subscapularis. Additionally, static restraint can be provided by an Achilles tendon allograft [19, 20]. There is no perfect reconstructive option in this situation, since no available transfer completely recreates the line of pull of the subscapularis muscle. At our institution, transfer of the pectoralis major with passage under the strap muscles is preferred. In smaller patients, the lower one-half or two-thirds of the pectoralis major is used. For most patients, especially if the muscle is robust, we prefer to only transfer the sternal head of the pectoralis major as this leaves the upper portion of the muscle improving cosmetic appearance of the axillary fold. This decision can be made intraoperatively after assessment of the muscular bulk of the pectoralis major. An anterior approach as described previously is used. The pectoralis major muscle is identified. Either the sternal head or the lower one-half to two-thirds of the muscle is detached of the humerus and mobilized (Figure 6.18A). It is important to detach the tendon as close as possible to the humeral shaft to obtain adequate length for the transfer. Care is taken to prevent injury to the biceps tendon. A window under the strap muscles is prepared using blunt dissection. Care is taken to prevent injury to the musculocutaneous nerve, normally passing about 5.6 cm inferior to the coracoid; this distance can be as short as 3.5 cm [21]. The pectoralis major tendon is mobilized circumferentially and advanced under the strap muscles (Figure 6.18B). Care is taken to avoid placing the musculocutaneous nerve on stretch. Debulking of the tendon may be required to eliminate undue tension on the nerve [22]. Passage of the tendon under the strap muscles better recreates the direction of pull of the subscapularis. It also allows the tendon to act as a sling for the humeral head, resisting anterior translation [22]. If extensive scar prevents passage of the tendon under strap muscles, transfer can be done over the strap muscles. This diminishes the recreation of physiologic muscle balance, but still provides a soft tissue buttress resisting anterior humeral translation [20]. The tendon is attached to the lesser tuberosity using heavy suture through bone tunnels or suture anchors (Figure 6.18C). If possible, the transferred pectoralis major muscle should also be fixed to the supraspinatus in the lateral aspect of the rotator interval. Medial rotator interval sutures lead to loss of external rotation. It is desirable to incorporate the remaining subscapularis muscle into the transfer.

Anterosuperior instability after shoulder arthroplasty is the result of a rotator cuff tear and an incompetent coracoacromial arch. This typically occurs in patients with previously failed rotator cuff repairs in which the coracoacromial ligament was violated and excessive bone was removed from the acromion. Unfortunately, no consistently reliable surgical options exist to treat anterosuperior instability at this time [23]. The reverse ball-and-socket prosthesis is a new option to address this problem. In theory, the reverse ball-and-socket design recreates the center of glenohumeral rotation. European studies report

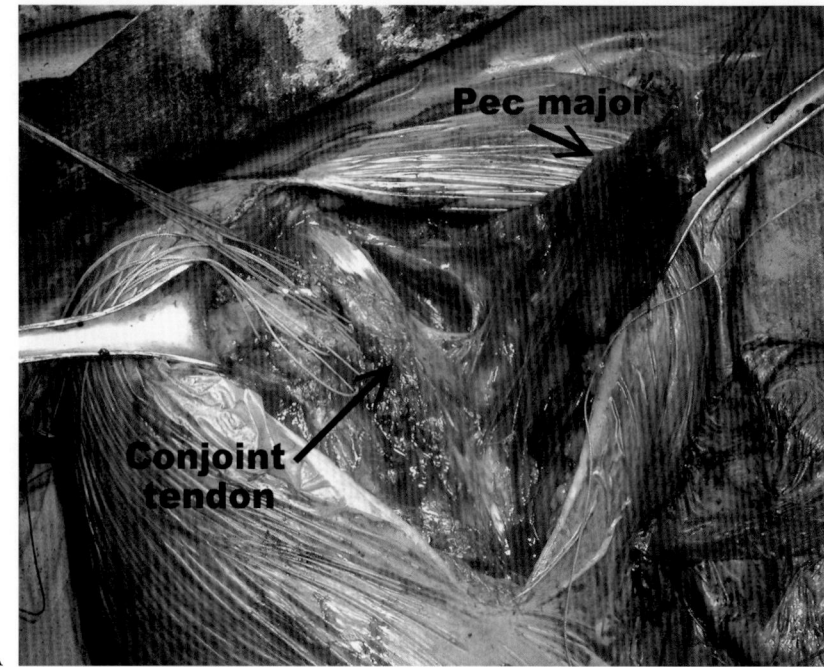

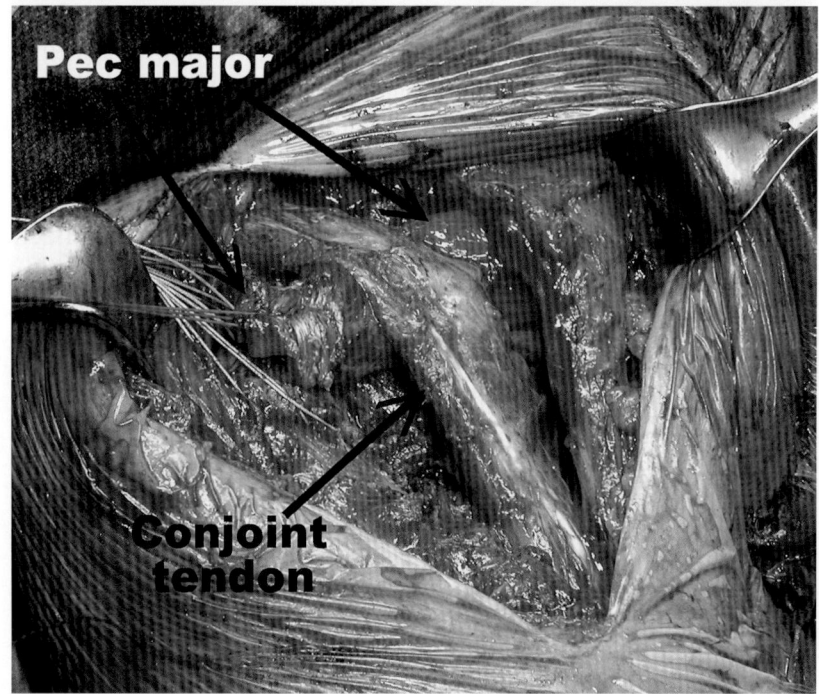

Figure 6.18. (A) Lower two-thirds of pectoralis major tendon mobilized for transfer. **(B)** Pectoralis major advanced under the strap muscles.

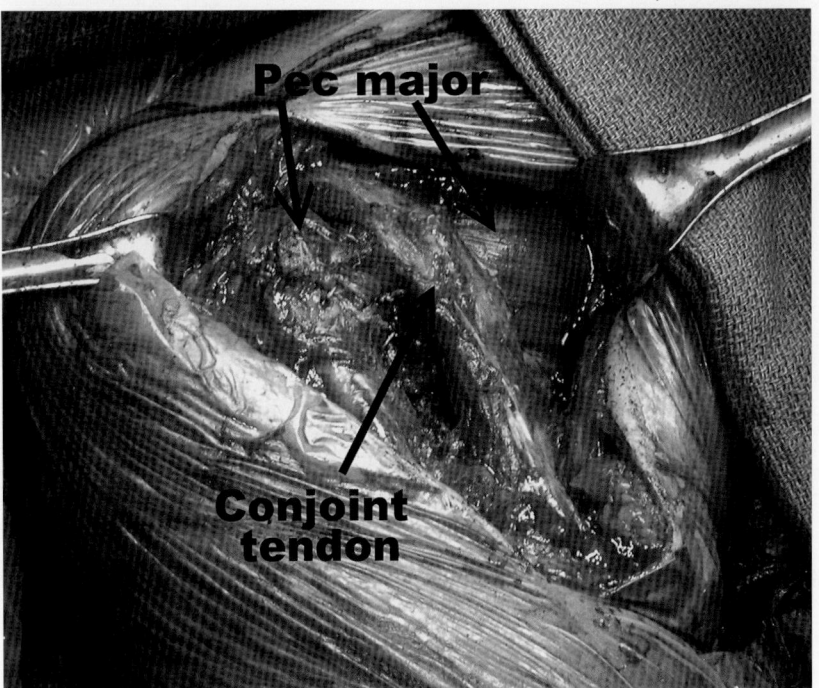

C

Figure 6.18. (*Continued*) **(C)** Pectoralis major transfer secured to the lesser tuberosity with transosseous sutures.

successful outcomes with use of this prosthesis, although clinical experience is limited in the United States and additional time and study are necessary before definitive recommendations on its use [24]. Also, more data are needed with respect to its use as a revision prosthesis, especially in a salvage situation. Figure 6.19A and 6.19B shows a custom reverse ball-and-socket prostheses performed for anterosuperior instability in a rotator cuff-deficient patient. There must be adequate bone stock to use this type of prosthetic design.

Superior instability after shoulder arthroplasty can result from rotator cuff deficiency, a humeral stem placed proud, or an inferiorly placed glenoid component. The humeral head is superiorly displaced but remains contained by the coracoacromial arch. Recentering of the humeral head on the glenoid is a challenging task. If glenoid component loosening is present, glenoid removal and rotator cuff repair is recommended. If insufficient rotator cuff tissue is present, the pectoralis major muscle can be advanced above the equator of the humeral head. This serves to augment humeral head depression and enhances shoulder function. A combined latisimusis dorsi and pectoralis major transfer is also an option; however, results of this extensive procedure are variable. Risks and benefits of this procedure must be carefully considered especially in frail older patients for whom the combined transfers are probably not indicated. Another option, described in detail in the section regarding arthroplasty in the rotator cuff deficient shoulder,

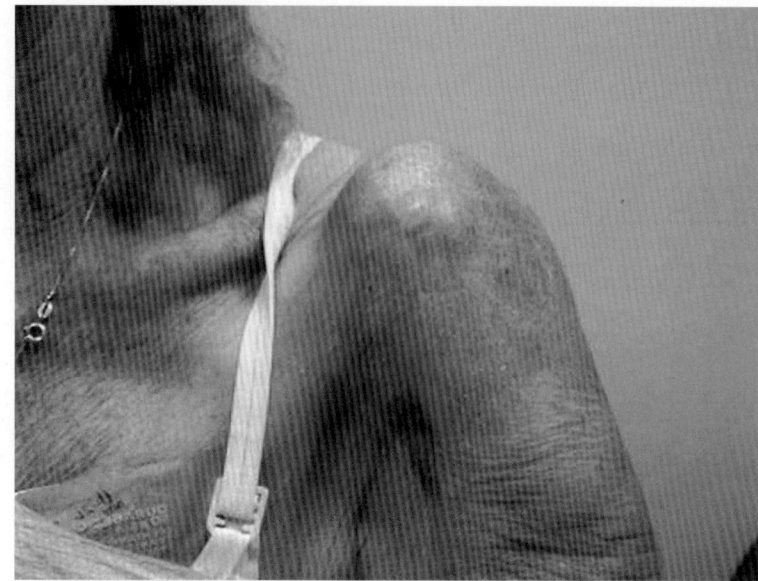

A

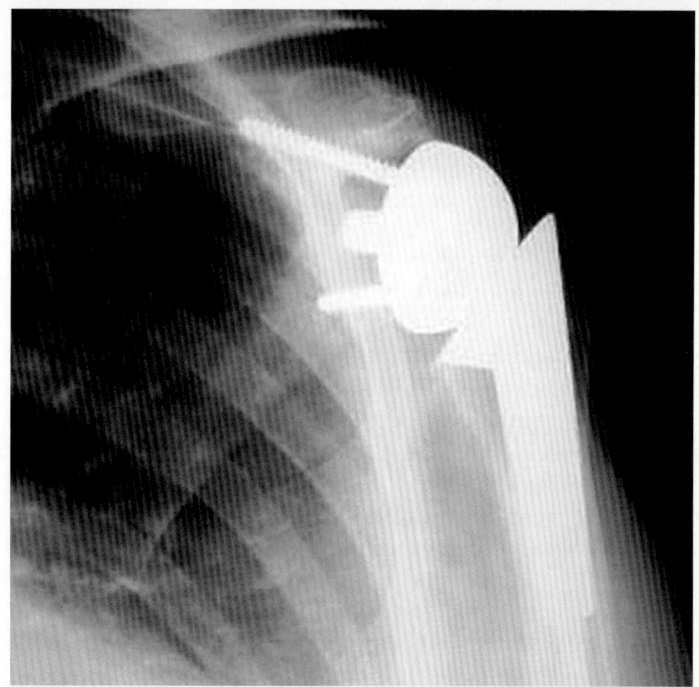

B

Figure 6.19. (A) Anterosuperior instability in a patient with massive rotator cuff tear and deficient coracoacromial arch. **(B)** Reverse-ball prostheses was used.

involves the use of a reverse ball-and-socket prosthesis to recreate the center of rotation of the glenohumeral joint.

Posterior instability is a challenging problem. Again contributory malposition of the glenoid and/or humeral components must be addressed using the aforementioned techniques (Figure 6.20). Often the glenoid component cannot be repositioned in appropriate version due

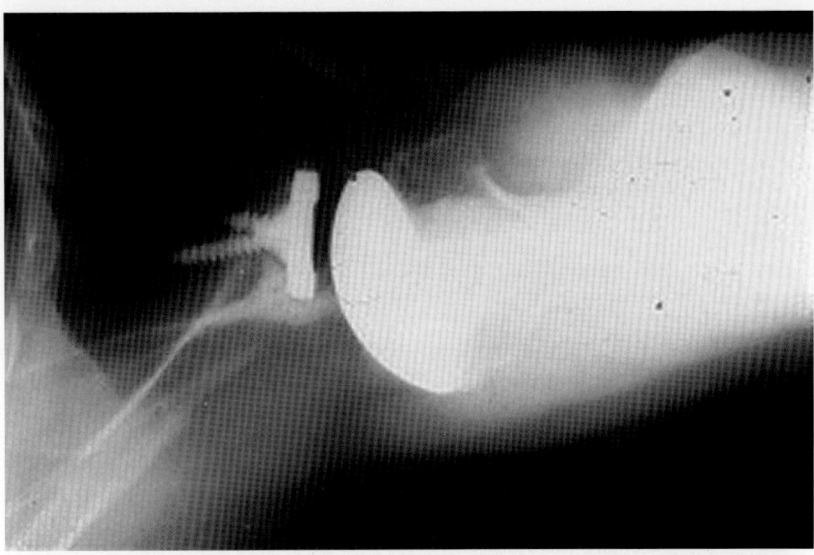

Figure 6.20. Axillary view demonstrating posterior humeral subluxation and retroverted glenoid component.

to limited bone stock and posterior wear. In such cases the humeral component should be placed in a relative anteverted position to compensate for the retroverted glenoid. Stability must be assessed intraoperatively, and experience with shoulder arthroplasty is essential in these cases. Failure to address posterior capsular redundancy during primary arthroplasty may be a cause of posterior instability. Deficient posterior soft tissue must be addressed during the revision surgery. Generally, component realignment and tightening of the posterior capsule can be accomplished through an anterior approach without the need for additional posterior incisions. Reduction of the posterior dislocation is performed through an anterior approach. If modular components were used, the humeral head is removed for better posterior capsule visualization. Posterior plication sutures are placed in a vertical direction. Vertical sutures are effective in decreasing the posterior capsular laxity and restoring the appropriate soft tissue balance. Sutures placed in a horizontal fashion tend to pull out or limit horizontal adduction of the shoulder. In some instances plication sutures may not be enough and a posterior capsular shift with infraspinatus shortening is indicated to balance the shoulder (Figure 6.21A–D). A combined anterior and posterior approach is necessary in the setting of a locked posterior dislocation. While this adds trauma to the posterior rotator cuff, it allows assessment and treatment of labral and capsular pathology.

Inferior instability usually results from inadequate restoration of the humeral height in the setting of arthroplasty after fracture. Humeral component revision to restore proper humeral height is performed as described in the section regarding the treatment of proximal humeral bone deficiency.

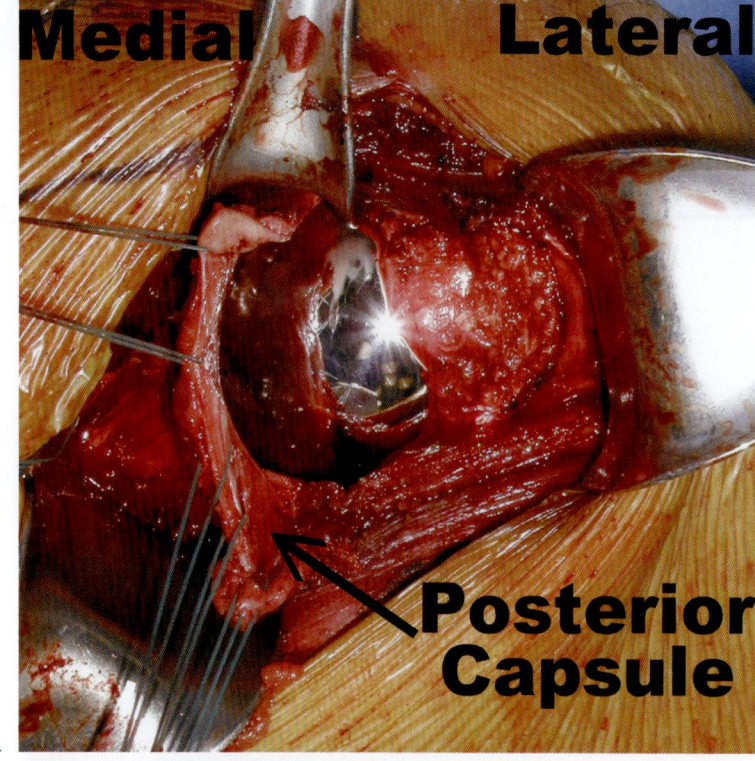

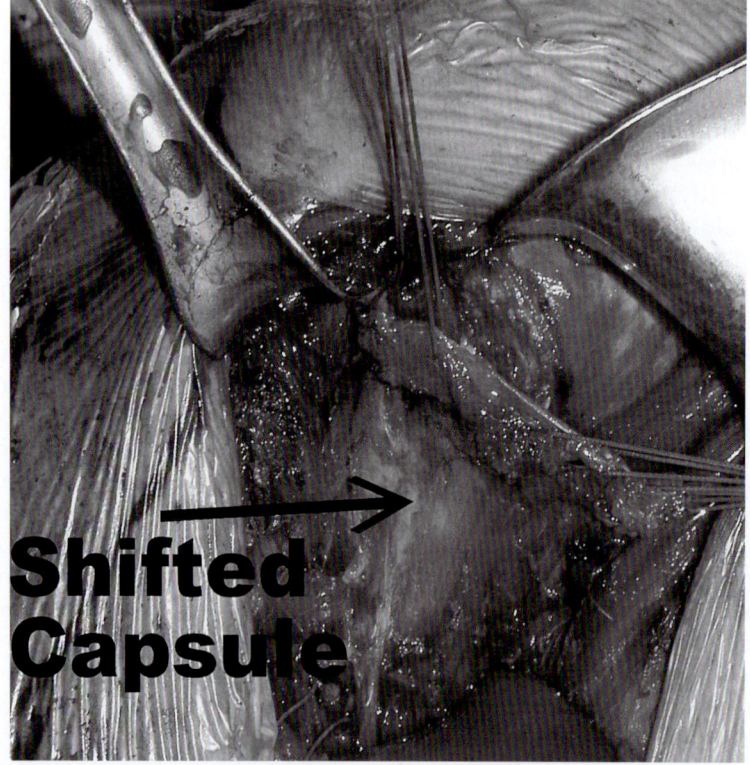

Figure 6.21. (A) Posterior capsular shift performed for posterior instability of TSA. Redundant and stretched out posterior capsule was identified. **(B)** Posterior capsule was advanced in lateral and superior direction.

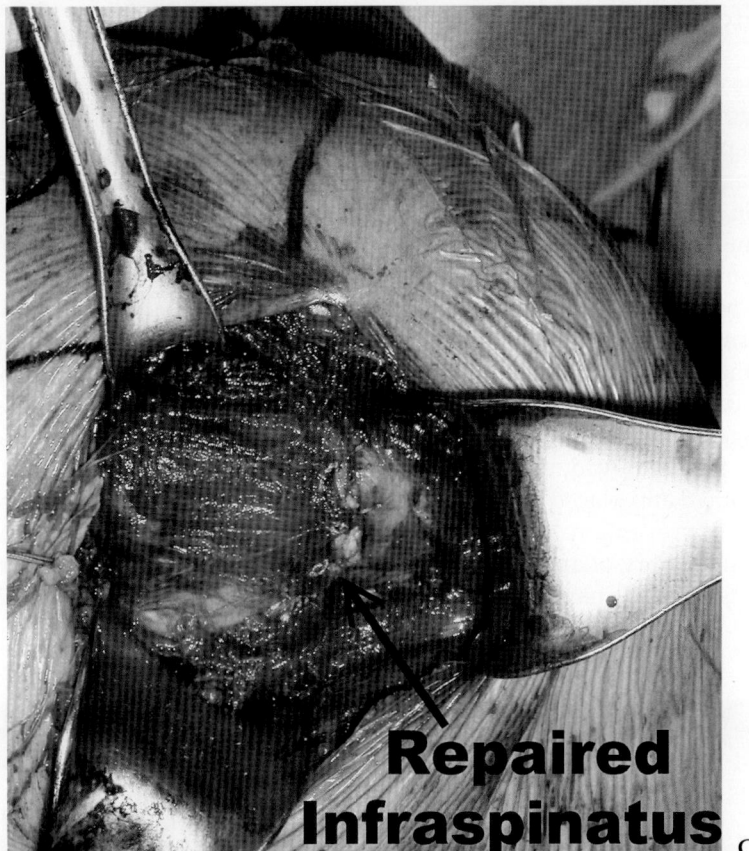

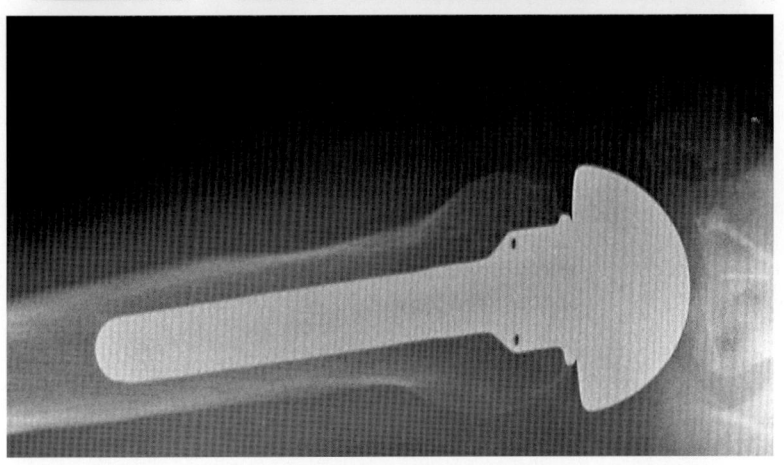

Figure 6.21. (*Continued*) **(C)** Infraspinatus was repaired and slightly imbricated. **(D)** Postoperative axillary view demonstrating well-centered humeral component and restoration of soft tissue balance.

Infection

The diagnosis of infection following shoulder arthroplasty is challenging. A high index of suspicion is essential, as most cases of chronic, deep infection may have minimal clinical symptoms except for pain. Diagnostic studies are often inconclusive. Eradication of chronic infection after arthroplasty requires removal of the prosthesis and all cement. Multiple deep cultures must be obtained for pathogen identification. Further surgical options depend on the virulence of the responsible organism. If the organism virulence is low, immediate reimplantation with new components using antibiotic-impregnated cement may be considered. However, the safest and surest option to eradicate infection and restore function in all situations involves a two-stage procedure. The infected prosthesis and any associated cement are first removed. An antibiotic-impregnated cement spacer can be sculpted and placed into the proximal humerus for preservation of joint space, prevention of extensive periarticular muscle contracture, and local delivery of antibiotic (Figure 6.22) [25]. Palacos cement (Zimmer, Warsaw, IN) may offer superior antibiotic elution properties [26].

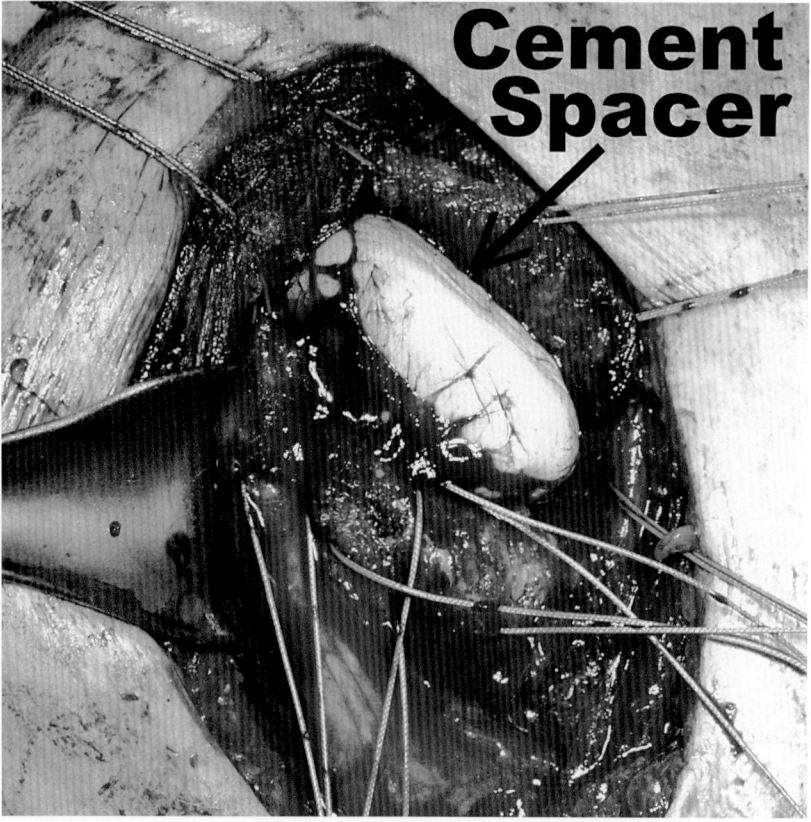

Figure 6.22. Antibiotic cement spacer is placed for preservation of soft tissue length and local antibiotic delivery.

Component reimplantation is performed in a subsequent procedure after 6 to 8 weeks, once the erythrocyte sedimentation rate, C-reactive protein, and white cell count have normalized. Needle aspiration to confirm resolution of infection may also be helpful before reimplantation. Intraoperatively tissue frozen section with analysis for organisms and lymphocyte count should precede component insertion. Antibiotic-impregnated cement should be used. We have used a trabecular metal humeral prosthesis for reimplantation after antibiotic cement spacer was removed. Not only excellent fixation of the humeral stem was achieved, but also impressive ingrowth of the greater tuberosity was achieved after chronic nonunion (Figure 6.23A). This patient achieved excellent function and is pain free without any signs of infection at 2-year follow-up (Figure 6.23B).

Periprosthetic Fracture

Satisfactory results have been reported following both surgical and nonsurgical treatment of periprosthetic fractures after shoulder arthroplasty [27, 28, 29]. If the fracture is minimally displaced and/or proximal to the tip of the prosthesis, conservative treatment is preferable. For fractures that are displaced, especially distal to the tip of the pros-

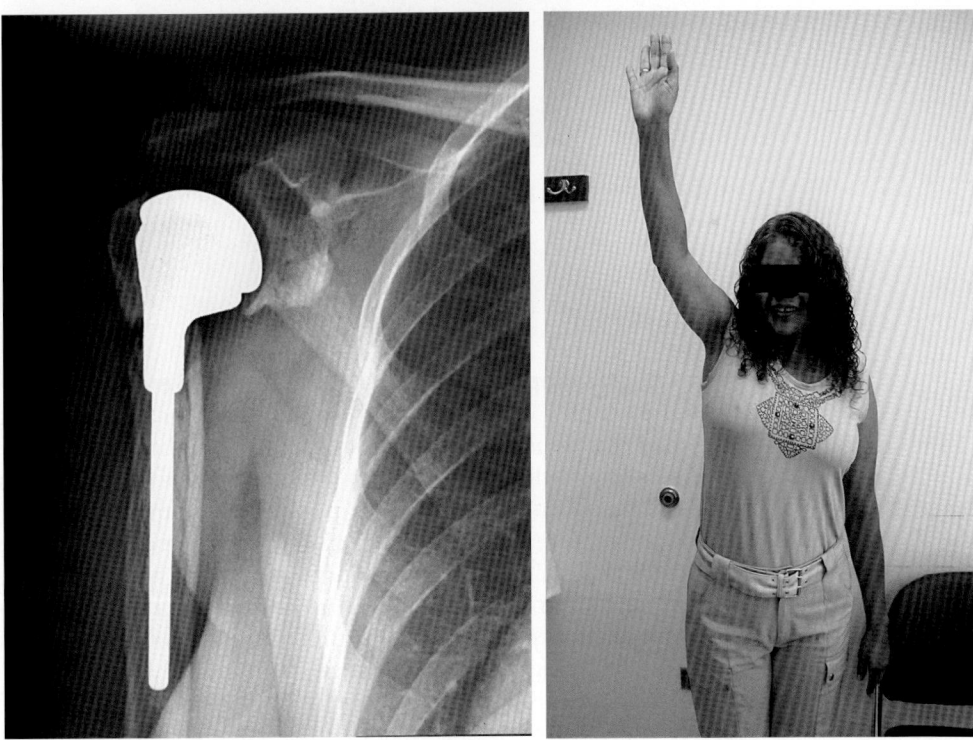

A   B

Figure 6.23. (A) Ingrowth of greater tuberosity into trabecular metal humeral stem. **(B)** Restoration of rotator cuff function after successful greater tuberosity ingrowth into humeral component resulted in excellent postoperative range of motion.

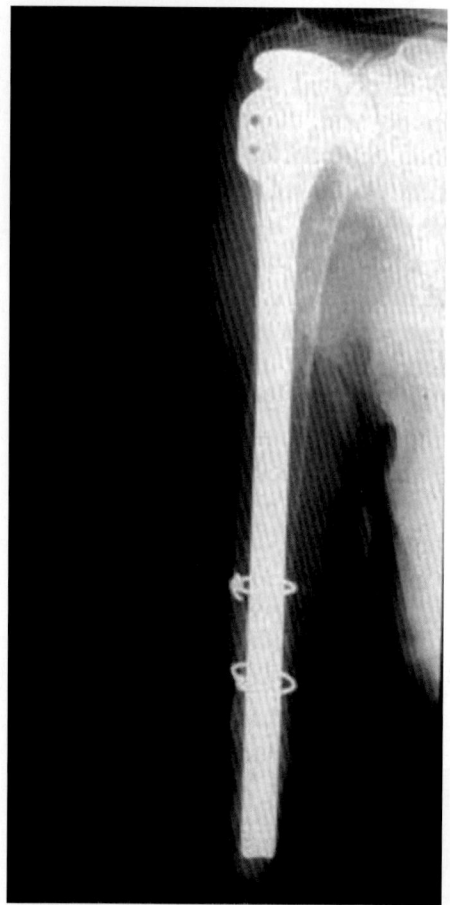

Figure 6.24. Long stem humeral stem placed for periprosthetic fracture.

thesis, we prefer operative management to achieve early, stable fixation and to enable early motion. Periprosthetic fractures can be categorized as intra-operative or post-operative. Wright and Cofield [29] classified periprosthetic humeral fractures into three types. This classification is based on the stability of the humeral component and location of the fracture relative to the tip of the humeral stem. Different methods of fixation can be used depending on the type of fracture. A standard deltopectoral approach is performed, with distal extension as required by the location of the fracture. If fixation of the prosthesis is compromised, removal of the humeral stem and revision to a longer, cemented prosthesis bypassing the fracture site by a distance twice the shaft diameter is recommended (Figure 6.24). If the fixation of the humeral stem is not disrupted, plate fixation is recommended with the use of screws distally and cerclage wires proximally. The addition of autogenous bone graft is recommended to augment healing.

Conclusion

Revision shoulder arthroplasty may represent the most difficult type of joint arthroplasty procedures [4, 5]. The relatively inferior results of revision surgery underscore the importance of proper technique when performing primary procedures. Multiple factors typically contribute to failure after primary shoulder arthroplasty. Scarred and/or insufficient soft tissues, bone loss, and the proximity of neurovascular structures present a multitude of technical challenges. Special equipment and extensive experience with primary shoulder arthroplasty are important to optimize outcomes. A systematic approach with recognition and address of all contributory pathology is essential for successful treatment.

References

1. Wirth MA, Rockwood CA Jr. Complications of shoulder arthroplasty. Clin Orthop 1994;307:47–69.
2. Wirth MA, Rockwood CA Jr. Complications of total shoulder-replacement arthroplasty. J Bone Joint Surg Am 1996;78(4):603–616.
3. Cofield RH, Edgerton BC. Total shoulder arthroplasty: complications and revision surgery. Instr Course Lect 1990;39:449–462.
4. Neer CS II, Kirby RM. Revision of humeral head and total shoulder arthroplasties. Clin Orthop 1982;170:189–195.
5. Neer CS II, Watson KC, Stanton FJ. Recent experience in total shoulder replacement. J Bone Joint Surg 1982;64A:319–337.
6. O'Driscoll SW, Petrie R, Torchia M. Arthroscopic glenoid removal for failed total shoulder arthroplasty. J Shoulder Elbow Surg 1999;8:665.
7. Torchia ME, Cofield RH, Settergren CR. Total shoulder arthroplasty with the Neer prosthesis: long-term results. J Shoulder Elbow Surg 1997;6(6): 495–505.
8. Sperling JW, Cofield RH. Revision total shoulder arthroplasty for the treatment of glenoid arthrosis. J Bone Joint Surg Am 1998;80(6):860–867.
9. Klimkiewicz JJ, Iannotti JP, Rubash HE, Shanbhag AS. Aseptic loosening of the humeral component in total shoulder arthroplasty. J Shoulder Elbow Surg 1998;7(4):422–426.
10. Wirth MA, Agrawal CM, Mabrey JD, et al. Isolation and characterization of polyethylene wear debris associated with osteolysis following total shoulder arthroplasty. J Bone Joint Surg Am 1999;81(1):29–37.
11. Edwards TB, Kadakia NR, Boulahia A, et al. A comparison of hemiarthroplasty and total shoulder arthroplasty in the treatment of primary glenohumeral osteoarthritis: results of a multicenter study. J Shoulder Elbow Surg 2003;12(3):207–213.
12. Orfaly RM, Rockwood CA Jr, Esenyel CZ, Wirth MA. A prospective functional outcome study of shoulder arthroplasty for osteoarthritis with an intact rotator cuff. J Shoulder Elbow Surg 2003;12(3):214–221.
13. Gartsman GMRT, Hammerman SM. Shoulder arthroplasty with or without resurfacing of the glenoid in patients who have osteoarthritis. J Bone Joint Surg Am 2000;82:26–34.
14. Franklin JL, Barrett WP, Jackins SE, Matsen FA III. Glenoid loosening in total shoulder arthroplasty. Association with rotator cuff deficiency. J Arthroplasty 1988;3(1):39–46.

15. Antuna S, Sperling JW, Cofield RH. Reimplantation of a glenoid component after component removal and allograft bone grafting: a report of 3 cases. J Shoulder Elbow Surg 2002;11(6):637–641.

16. Latarjet M. Techniques chirurgucales dans le traitement de la luxation anteriointerne recidivante de l'epule. Lyon Chir 1965;61:313–318.

17. Allaine J, Goutallier D, Glorion C. Long term results of the Latarjet procedure for the treatment of anterior instability of the shoulder. J Bone Joint Surg Am 1998;80:841–852.

18. Burkhead WZ Jr, Hutton KS. Biologic resurfacing of the glenoid with hemiarthroplasty of the shoulder. J Shoulder Elbow Surg 1995;4(4):263–270.

19. Moeckel BH, Altchek DW, Warren RF, Wickiewicz TL, Dines DM. Instability of the shoulder after arthroplasty. J Bone Joint Surg Am 1993;75(4): 492–497.

20. Jost B, Puskas GJ, Lustenberger A, Gerber C. Outcome of pectoralis major transfer for the treatment of irreparable subscapularis tears. J Bone Joint Surg Am 2003;85-A(10):1944–1951.

21. Flatow EL, Bigliani LU, April EW. An anatomic study of the musculocutaneous nerve and its relationship to the coracoid process. Clin Orthop 1989; 244:166–171.

22. Resch H, Povacz P, Ritter E, Matschi W. Transfer of the pectoralis major muscle for the treatment of irreparable rupture of the subscapularis tendon. J Bone Joint Surg Am 2000;82(3):372–382.

23. Flatow ELC, Levine WN, Arroyo JS, Pollock RG, Bigliani LU. Coracoacromial arch reconstruction for anterosuperior subluxation after failed rotator cuff surgery: a preliminary report. J Shoulder Elbow Surg 1997;6.

24. Rittmeister M, Kerschbaumer F. Grammont reverse total shoulder arthroplasty in patients with rheumatoid arthritis and nonreconstructible rotator cuff lesions. J Shoulder Elbow Surg 2001;10(1):17–22.

25. Ramsey ML, Fenlin JM Jr. Use of an antibiotic-impregnated bone cement block in the revision of an infected shoulder arthroplasty. J Shoulder Elbow Surg 1996;5(6):479–482.

26. Duncan CP, Masri BA. The role of antibiotic-loaded cement in the treatment of an infection after a hip replacement. J Bone Joint Surg Am 76: 1742–1751.

27. Campbell JT, Moore RS, Iannotti JP, Norris TR, Williams GR. Periprosthetic humeral fractures: mechanisms of fracture and treatment options. J Shoulder Elbow Surg 1998;7(4):406–413.

28. Boyd AD Jr, Thornhill TS, Barnes CL. Fractures adjacent to humeral prostheses. J Bone Joint Surg Am 1992;74(10):1498–1504.

29. Wright TW, Cofield RH. Humeral fractures after shoulder arthroplasty. J Bone Joint Surg Am 1995;77(9):1340–1346.

Chapter 7

Arthroplasty and Rotator Cuff Deficiency

Gregory P. Nicholson

Rotator cuff deficient shoulders with degenerative joint disease are a treatment challenge. Most patients present primarily due to shoulder pain. Shoulder function can be variable even with significant chronic rotator cuff deficiency. The arthritic condition of the shoulder due to a chronic rotator cuff tear has been termed *cuff-tear arthropathy* [1]. This is characterized clinically by pain and poor active motion, but with near normal passive motion. Within the shoulder there is crepitus and occasional significant fluid production seen under the deltoid. On manual muscle testing, there is significant weakness of elevation and external rotation. Radiographically, this condition is characterized by elevation of the humeral head. There is loss of joint space at the glenohumeral joint and adaptive changes on the acromion and humeral heads. Typically a new *acromiohumeral* articulation has been formed (Figure 7.1). In advanced conditions, there can be collapse of the humeral head and significant incongruity between the humeral head and the superior glenoid, and between the humeral head and the undersurface of acromion.

Radiographically, there can be a pattern of more superior wear with significant adaptive changes and concavity of the acromion (Figure 7.2). There can be a centralized wear pattern between the humeral head and significant loss of glenoid bone stock (Figure 7.3). There can also be seen a more massive destructive arthropathy between the humeral head, glenoid and acromion (Figure 7.4A and 7.4B). It is unclear at this time if these are three different points on the time line of degeneration; or if the shoulder responds differently with differing degenerative patterns to the chronic cuff deficiency. There has been no staging or classification of these radiographic changes or of clinical function. To make matters more confusing, not every shoulder with an irreparable rotator cuff tear goes on to painful, symptomatic cuff tear arthropathy.

An attempt to classify the changes on the acromion and on the glenoid seen radiographically has recently been attempted [2]. This radiographic evaluation was performed in France to try to determine prognostic factors for treatment in the differing patterns of the degenerative change seen in cuff tear arthropathy. Patients were treated with

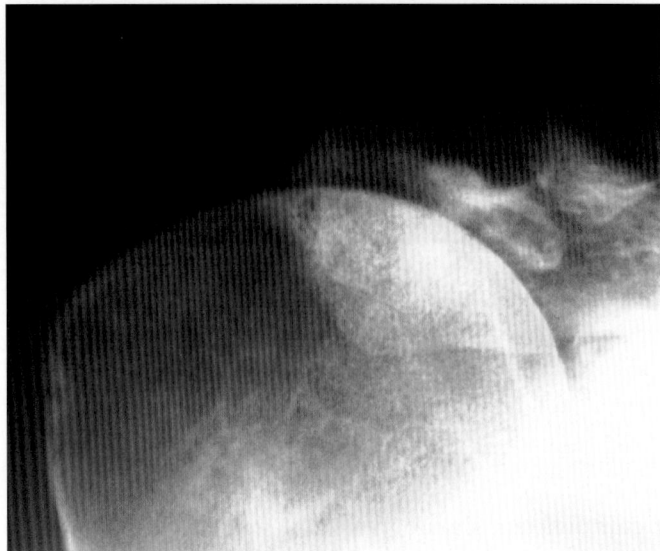

Figure 7.1. Characteristic adaptative changes in a right shoulder with cuff deficient arthritis. Note the concave acromion and the *new* acromiohumeral articulation. The greater tuberosity has *rounded off* also.

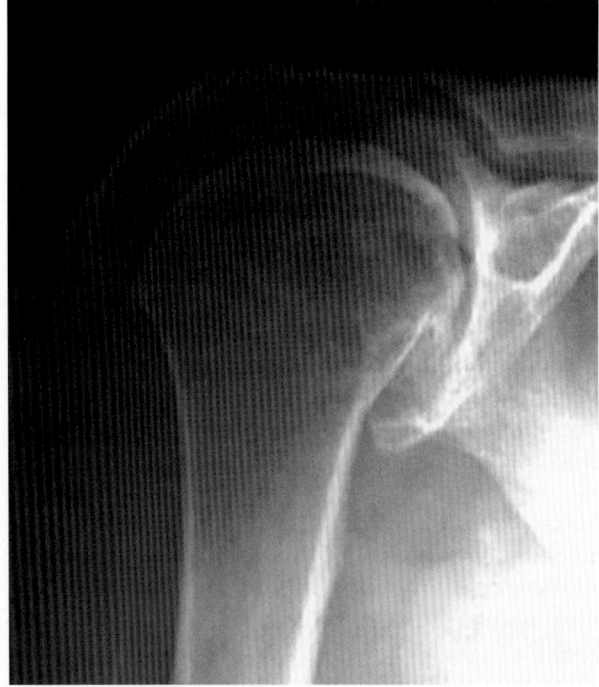

Figure 7.2. This shoulder exhibits a superior wear pattern. Note the extensive thinning of the acromion and the matching concave surfaces between the acromion and humeral head.

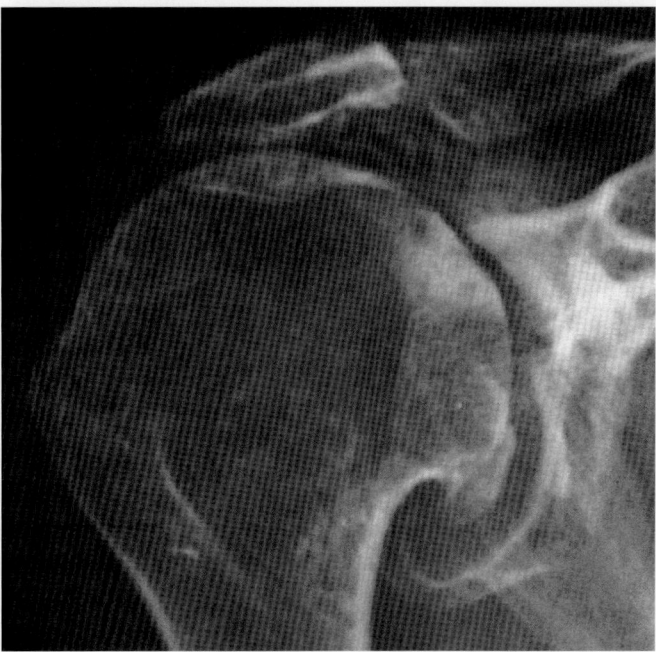

Figure 7.3. This shoulder exhibits a more central pattern of degenerative change. Note the narrowed acromiohumeral distance, but little concavity to the acromion. However, there are glenohumeral joint changes with irregularity, sclerosis, and glenoid bone erosion.

either hemi-arthroplasty or, then available only in Europe, a reverse prosthesis. Four differing patterns of wear of the acromion and four different patterns on the glenoid side were identified. Risk factors for a poor result were found in patients with a so-called E2 glenoid. This is a glenoid that has significant superior wear and thus, on an AP X-ray, shows significant superior slope (Figure 7.5). In both hemi-arthroplasty and reverse shoulder prosthesis, this superior slope glenoid had poor results. On the acromial side, significant thinning with either an impending fracture or evidence of an insufficiency fracture of the acromion led to very poor results with hemi-arthroplasty. This was the first type of any classification to determine any prognostic significance to the degenerative changes seen in cuff tear arthropathy. Certainly more detailed analyses and follow-up will be necessary to conclusively determine prognostic factors in this disease process.

As the population is getting older and staying more mentally and physically active, cuff deficiency with arthritis will be a problem that orthopedic surgeons will have to deal with, and the more detailed analysis and information on cuff tear arthropathy can only lead to better treatment. When evaluating an elderly patient with shoulder problems, a history and physical examination, as in any condition, is of paramount importance. History of previous surgery around the shoulder, especially earlier attempts at rotator cuff repair, is extremely important to know. A history of trauma such as previous falls, dislocations, or fractures needs to be known. Also the type of medication

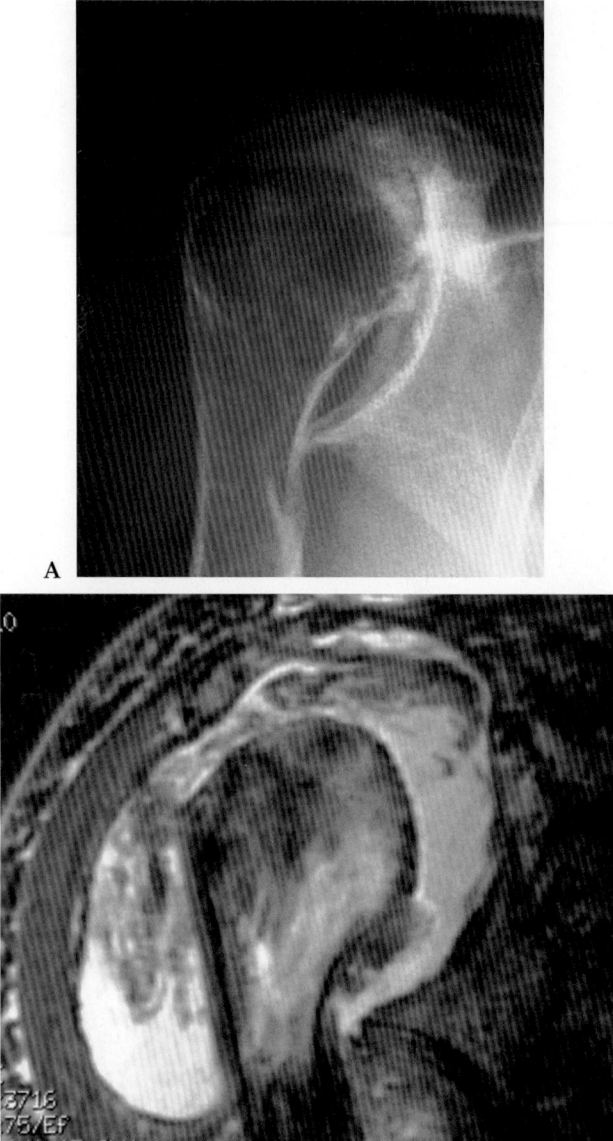

Figure 7.4. Severe destructive arthropathy of a right shoulder. The AP radiograph shows superior and medial migration of the humeral head **(A)**. The MRI reveals tremendous fluid accumulation under the deltoid **(B)**.

the patient is on, especially anti-metabolites or corticosteroids, is extremely important to document.

Physical Examination

On physical examination, one of the hallmarks of cuff tear arthropathy is the fact that passive motion of the shoulder is near normal but usually painful and has some crepitus associated with it. However, active motion of the shoulder is usually very restricted, and with

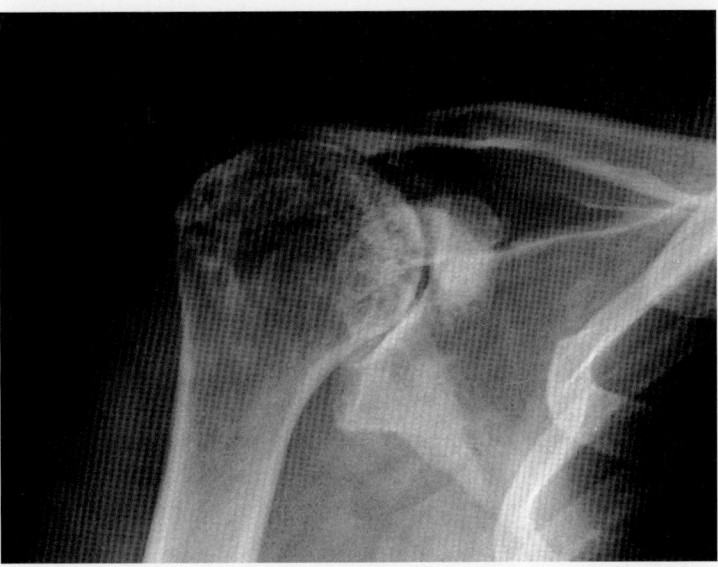

Figure 7.5. An example of the glenoid wear pattern categorized as E2, with significant superior glenoid bone erosion, creating a superior slope to the glenoid joint surface. Note that the medial humeral shaft is almost impacting on the inferior glenoid rim.

attempted active elevation, the scapula will shrug. In advanced arthropathy there will even be an internal rotation drop sign, with the forearm not being able to be held against gravity in external rotation. If viewed from the posterior aspect, most patients show atrophy of the supraspinatus and infraspinatus fossae. Typically, the deltoid is not atrophic but actually sometimes shows a bulge because of the fluid production and fluid collection under the deltoid that can occur (Figure 7.6). Occasionally, the shoulder seems very squared-off at the acromion because of the medialization of the glenohumeral joint line bringing the acromion into relief laterally. Careful evaluation on how the patient tends to elevate his or her arm is important. If with attempted active elevation there is anterior superior instability with the humeral head riding out from underneath the coracoacromial arch, either from previous coracoacromial arch surgery or significant loss of bone and soft tissue, this is a very poor prognostic sign for hemi-arthroplasty.

Imaging studies with plain X-rays are essential. The views obtained should be a true AP of the glenohumeral joint, an axillary view, and a scapular Y view. In patients without advanced osseous changes, a CT or MRI scan can be considered. This gives a quantitative and qualitative impression of the size and location of the rotator cuff tear and, more importantly, the status of the muscle bellies of the supraspinatus, infraspinatus, subscapularis, and teres minor. These studies can provide the surgeon with an assessment of the reparability of a rotator cuff tear with minimal degenerative changes as opposed to a long-standing rotator cuff tear with significant atrophy of the muscle bellies and fatty infiltration of the muscle bellies, which would indicate a technically challenging surgery and one in which functional restoration will not occur [3–7]. Most patients with advanced rotator

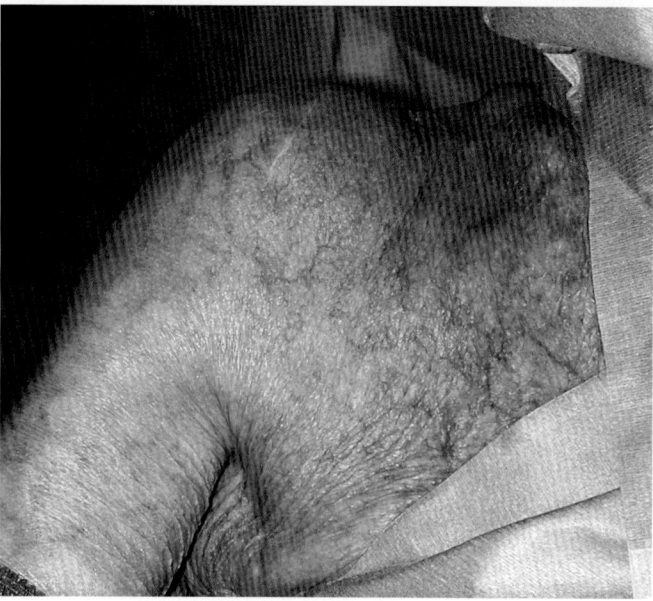

Figure 7.6. A right shoulder with an *inflated* appearance due to significant fluid accumulation under the deltoid.

cuff tear arthropathy with adaptive and degenerative changes seen on plain films do not require advanced imaging studies such as CT scan or MRI, however.

Indications

Indications for surgical intervention in a patient with significant shoulder pain and advanced degenerative changes consistent with rotator cuff tear arthropathy are primarily for pain relief. As stated previously, the active forward elevation and shoulder function ability of patients in this disease process can be somewhat variable. Patients can have significant ability to raise the arm above horizontal and have dramatic radiographic changes and minimal pain. This patient should be treated conservatively. Some patients have almost no pain but extremely poor function with the inability to actively elevate above the horizontal or even use the hand away from the body at waist height. These patients are much more of a challenge because they have a painless *pseudoparalysis* of the shoulder. Hemi-arthroplasty does not restore active elevation ability in a patient who has pseudoparalysis. Prior to considering arthroplasty, an assessment of the patient's goals and needs should be made. Any surgery on cuff tear arthropathy is a limited goal procedure for pain relief and improved function of the shoulder for activities of daily living. The ability to actively elevate above the horizontal will be extremely unpredictable. Conservative management would include a corticosteroid injection to decrease the inflammation and fluid production and to control the pain and allow the patient to rehabilitate. Physical therapy would have to focus on the structures that are left, which are typically some of the external rotators, some of the internal rotators, and the anterior deltoid. This can help patients gain another 5, 10, or 15 degrees of motion and stability. This can be a significant gain for these patients with regard to using the hand away from the body. If pain relief can be maintained, patients can be quite satisfied with these gains.

For the patient with cuff-tear arthropathy who has pain that is unresponsive to conservative management, no previous coracoacromial arch surgery, and no pseudoparalysis, hemi-arthroplasty is a reliable treatment. There appears to be no advantage to total shoulder arthroplasty (TSA) with resurfacing of the glenoid in an unconstrained shoulder design as there have been reports of longer operating room time, no advantage with regard to pain relief, and the risk of glenoid loosening because of the eccentric load of the humeral head on the glenoid component in rotator cuff-deficient patients [8, 9]. Bipolar shoulder hemi-arthroplasty has been advocated as a potential advancement for cuff tear arthropathy [10]. However, there has been no advantage to active forward elevation with the use of the bipolar and, in fact, in a published study, there was actually poorer active elevation ability than in other studies using hemi-arthroplasty.

Hemi-arthroplasty has shown the ability to predictably relieve pain in cuff tear arthropathy. Functional ability, specifically active elevation has been less predictable, however. At best, patients and surgeons should expect active elevation on the average to be approximately 90 degrees [9, 11–16]. It is unclear why some patients do better than others with regard to active elevation and shoulder function. No prognostic factor has been identified to correlate with a better functional result [11]. However, it is quite clear that poorer results are associated with those patients who had prior rotator cuff surgery, coracoacromial arch violation, or the use, as discussed earlier, of a total shoulder [9, 11, 13, 14].

Operative Technique

The operative technique for arthroplasty in cuff tear arthropathy begins with a thorough preoperative evaluation. The vast majority of these patients are elderly, over the age of 62, and have comorbidities. These should be thoroughly evaluated by both the orthopedic surgeon and the patient's primary care physician. An anesthesia consult preoperatively can also be beneficial. We discuss the technical aspects of hemi-arthroplasty in this section.

Anesthesia can be provided with a scalene regional block. This provides excellent intraoperative pain relief and postoperative pain relief. The operation can be done completely under scalene regional anesthesia with sedation if desired or medically indicated. The procedure can also be done under a combined technique with a light general anesthetic in combination with the scalene regional block. This technique provides control of the airway and less requirement for intraoperative anesthesia because of the concomitant regional anesthetic and may be less stressful to the elderly patient.

Positioning is extremely important. The patient should be moved to the lateral edge of the operating room table. The operative arm should be able to be brought off the side of the table for gentle extension, external rotation, and adduction to dislocate the humeral head forward. The head and neck need to be supported. Because of the elderly nature of these patients, many of them have kyphosis of the thoracic spine and other cervical disease. A headrest that can extend or lengthen from the level of the back to the position on the occiput is helpful so as not to place these elderly patients in extension at the neck. A movable arm board, preferably a short arm board, is extremely important on the side of the table so that it can support the upper arm during the procedure but also slide down out of the way for the time when the arm needs to be dislocated off the side of the table. The shoulder and arm are draped free for maximum flexibility and position.

A deltopectoral approach is used so as not to violate the anterior deltoid (Figure 7.7). Typically the anterior deltoid is one of the few

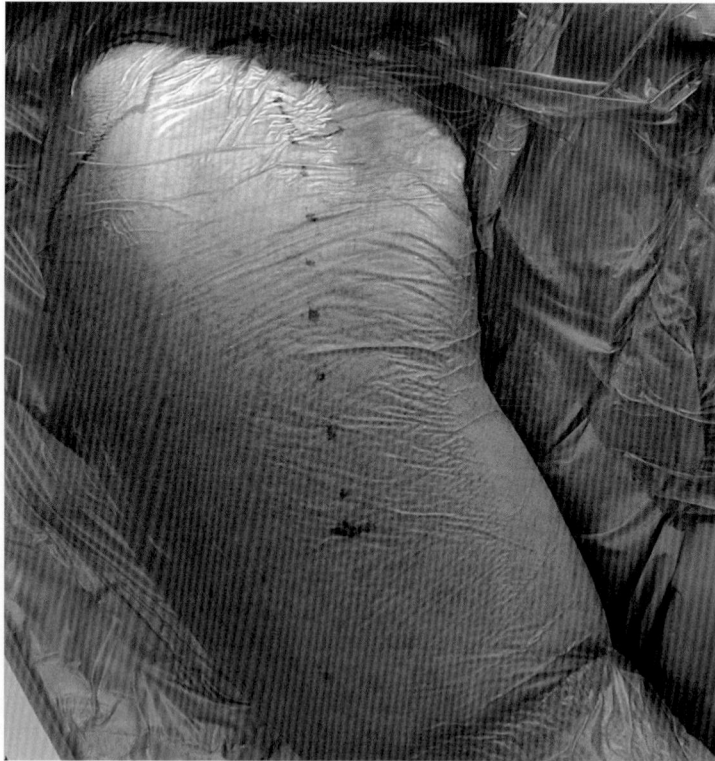

Figure 7.7. A right shoulder with the deltopectoral incision marked out on the skin.

remaining functional muscles. Certainly before performing shoulder arthroplasty, an assessment of deltoid function needs to be made. If the deltoid has been denervated or is not functioning, hemi-arthroplasty is not indicated. The cephalic vein can be taken laterally with the deltoid or medially with the pectoralis major; it is a surgeon's choice. Typically after exploring the deltopectoral interval, extensive bursal material is encountered under the deltoid and under the clavipectoral fascia lateral to the strap muscles off the coracoid. This material can be quite extensive and can be found in an *onion skin* layering that can contain a significant volume of fluid in each layer. On first look the surgeon may think that they are cutting the subscapularis because of the robust nature of this material. With internal and external rotation of the humerus and forearm, the remnant of the subscapularis rotates with the humeral head. Thus, material that moves with shoulder and arm movement is the attached remnant of the subscapularis. Material that does not move is adaptive bursal material and this material should be debrided. Once the subscapularis is identified, the anterior circumflex vessels identify the inferior border of the subscapularis and are almost always present even in almost complete subscapularis deficiency. Whether there is significant subscapularis available or very minimal subscapularis available, the subscapularis should be incised off the lesser tuberosity. The author prefers a needle tip Bovie cautery and begins almost in the biceps groove and comes up over the top of the lesser tuberosity and takes the subscapularis off in a full thickness fashion in an attempt to preserve length.

The humeral head most typically has found a new superior and medial location, and thus the subscapularis attachment is more superior within the shoulder and within the incision than seen in a typical shoulder operation. The axillary nerve should be palpated along the inferior border of the subscapularis and protected as the subscapularis is incised off the humerus. Placing the arm in adduction, external rotation brings the insertion of the subscapularis laterally away from the axillary nerve. Also, placing a Fukuda humeral head retractor within the glenohumeral joint places the axillary nerve on gentle stretch, allowing easier palpation and protection while incising the subscapularis.

Because of the superior location of the humeral head, the inferior capsule can be quite contracted. This inferior capsule needs to be released off the inferior neck of the humerus so that the humeral head can come down and be dislocated. This can be done safely with a blunt elevator and the capsule can be pushed off the inferior aspect of the neck of the humerus safely. The subscapularis should be tagged with sutures and reflected medially. There will be a variable quality to the subscapularis tendon and muscle belly in these patients. The subscapularis can be contracted to the anterior glenoid rim and the anterior capsule should be judiciously released from this area and the subscapularis also released from the undersurface of the base of the coracoid. This allows maximum excursion and a good *bounce* to the muscle belly. If the subscapularis is completely deficient, consideration can be given to a pectoralis major transfer. This can take the form of transferring the whole pectoralis major superiorly. Alternatively, the sternal head of the pectoralis major can be harvested and brought under the clavicular head and brought up, or the pectoralis major could be placed in a subcoracoid position for subscapularis substitution [17, 18].

Again, these are elderly patients and an assessment of the surgeon's ability to perform this part of the operation should be critically evaluated. Pectoralis major transfer in cuff tear arthropathy in addition to the utilization of a hemi-arthroplasty has not been a common combination. The advantage of pectoralis major transfer with hemi-arthroplasty has not been determined at this time.

At this point, the humeral head is gently dislocated. These patients have contracture as stated and are typically women over the age of 65 with osteopenic bone. Great care should be taken to gently distract the arm and put a flat retractor behind the humeral head. This should be the majority of the lever placed on the humerus, and then the arm carefully positioned in extension, adduction, and external rotation to bring the humeral head forward. It is hoped that these maneuvers will prevent any type of intraoperative fracture from occurring. The humeral head will be markedly deformed with a complete loss of supraspinatus tendon substance (Figure 7.8). Adaptive changes of the

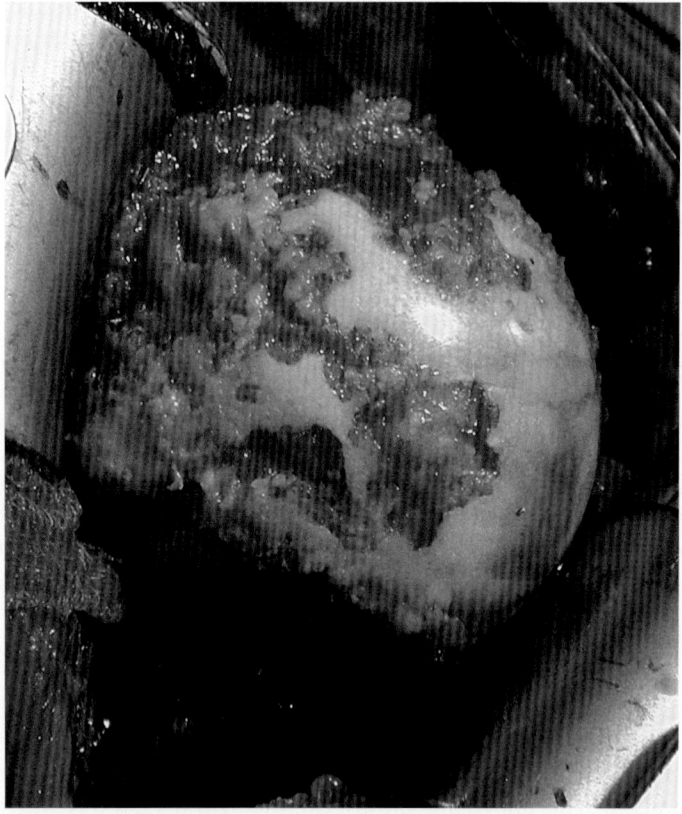

Figure 7.8. An intraoperative photo of a right shoulder with cuff tear arthropathy. Note the severe deformity and erosions of the articular surface. Landmarks such as the biceps groove, greater and lesser tuberosities are not discernible.

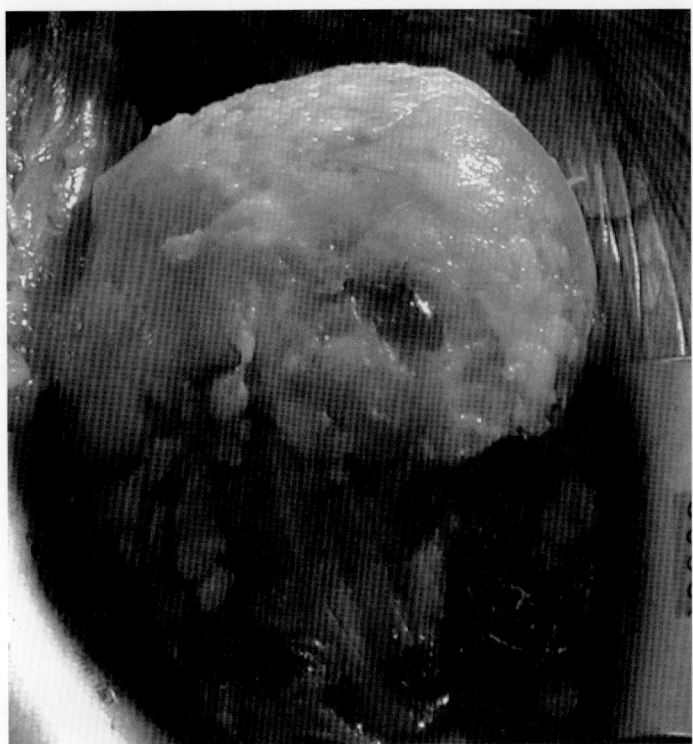

Figure 7.9. This right shoulder is much more sclerotic, but so deformed it is difficult to determine medial or lateral orientation to the humeral head.

greater tuberosity that obscures the biceps groove and deforms the humeral head itself may leave no visible normal contour of the humeral head. The humeral head itself may look more like the ball on top of a flagpole than the more typical angled articular surface (Figure 7.9). Depending on what prosthetic system the surgeon is using, extramedullary or intramedullary cutting guides can be used to mark humeral head osteotomy angle and location. The humeral head should be osteotomized with an oscillating saw with protection of the soft tissues. Once the humeral head has been osteotomized, the humeral canal is prepared with a selection of reamers and broaches as determined by the specific humeral implant that is being used. Careful reaming should be performed as again this can be very thin osteopenic bone. It is the author's preference to cement the humeral stem into place in the vast majority of these cases. The ability to get a press-fit within a very osteoporotic humerus with endosteal erosion can be difficult and can lead to intraoperative fracture. Also, cement stabilizes the proximal aspect of the humerus and supports sutures that are placed through the anterior anatomic neck for subscapularis reattachment without the risk of these sutures pulling through osteopenic bone.

One of the most problematic aspects of this operation for the surgeon is prosthetic humeral head size and position. Because the anatomy is so distorted, the restoration of normal glenohumeral joint relationships does not apply. General guidelines can be thought of as choosing a

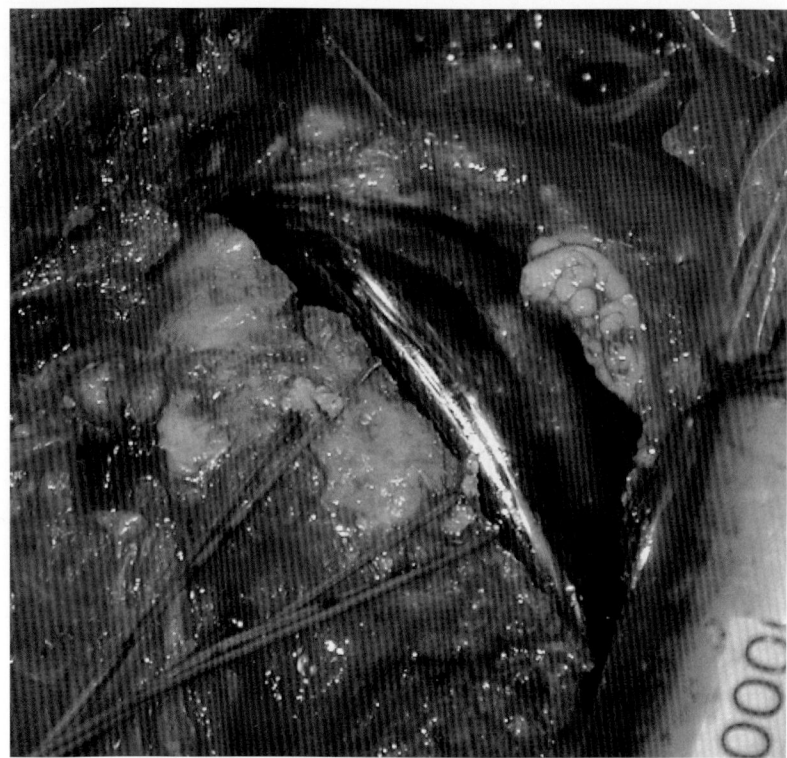

Figure 7.10. The prosthetic head of the hemiarthroplasty has been sized to fit and fill the coracoacromial arch without overstuffing the joint. The sutures are for subscapularis reattachment.

humeral head size that will fill the existing coracoacromial arch. This should not be overstuffed, but should fill the coracoacromial arch because this is the new adaptive joint the patient has created (Figure 7.10). It is helpful to have a prosthetic head that allows approximately 50% of posterior translation on the glenoid. With the arm in approximately 70 degrees of abduction, at least 40 degrees of internal rotation of the arm should occur. This avoids overstuffing the glenohumeral joint cavity and creating the potential for posterior capsular tightness, anterior translation, and subsequent anterior and superior instability. This also avoids overstretching the subscapularis that needs to be repaired in some fashion at the end of the procedure. Thus, once the trial stem is in place and the trial humeral head in place, the surgeon should evaluate to make sure that the subscapularis can be repaired with the arm at approximately 30 degrees of external rotation, that the humeral head is stable underneath the coracoacromial arch, and that internal rotation is not significantly tethered. If there is adequate subscapularis material from superior to inferior, then the subscapularis can be translated superiorly to try to repair the upper centimeter of this to the anterior greater tuberosity. Any available posterior rotator cuff that can be identified and mobilized should be repaired to the greater tuberosity. However, no heroic repairs or tendon transfers should be attempted. They show no advantage for pain relief or the restoration of active motion for the increased surgical time. All the soft tissue and rotator cuff mobilization should be done with the humeral trial head removed to maximize exposure and mobilization of this tissue.

Prior to cementing the hemi-arthroplasty stem in place, heavy non-absorbable sutures should be placed through the greater tuberosity if there is posterior rotator cuff to be repaired, and through the anatomic neck anteriorly for subscapularis reattachment. When cementing a cement restrictor plug should be used, the canal gently pulse lavaged of all fatty material, and poly methylmethacrylate cement mixed and placed down the canal. It is unnecessary and possibly dangerous to use a cement gun in the way that femurs are pressurized. Again, this is thin bone and, with pressurization, the cement can actually be pushed through a defect in the humerus. A Toomey syringe is an excellent way to place cement down the canal of the humerus, still provide an excellent cement mantle and control the cement technique. The humeral stem is then cemented into place in the determined position of height and retroversion. Depending on the system being used, the prosthetic humeral head may be placed on the stem before implantation or after the cement has hardened. Once the head is in place, the humerus is relocated in the glenohumeral joint cavity underneath the coracoacromial arch. The subscapularis is repaired to the lesser tuberosity. A drain may or may not be used underneath the deltoid. In many patients, because of the amount of bursal material and fluid production that needed to be debrided, there can be significant dead space. A drain for 24 hours may prevent a collection of a hematoma.

The deltopectoral interval is then tacked closed with absorbable sutures. The subcutaneous tissue is closed with absorbable sutures and then the skin closed by surgeon preference. A supportive sling and swathe device can be applied. If a scalene regional block has been used, the arm will have no muscle power and the swathe will control the arm at the side. It is also recommended that a pillow be placed behind the elbow postoperatively so that the arm, even though it is in a sling, cannot fall into an obligate extension position with the elbow at the level of the patient's back. It is much more comfortable to have the elbow at the level of the patient's anterior border along the stomach than having it fall back to the level of the back along the level of the mattress.

What about the glenoid? We had discussed that a superior sloping glenoid can be a cause for poorer results. With hemi-arthroplasty this allows the prosthetic head to slide superiorly and medially and continues significant bony erosion. Function is poor and the inferior aspect of the glenoid can actually impact the medial aspect of the humeral shaft. In these cases, with a severe superiorly sloped glenoid, consideration can be made for judiciously resculpting the glenoid with a reamer. The goal is to lessen the superior slope and try to provide a more concentric bearing surface on the glenoid side. This needs to be undertaken with great care as there can be very minimal bone stock in extremely soft bone. Authors have advocated superior glenoid bone grafting but, in these elderly patients, it can be a difficult operation. Results of this type of procedure have been performed in a limited number of patients and a clear advantage has not been seen [19]. Hooded glenoid components to try to prevent this superior migration have been attempted but have universally failed due to loosening [20]. The best option is to identify the problem preoperatively with good radiographs and discuss with the patient that the goals of the surgery are pain relief, that function is going to be unpredictable, and that there can be progressive bony erosion from hemi-arthroplasty in these types of severe degenerative changes of the glenoid and acromion, which can lead to later pain and diminished function [14].

Postoperative Care

Patients after hemi-arthroplasty for cuff tear arthropathy should be supported in a sling. Other co-morbidities such as lower extremity mobility problems from other types of arthritis need to be identified preoperatively. Many patients rely on their upper extremities to help support themselves during ambulation. This should be avoided in the early postoperative period. Passive range of motion should begin on the first postoperative day with pendulum exercises. Passive external rotation with a limit of 30 degrees, passive forward elevation with a limit of approximately 90 degrees and pulley exercises should be instituted. The patient is encouraged to use the hand, wrist, and elbow for activities of daily living within the sling. Aggressive stretching and attempts at improving range of motion are typically detrimental early on. After one month, the sling can be discontinued and active assisted range of motion can begin. The patient is encouraged to use the arm for activities of daily living and isometric strengthening for the muscle groups that are still workable are instituted. This would include the external rotators, all three heads of the deltoid and the scapular rotators. Any resistance to the internal rotators, specifically the subscapularis, should be avoided for approximately six weeks. At the end of two months, light resistive exercises with resistive exercise bands should be instituted for the external rotators, the internal rotators and all three heads of the deltoid. The patient should be informed both preoperatively and postoperatively that this will be a prolonged and slow rehabilitation. They will not reach their best or maximum potential for approximately six months after the operation.

Results

Multiple studies have documented the predictable pain relief that hemi-arthroplasty can provide to patients who have unremitting pain from the degenerative changes of arthritis with cuff deficiency. This has also been shown to be the most consistent when there have not been previous attempts at rotator cuff repair or acromioplasty-coracoacromial arch violation type surgery. The average active forward elevation that patients can expect from a hemi-arthroplasty for cuff tear arthropathy is approximately 90 degrees [9, 11–16, 21]. If patients have the so-called pseudoparalysis of the arm in which there is an extremely poor active elevation ability, a hemi-arthroplasty will not immediately restore active elevation. In these patients with poor preoperative active forward elevation, the hemi-arthroplasty provides pain relief, but the patient still may struggle with active elevation below the horizontal. It is extremely important that the surgeon reiterates to the patient and family, both preoperatively and postoperatively, realistic expectations for function. Once patients have obtained significant pain relief, they are typically disappointed that their active elevation and corresponding strength are still poor. Long-term results of hemi-arthroplasty have not been reported with regularity. Most studies have two-year followup, but longer term follow-up studies are being reported. These studies show that there is progressive bony erosion of the acromion and superior glenoid and that these erosions correlate with pain and decreasing function over the longer periods of time [14, 21].

Thus, it is extremely important to counsel the patients and the family about realistic expectations for pain relief, function, active elevation ability, and the fact that this is a limited goals procedure for pain relief and activities of daily living. It is also extremely important to counsel the patient that if he or she had previous acromioplasty surgery, hemiarthroplasty, while the only option to restore concentric joint surface for the most part, will potentially be an ultimate failure because of the violation of the coracoacromial arch. In almost every report, those patients that have had previous acromioplasty surgery have gone on to anterior superior instability, poor active motion, and pain and have had a substantially worse result than those patients with no prior acromioplasty [11, 13, 14, 16]. The author does not recommend hemiarthroplasty in those patients with prior acromioplasty surgery and evidence of anterior superior instability. Semiconstrained reverse shoulder arthroplasty is a better management option for patients with coracoacromial arch violation due to the predictable failure of hemiarthroplasty in that clinical scenario. The reverse shoulder arthroplasty will eliminate anterosuperior instability and provide the potential for better active elevation.

Complications

As discussed previously, the complications of hemi-arthroplasty for cuff deficiency begin with the fact that these are elderly patients and have co-morbidities. Cardiopulmonary side effects of the surgery can certainly occur. Medical problems can be exacerbated by surgery in the elderly. The unpredictable function results, especially with regard to strength and active forward elevation, make it imperative that a discussion occurs preoperatively and then postoperatively with the patient to avoid unrealistic expectations. One of the complications that has recently been seen after 4 to 5 year follow-up is the bone erosion that is progressive at the superior glenoid and the under-surface of the acromion that correlates with increasing pain and decreasing function [14, 21]. Anterior superior instability, as discussed in the previous section, is a difficult problem. A hemi-arthroplasty will not solve this problem and actually will create a much more diffi-cult problem to manage with resultant anterosuperior instability. Excessive retroversion of the humeral component and attempted coracoacromial arch reconstruction has not stopped the anterior supe-rior instability [13, 14, 21–23]. Dynamic muscle transfer, such as pec-toralis major transfer, have been advocated and, in small experience, have improved function of the hand away from the body at waist height [17].

If there is anterior superior instability for whatever reason and the coracoacromial arch has been violated, the best option at this particu-lar time in these elderly patients would appear to be semiconstrained reverse shoulder arthroplasty. An update on the older concept of reverse shoulder arthroplasty was provided by Grammont and has been used in Europe for the past eight years [24]. Early results of the reverse prosthesis in elderly patients with cuff tear arthropathy have shown excellent pain relief, elimination of anterior superior instability, and superior motion for active elevation as compared with traditional hemi-arthroplasty [25, 26]. In a comparison study with follow-up greater than three years, patients with no prior shoulder surgery and cuff tear arthropathy were treated either with hemi-arthroplasty or reverse shoulder arthroplasty. The patients with reverse shoulder arthroplasty had 40 degrees greater active forward elevation for an average of 138 degrees; and the Constant Score was 20 points higher than those patients with hemi-arthroplasty [27]. There were no cases of glenoid loosening requiring revision. The hemi-arthroplasties had over one third of the cases with progressive bone erosion in the superior glenoid and acromion with increasing pain.

Reverse shoulder arthroplasty has been used on a custom basis for patients with anterior superior instability in the United States and has shown the ability to prevent anterior superior instability and provide shoulder stability with good active elevation (see Figure 6.19). The scapula is able to function in a much more normal ratio and provide the patients with consistent ability to use the hand away from the body between waist and shoulder height and, in most cases, above shoulder height [23, 28]. Reverse shoulder arthroplasty has just become available in the United States. Critical evaluation of the European experience allows us to say, while not a perfect solution, reverse shoulder arthroplasty certainly should be in the armamentarium of the shoulder surgeon to treat patients with cuff deficiency in advanced shoulder arthritis. This should primarily be reserved for those patients who have had multiple failed rotator cuff repair attempts with viola-tion of the coracoacromial arch and anterior superior instability. It should also be considered in those patients with the pseudoparalysis and extremely poor active motion. Those patients with an extremely thin acromion or an acromial insufficiency fracture should also be con-sidered candidates for reverse shoulder arthroplasty.

Summary

Cuff tear arthroplasty is a disabling condition of the shoulder found in elderly patients. It is variable in its presentation with regard to the extent of degenerative osseous change in the glenoid, humeral head, and acromion. It is variable in its presentation with regard to preoperative active elevation ability and pain level. The overriding indication for hemi-arthroplasty in cuff tear arthropathy is pain relief. Reverse shoulder arthroplasty, now available in the United States, may provide improved active elevation in select patients.

References

1. Neer CS II, Craig EV, Fukuda H. Cuff-Tear Arthropathy. J Bone Joint Surg 1983;65A:1232–1244.
2. Huguet D, Favard L, Lautman S, et al. Epidemiologie, Imagerie, Classification. P de Boileau, Mole D, Editor: 2000 Shoulder Prostheses . . . two to ten year follow-up. Sauramps Medical, Montpelier, France, 2001;233–240. L'Omarthose avec rupture massive et non reparable de la coiffe.
3. Zanetti M, Gerber C, Hodler J. Qualitative assessment of the muscles of the rotator cuff with MR imaging. Invest Radiol 1998;33:163–170.
4. Thomazeau H, Rolland Y, Lucas C, et al. Atrophy of the supraspinatus belly. Assessment by MRI in 55 patients with rotator cuff pathology. Acta Orthop Scand 1996;67:264–268.
5. Thomazeau H, Boukobza E, Morcet N, et al. Prediction of rotator cuff repair results by magnetic resonance imaging. Clin Orthop 1997;344:275–283.
6. Fuchs B, Weishaupt D, Zanetti M, et al. Fatty Degeneration of the muscles of the rotator cuff: assessment by computed tomography versus magnetic resonance imaging. J Shoulder Elbow Surg 1998;8:599–605.
7. Goutallier D, Postel JM, Bernageau J, et al. Fatty muscle degeneration in cuff ruptures: pre and post-operative evaluation by CT-scan. Clin Orthop 1994;304:78–83.
8. Franklin J, Barrett W, Jackins SE, et al. Glenoid loosening in total shoulder arthroplasty. Association with rotator cuff deficiency. J Arthroplasty 1988; 3:39–46.
9. Pollock RG, Deliz ED, McIlveen SJ, et al. Prosthetic replacement in rotator cuff-deficient shoulders. J Shoulder Elbow Surg 1992;1:173–186.
10. Worland RL, Jessup DE, Arrendondo J, et al. Bipolar shoulder arthroplasty for rotator cuff arthropathy. J Shoulder Elbow Surg 1997;6:512–515.
11. Nicholson GP, Kunkel SS: Prospective evaluation of shoulder hemiarthroplasty for cuff tear arthropathy. J Shoulder Elbow Surg 1999;8(5):537.
12. Williams GR Jr, Rockwood CA Jr. Hemiarthroplasty in rotator cuff deficient shoulders. J Shoulder Elbow Surg 1996;5:362–367.
13. Field LD, Dines DM, Zabrinski SJ, et al. Hemiarthroplasty of the shoulder for rotator cuff arthropathy. J Shoulder Elbow Surg 1997;6:18–23.
14. Sanchez-Sotelo J, Cofield RH, Rowland CM. Shoulder hemiarthroplasty for glenohumeral arthritis associated with severe rotator cuff deficiency. J Bone Joint Surg 2001;83A:1814–1822.
15. Arntz CT, Jackins S, Matsen FA III. Prosthetic replacement of the shoulder for the treatment of defects in the rotator cuff and the surface of the glenohumeral joint. J Bone Joint Surg Am 1993;75:485–491.
16. Zuckerman JD, Scott AJ, Gallagher MA. Hemiarthroplasty for cuff tear arthropathy. J Shoulder Elbow Surg 2000;9:69–172.

17. Klepps SJ, Goldfarb MD, Flatow EF, et al. Anatomic evaluation of the sub-caroacoid pectoralis major transfers in human cadavers. J Shoulder Elbow Surg 2001;10:453–459.

18. Resch H, Povacz P, Ritter E. Transfer of the pectoralis major muscle for the treatment of irreparable rupture of the subscapularis tendon. J Bone Joint Surg Am 2000;82:372–382.

19. Cantrell JS, Itamura JM, Burkhead WZ Jr. Rotator Cuff Tear Arthropathy. Chapter 24 in Complex and Revision Problems in Shoulder Surgery, JJP Warner, Iannotti JP, Gerber C, Editors. Philadelphia: Lippincott-Raven, 1997;303–318.

20. Nwakama AC, Cofield RC, Kavanaugh BF, et al. Semiconstrained total shoulder arthroplasty for glenohumeral arthritis and massive rotator cuff tearing. J Shoulder Elbow Surg 2000;9:302–307.

21. Favard L, Lautmann S, Sirveaux F, et al. Hemiarthroplasty versus reverse arthroplasty in the treatment of osteoarthritis with massive rotator cuff tear. In 2000 Shoulder Prostheses: Two to Ten Year Follow-up, G Walch, Boileau P, Mole D, Editors. Montpelier, France: Sauramps Medical, 2001;261–268.

22. Wiley AM. Superior humeral dislocation. A complication following decompression and debridement for rotator cuff tears. Clin Orthop 1991;263: 135–141.

23. Nicholson GP. Treatment of anterior superior shoulder instability with a reverse ball and socket prosthesis. Operative Techniques in Orthopaedics 2003;13:235–241.

24. Grammont PM, Baulot E. Delta shoulder prosthesis for rotator cuff rupture. Orthopedics 1993;16:65–68.

25. Boulahia A, Edwards TB, Walch G, et al. Early results of a reverse design prosthesis in the treatment of arthritis of the shoulder in elderly patients with a large rotator cuff tear. Orthopedics 2002;25:129–133.

26. Valenti PH, Boutens D, Nerot C, et al. Delta 3 Reversed Prosthesis for Osteoarthritis with Massive Rotator Cuff Tear: Long Term Results (>5 Years). In "2000 Shoulder Prostheses . . . two to ten year follow-up," G Walch, Boileau P, Mole D, Editors. Montpelier, France: Sauramps Medical, 2001;253–259.

27. Constant CR, Murley AH. A clinical method of functional assessment of the shoulder. Clin Orthop 1987;214:160–164.

28. Nicholson GP. Reverse Ball and Socket Shoulder Arthroplasty for Rotator Cuff Deficient Shoulders with Anterosuperior Instability. Preliminary Results. Presented at the 18th American Shoulder and Elbow Surgeons Meeting, Napa, CA, October, 2001.

Chapter 8

Rehabilitation of Shoulder Arthroplasty

John Basti

Humeral head replacement and nonconstrained total shoulder arthroplasty (TSA) have become more commonly performed procedures for eliminating pain and increasing function for an array of traumatic and arthritic conditions that involve the destruction of one or both surfaces of the glenohumeral joint [1–7]. Optimizing a patient's response to arthroplasty is the combination of a positive surgical experience and a well-planned postoperative rehabilitation program. Successful shoulder arthroplasty is dependent on several factors: the pathological condition of the joint, the quality of the bone and soft tissues, the status of the deltoid and rotator cuff, the overall condition of the patient, and the surgical procedure. The application of the postoperative rehabilitation and patient compliance is of paramount importance. This program requires a team approach involving the surgeon, patient, and therapist all interacting to develop and implement a well-designed progression of postoperative rehabilitation.

Rehabilitation of the shoulder joint can be challenging and more difficult than any other joint in the body. The glenohumeral joint has little bony stability and relies on the surrounding soft tissues, the capsule, ligaments, rotator cuff, and deltoid and periscapular muscles to provide static as well as dynamic stability for optimal function of the upper extremity. Recognition of the importance of the soft tissue structures affecting functional outcome is essential to achieve a high percentage of successful results. The challenge lies in establishing normal motion, dynamic stability, and strength. Therefore, an adaptive and progressive system of rehabilitation consisting of appropriate applications of range of motion and strengthening is required. The preferred rehabilitation program is designed to protect certain structures early in the recovery phase and then maximize motion and strength as healing occurs. Within that process, the therapist tailors the treatment program as directed by the surgeon, gradually introducing certain exercises according to the signs and symptoms of the patient and the patient's response to treatment. The treatment program is designed to encourage active participation of the patient through team support, education, and on-going communication. The material developed and presented in this chapter has been successful in helping our patients achieve optimal results.

Indications for Shoulder Arthroplasty

The indications for shoulder arthroplasty have been well interpreted. The most common indications for shoulder arthroplasty is osteoarthritis; rheumatoid arthritis follows second [8, 9]. The most prevalent indication for humeral head replacement continues to be trauma, including three and four-part fractures of the proximal humerus [6, 10, 11]. Other clinical problems that are often treated with shoulder arthroplasty include traumatic arthritis, avascular necrosis, arthritis of instability, and rotator cuff tear arthropathy. Participation of the patient with appropriate motivation and realistic demands who will commit to a time-consuming, sometimes lengthy, rehabilitation program are positive criteria for joint replacement. Lack of these criteria is considered a potential contraindication to surgical intervention [12].

Shoulder Pathology: Implications in Rehabilitation

Proximal Humerus Fractures

Patients who sustain acute trauma are considered candidates for humeral head replacement if they have incurred a four-part fracture, some three-part fractures, fracture dislocation in which the head segment is detached, humeral head impression fractures greater then 40%, and head-splitting fractures [11, 13–16]. Older individuals with poor bone quality have the highest incidence of humeral fractures. Women having a higher percentage of occurrence than men [11]. Falling on an outstretched hand is a common mechanism of injury [14, 17]. In the younger population, proximal humeral fractures and fracture dislocation are more likely to be the result of high-velocity trauma [14]. The acute trauma and possible neurovascular injury, followed by surgical reduction, influence the rate and progression of rehabilitation and recovery. Bigliani, McCluskey, and Fisher [18] reported two major complications affecting outcome that were directly related to inappropriate postoperative rehabilitation: stiffness due to delayed rehabilitation and tuberosity pull-off due to overaggressive early active motion. The exercise program must be designed to allow for appropriate healing without disruption, while early safe motion is applied to prevent contracture. Pain relief is fairly predictable with excellent to satisfactory results, however, functional outcome is not as optimistic with limitations in functional recovery [6, 19]. Several factors, including adequate fracture reduction, an appropriate rehabilitation progression, and a cooperative, motivated patient make results more predictable [11, 17, 20–22]. It should be understood that maximum recovery can be a lengthy process taking place anywhere from six post-injury months to a year [17, 22, 23].

Osteoarthritis and Rheumatoid Arthritis

Clinically, osteoarthritic patients often present with global limitations in range of motion, particularly external rotation. These patients, however, have a low incidence of rotator cuff tears. Of those patients who have small full-thickness tears of 1 cm or less, rotator cuff strength following surgery is fairly normal with no adverse affect to functional outcome {24–26]. Patients tend to be stiff, especially in external rotation due to long-standing limitation of motion. In these cases, close attention is paid to range of motion and stretching in the postoperative rehabilitation program, with strengthening emphasized as range of motion and flexibility improves.

Patients with rheumatoid arthritis are usually younger, with a higher incidence in female subjects [24]. The systemic disease affects multiple joints with associated periarticular soft tissue involvement. These patients often present with atrophy and significant weakness. Weakness is most often due to underlying rotator cuff tears or significant attrition of the rotator cuff that is commonly found in conjunction with the disease [27]. Full-thickness rotator cuff tears have been reported in 20% to 42% of patients with rheumatoid disease [28]. Pain and dysfunction of other multiple joints requires key planning in the timing of their surgery. Special consideration with respect to the patient's general condition, mobility, opposite extremity function, and cervical spine must be planned for in postoperative rehabilitation to maximize exercise and avoid complication following surgery.

Avascular Necrosis

Avascular necrosis can be idiopathic or caused by a number of processes including trauma, corticoid steroid use, alcoholism, systemic lupus erythematousis, and other less frequent disorders [29, 30]. Although less common, these patients, similar to those with underlying arthritis, often present with progressive pain and disability in the shoulder region. Often, passive range of motion is fairly well maintained unless the patient has advanced disease that secondarily involves the glenoid articular surface. Clinically, the rotator cuff in these patients is almost always intact. Therefore, they have the potential to develop normal cuff strength following surgery.

Arthritis of Instability

Arthritis of instability falls into two groups, patients who have chronic recurrent dislocation or subluxation and those who have had a previous surgical procedure for instability. These patients tend to be of a younger age with a more common occurrence in male subjects [24]. In a case controlled study, Marx et al. [31] found that patients who have had one or more dislocation are at a greater risk of developing arthrosis.

Surgery for instability attempts to reestablish the balance of the soft tissue envelope surrounding the glenohumeral joint. Failed attempts can result in articular cartilage damage, requiring shoulder arthroplasty. In some procedures when staples or screws are used, improper positioning or migration of the metal implants results in articular cartilage damage [32]. In another instance, overtightening the soft tissues in an attempt to restore stability to either side of the glenohumeral joint, for anterior instability or missed multidirectional instability, results in displacement of the humeral head to the unaddressed side [33, 34]. This results in a chronically subluxed humeral head, away from the repaired side with the consequence of disabling pain, soft tissue contracture, progressive cartilage wear, bone loss and loss of motion. Van der Zwaag et al. [35] found an increase in glenohumeral arthrosis in patients who had undergone a Putti-Platt procedure for recurrent anterior dislocation. A correlation between arthrosis and length of time from surgery was also noted. Bigliani et al. [36] reported on 17 patients with osteoarthritis after surgery for instability. Thirteen men and four women at an average age of 43 had a prosthetic replacement at an average of 16 years from the time of their instability repair. All patients had pain and severe functional disability with loss of motion, especially in external rotation. Pain relief was accomplished in 94% of the patients with an average increase in range of motion to 37 degrees of elevation and 53 degrees of external rotation. Each individual surgery is unique and may require special alterations in the rehabilitation program. Altered anatomy, soft tissue loss and contracture, as well as excessive bone loss influence the rehabilitation strategy. With soft tissue repair, reconstructed areas can be put at risk just by improperly positioning a patient during exercise. For instance, it may be inadvisable to exercise patients with posterior soft tissue reconstruction in a supine position because of the tendency of the humeral head to move posteriorly with forward elevation. The force generated in the supine position by the weight of the arm as it approaches 90 degrees pushes the head posteriorly. Exercise in the prone or sitting position may be better suited in this instance. Anterior reconstructions require limitation in external rotation to allow healing and subsequently maintain the humeral head centered on the glenoid. On one end of the spectrum, excessive rotation can disrupt the repaired anterior reconstruction prior to adequate healing. On the other hand, too little motion can result in contracture of the same tissue, resulting in an excessive posterior directed force at the glenohumeral joint. Establishing and maintaining a balance of the periarticular soft tissue is the goal of the surgery and postoperative rehabilitation program. These patients are often of a young age, active and athletic. They can be stiff and/or weak, requiring appropriate stretching, then strengthening with the ultimate goal of restoring scapulo-humeral synchronous motion and good function of the shoulder and upper extremity.

Balancing the need for early motion and healing while maintaining stability requires explicit instruction from the surgeon, an informed therapist, and an educated cooperative patient, when encountering these usually complex re-repairs.

Rotator Cuff Tear Arthropathy

Patients with massive rotator cuff deficiency and associated glenohumeral arthritis tend to be elderly with an increased prevalence in the female patients who experience unrelenting pain at rest, which is intensified by activities of daily living. Neer's theory on the etiology of cuff tear arthropathy suggests that a combination of nutritional factors and mechanical factors are the roots of its development. Cuff tear arthropathy (CTA) was introduced by Neer in 1975. Massive rotator cuff tear, rupture, or dislocation of the long head of the bicep; collapse of the osteoporotic subchondral bone; distortion of the articular surfaces leading to erosion and medialization; with the ascent of the humeral head and gross anterior and posterior instability describes this debilitating progression of destruction. With massive rotator cuff tears, extensive weakness, instability and severe limitations in the use of the upper extremity are usually present. Assessment of deltoid function in these patients is an important indicator of success or failure of the surgery. If progressive deltoid dysfunction is present, these patients may not be candidates for the surgical procedure. However, Neer advocates this pain-sparing procedure in these severely involved patients [12]. The remaining soft tissue envelop and all viable tissue is repaired to provide as much soft tissue support for stability and function. Rehabilitation is modified and focuses on comfort and function below the horizontal.

Rehabilitation Principles

Treatment principles form the foundation of any well-defined rehabilitation program. The concept of early passive motion tailored to the surgical repair has been advocated in the literature to limit the effect of postsurgical soft tissue scarring and adhesions [3, 8, 11, 12, 30, 33, 36–42]. The principles of early passive motion are effective in establishing motion before maturation of adhesions. Active exercises are deferred to a later point in treatment since they may cause increased reactivity and muscle soreness, which will interfere with recovery of motion. Strengthening exercises are more effective when good range of motion has been established and reactivity has diminished after surgery [12].

The scapular plane has been defined as the plane of maximal elevation [12] (Figure 8.1). This position allows the humeral head to be centered on the glenoid, and the capsule to be relaxed with appropriate tension on the ligaments and muscles. Maintaining the upper extremity in this plane renders more comfort postoperatively, avoids overstretching of repaired structures, and maximizes functional elevation.

Proximal and distal joints should be incorporated into the rehabilitation program. Stability from the proximal musculature is required for proper function of the glenohumeral joint and should be addressed at an appropriate time during the program. Elbow and hand range of motion facilitates improved circulation, reduced edema, and less stiffness.

Appropriate analgesics and pain medication should be incorporated and administered prior to exercise to help control pain and muscle spasm.

The success of the program relies heavily on patient education, compliance, and the ability to participate in a home exercise program. The

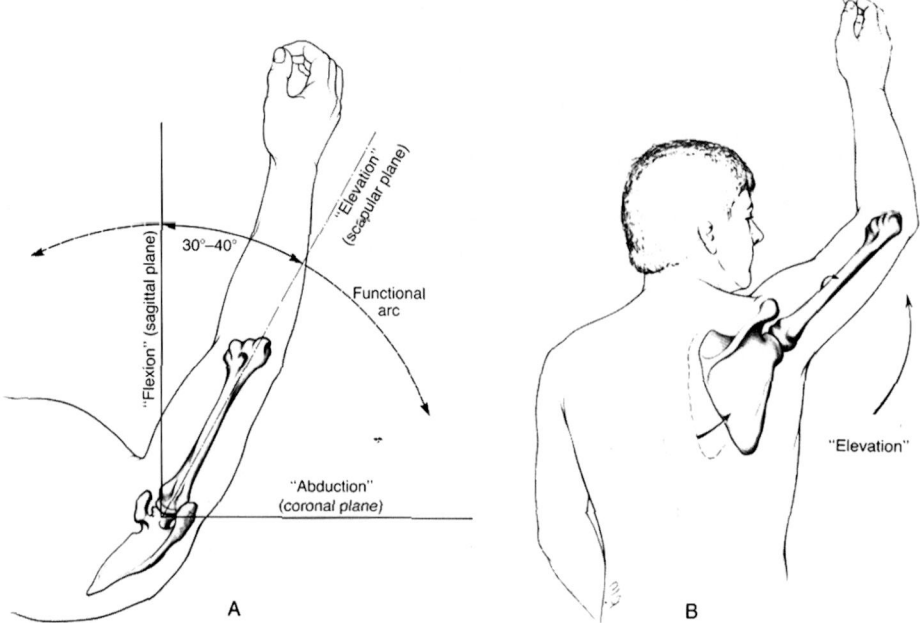

Figure 8.1. The plane of maximal elevation is centered on the scapular plane, rather than the coronal plane (abduction) or sagittal plane (flexion). Shoulder movements should be thought to be centered on this plane because (**A**) the capsule of the glenohumeral joint is most relaxed in the scapular plane, allowing the highest upward excision, with the greatest ease and freedom of movement; and (**B**) the glenohumeral joint is most often used in this plane. Movements here occur more naturally and with less effort. The body may be rotated to cause the arm to be raised in the scapular plane rather than the coronal plane. The concept is stressed in the postoperative exercise program. (From Neer [12], by permission of WB Saunders.)

home program consists of instruction in the use of medication, the application of heat or ice, instruction for family members and friends, and positioning for comfort in preparation for a concise exercise program and less complicated recovery.

Understanding the surgical procedure, and thus the reasons for doing specific exercises in a certain progression, helps the therapist tailor the rehabilitation program to the patient. The exercise program is composed of a progression of passive range of motion, active assistive range of motion, isometrics, active exercise (which initiates strengthening), advanced stretching, and progressive resistive exercise. The program incorporates the design progression of intensity of exercise over time determined by the pathology, surgery, bone, and soft tissue healing (Figure 8.2). Written instructions and illustrations should be given to the patient that provide a clear understanding of the program.

Rehabilitation Program

The postoperative program is initiated on the same day as surgery unless a special consideration determined at the time of surgery necessitates a delay. The surgeon and/or therapist will be able to move the

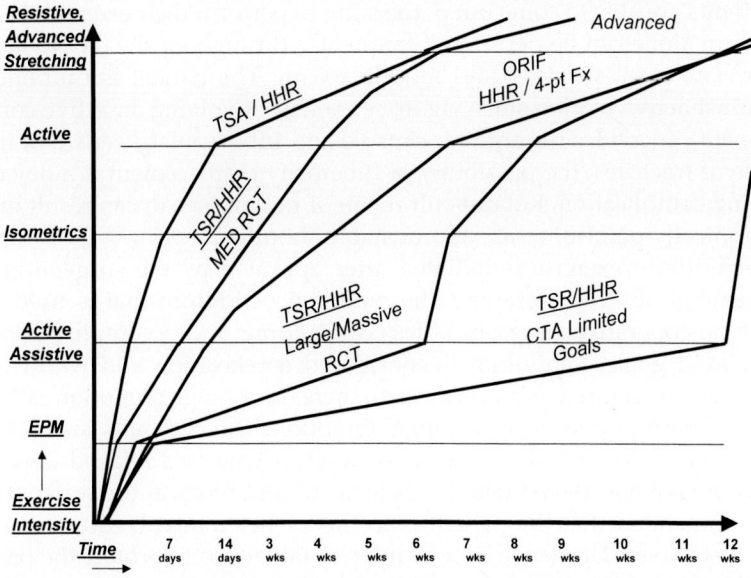

Figure 8.2. The graph demonstrates the rehabilitation progression design and the relationships between intensity of exercise over time and the surgical repair. Arthroplasty for OA moves much quicker through the exercise progression. While arthroplasty with repair of large or massive rotator cuff tears move at a slower pace due to the healing requirements of the repaired tissue.

shoulder, comfortably and without pain, to the passive limits set since the regional anesthesia (interscalene block) is still in effect. Several authors believe that early passive motion tailored to the surgical procedure is the cornerstone to a successful outcome, provided the bony repair and soft tissues are not overstressed and adequate pain control is achieved [3, 8, 11, 12, 30, 33, 36–42]. McCann et al, [43], in their electromyographic study of shoulder rehabilitation exercises, found that in the supine position, passive exercise of forward elevation and external rotation generated the least electrical activity of the rotator cuff and deltoid muscles. They also noted significantly less activity in the middle deltoid and supraspinatus during elevation in the scapular plane with the elbow bent, compared with elevation with the elbow straight. This study supports the risk/benefits of early motion and protection of repaired soft tissues postsurgery. Passive limits of motion are usually set, unless otherwise specified, to 30 degrees of external rotation and 130 degrees of forward elevation in the plane of the scapula. Passive motion, with the interscalede block in place, demonstrates to the patient how freely the shoulder joint moves with the new replacement and pain alleviated. As the block wears off, usually the following day, the patient begins to regain feeling. They are instructed to frequently take their arm out of the sling and begin flexing and extending their elbow, wrist, and fingers for a few minutes throughout the day. The patient is usually protected in a sling for 2 weeks unless there is a fracture or rotator cuff tear. In these cases, protection in the sling is longer, usually 4 to 6 weeks depending on the pathology and repair.

Patients are able to come out of the sling to perform their exercise. Pendulum alone can be performed frequently throughout the day to help alleviate pain, stiffness, and muscle spasm. The patient is cautioned against active motion since vigorous exercise involving an active component can avulse the anterior capsule and subscapularis repair. In the case of fractures, the possibility of tuberosity displacement is a devastating complication. Rotator cuff repair, if not protected, can result in a chronically painful, weak, and unstable shoulder.

Pendulum exercise is initiated after approval by the surgeon and instruction by the therapist. The modified pendulum that is used in our postoperative program is less demanding and accomplishes the intended goals. Pendulum is considered a relaxation and warm up exercise, therefore it is a precursor to increasing range of motion rather than an exercise to increase range of motion. The patient is instructed to allow the operated extremity to slowly swing to a relaxed dependent position as the patient bends forward and flexes at the waist. It is recommended that the patient place his or her uninvolved extremity on a stable surface (such as a counter or table top) to protect the back and to enhance proximal stability for relaxation. The slight traction created by the weight of the extremity facilitates a gentle stretch, which is effective in relaxing the sometimes tight periscapular, rotator cuff, and deltoid muscles. Small circles clockwise and counterclockwise initiated by the patient rocking his or her body creates a gentle momentum, allowing for easy stress-less circular motion. The rotational component at the glenohumeral joint and scapulothoracic articulation further enhances the relaxation and movement between the soft tissues. Following pendulum passive exercise is initiated by the therapist. The patient is placed in a supine position with a pillow placed under the arm to avoid extension. While the upper extremity is supported at the elbow and held at the wrist, gentle small circular rotation of the extremity for muscle relaxation is performed prior to external rotation of the shoulder to 30 degrees as specified by the surgeon. Slow, gentle motion to the point of stiffness is initially undertaken. Forward elevation is accomplished in the same manner, with the arc of motion in the plane of the scapula proceeding no higher than 130 degrees (Figure 8.3). The patient must receive constant verbal cues to relax during the exercise period to ensure that the exercise is truly passive [37]. The therapist should proceed slowly and ask for patient feedback as they progress through the exercise. In some instances patients feel more comfortable in the sitting position when passive exercise is performed. It is important to proceed very carefully when forward elevation is performed. Once you have elevated the arm to 130 degrees in the sitting position, it may be difficult to bring the extremity back down, since some patients tend to actively guard if they begin to feel discomfort. Verbal cues to "let the shoulder go" are important at this point. Relaxation is vital in this situation since passive exercise converts to an eccentric exercise putting cuff repair and tuberosity fixation at risk. If relaxation can not be accomplished the supine position is reverted to.

The establishment of trust between the therapist and patient is initiated on first meeting and cannot be overemphasized. Making the

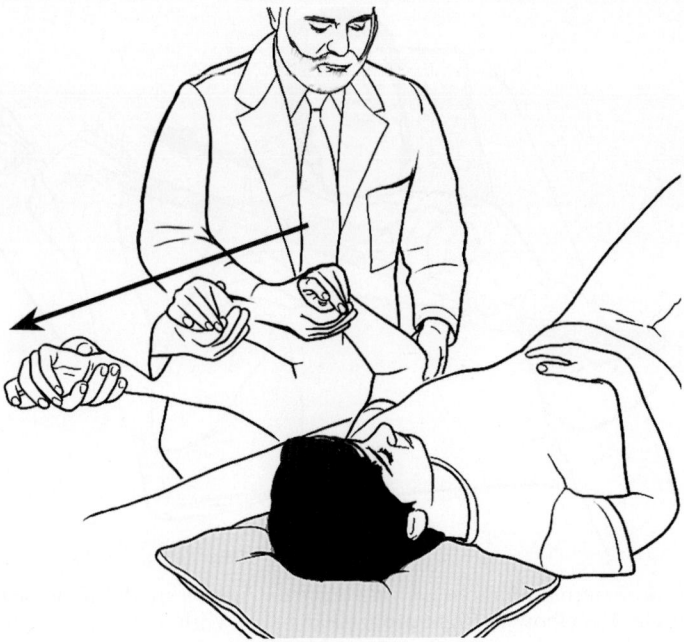

Figure 8.3. Passive forward flexion, supine. Lie on your back, with your affected elbow cushioned. Relax your arm completely. The therapist supports your wrist and arm, and repeats the passive forward flexion exercises.

patient aware of the intended goals of treatment and the therapist being responsive to their feedback will ensure an ongoing patient/therapist working relationship. As the patient becomes more familiar with the passive exercise, and if their surgical procedure permits, active assistive supine external rotation with a stick is initiated (Figure 8.4) and assistive supine forward elevation are initiated. It is important to instruct the patient to put a folded towel or bolster under the arm at a comfortable distance from the trunk (approximately 15–20 degrees) while in this position. This facilitates a neutral position at the glenohumeral joint, allowing the exercise to start in the plane of the scapula. The supine position, rather than erect sitting, allows the patient to be more relaxed and is helpful in isolating motion at the glenohumeral joint while limiting trunk and scapula substitution. The patient is instructed to grasp the wrist of their operated extremity and use the force of their opposite extremity to elevate the arm. It is helpful to give the patient a point of reference to go to for instance a headboard on a bed. The upper extremity is moving to a gravity-eliminated position when approaching 90 to 130 degrees of forward elevation, which appears to facilitate muscle relaxation and more comfortable motion under the coracoacromial arch [44]. The hospital stay can vary from 2 to 3 days with the primary goals of early motion limits, pain control, and establishment of an independent home program. Due to the establishment of this home program, it is important that patient and family members have a good understanding of the exercises. Performing the

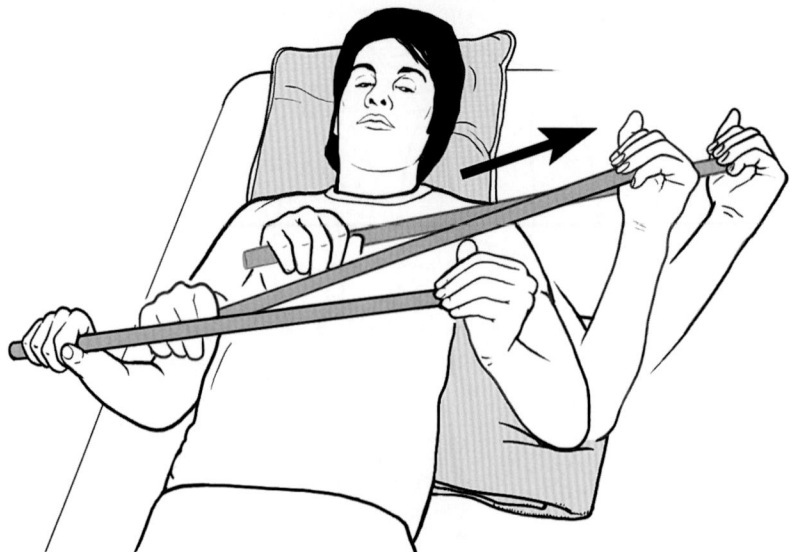

Figure 8.4. External rotation. Lie on your back, with a small pillow or folded towel under the elbow as illustrated. Hold a stick with one end in each hand. Use your good hand to push the affected hand gently outward with the stick, and then return to the starting position.

exercises independently in the hospital ensures a smooth transition to a home program. Patients are instructed to call the surgeon if they develop a fever greater than 101 degrees Fahrenheit, severe pain unrelieved by the pain medication, inability to tolerate the pain medication, excessive bleeding from the surgical site, and with any additional questions they may have concerning their post surgical course.

Outpatient Therapy

Obtaining a detailed history and performing an appropriate physical examination of the patient directs the establishment of realistic goals during continued rehabilitation. The functional requirements of each individual vary depending on their lifestyle, occupation, age, medical history, and participation in leisurely activities and sports. Communication with the surgeon, in addition to an operative report, further ensures the proper care and progression of the patient, developing an appropriate postoperative program. Special care early on should be taken to observe the surgical site, the amount of swelling, and any discoloration of the shoulder and upper extremity. Development of redness around the border of the suture line should be suspect of an underlying infection and should be reported to the surgeon. It is also important to remind the patient that coordinating pain medication with exercise will facilitate a more comfortable accomplishment of the goals set during the exercise program. Following the evaluation, a review of the patient's home program is important to establish a baseline and redirect the patient if they are having difficulty with a particular exercise. Many times patients complain of positional discomfort at home, especially if they attempt to sleep in the supine position. It is our experience that a semireclined position with a pillow under the arm combined with the application of ice or heat and pain medication allows the patient to have adequate rest during early recovery. Modalities for control of postoperative discomfort, edema, and muscle spasm are helpful in preparing for the exercise program. Later in the program, in the subacute stage, when adequate healing of the suture line has occurred and postoperative swelling has diminished, a combination of heat, gentle soft tissue mobilization, and therapeutic massage followed by gentle mobility exercise have been effective in making the patient more comfortable, allowing the patient to have a more positive experience during the program.

Active Assistive Exercise (ROM): Active assistive exercise continues for 6 weeks, including pendulum, supine external rotation with a stick to 30 degrees, and supine forward elevation to 130 degrees (see Table 8.1) Patients are always instructed to relax the involved extremity, move their arm to the point of stiffness, continue a slight amount and hold that position for the count of five, and finally return to the resting position. The exercise should be repeated 3 to 4 times daily with 5 repetitions as tolerated per exercise increasing to 10 repetitions as healing and comfort allow. The pulley exercise can be initiated on the 3rd postoperative day with the limit of 130 degrees of FE (Figure 8.5). McCann et

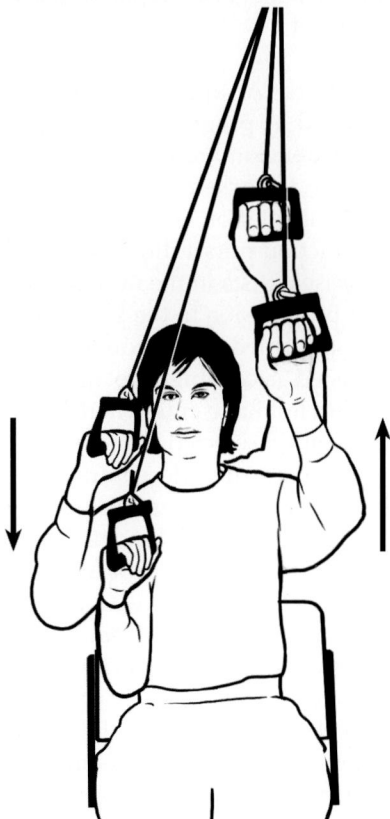

Figure 8.5. Sit on a chair and hold the handles of the pulley system. Relax your involved arm and use your good arm to pull the involved arm gently above your head. Gently lower the arm to your starting position, and then repeat.

al. [43] noted a significant increase in EMG activity of the deltoid and spinati muscles with pulley exercise. With a large or massive rotator cuff repair or a proximal humeral fracture, pulleys are started later, at approximately 6 weeks, when the repairs are stable (see Tables 8.2 and 8.3). The patient is instructed to place the pulley over the operated shoulder (this keeps the line of the scapular plane) while pulling the extremity up with the opposite hand to the limit of 130 degrees. The sitting position with a backed chair limits trunk substitution and rotation when performing this exercise. Patients tend to do well with this exercise since it is a closed loop patient-controlled activity. It involves considerable movement of both upper quarters in a reciprocal pattern, initiating comfortable neuromuscular reeducation, yet is protective within the limits of surgery. Active assistive extension with the stick is performed by grasping a stick with both hands, behind the back, at shoulder width, arms straight, and palms facing backward. To avoid substitution by flexing at the trunk, patients are asked to face a wall or a door. Active assistive internal rotation is performed by grasping the wrist of the operated extremity and sliding it up the center of the back along the spine. These exercises put stress across the subscapularis repair and are not started until adequate healing has occurred at the sixth postoperative week. Additionally, extension and internal rotation put unwanted tension on the repaired rotator cuff tendon and tuberosity fixation after proximal humeral fracture. These motions are also avoided for 6 weeks until adequate healing has occurred.

Isometrics: At approximately 6 to 9 days, submaximal isometrics are initiated. A progression of gentle external rotation, flexion, abduction, and extension are sequentially introduced. Isometric exercise demonstrated a marked increase in activity when evaluated by EMG [43]. Internal rotation is therefore avoided for 6 weeks since active muscle contraction puts a direct pull across the subscapularis repair. Isometric exercise assists in the initiation of muscle reeducation and is an important progression in the program. It is recommended that the isometrics be performed submaximally and gradually increased to maximum, adjusted accordingly to the patient response and reactivity. Patients should not have pain when performing this exercise. Isolation and contraction of selected muscles helps the patient identify and initiate a comfortable muscle contraction that may have been difficult to do before surgery. Usually, younger patients and patients with good strength and control move quickly through this step. With some older individuals, the concept and execution of the isometric exercise may require repeated instruction. In patients with small to medium rotator cuff repair, isometrics can be initiated at 2 to 3 weeks. With large or massive repairs, isometrics are started at approximately 6 to 8 weeks. With four-part fractures, submaximal isometrics can be initiated at 3 to 4 weeks, depending on the degree of healing and callous formation as determined by the surgeon. Patients who demonstrate considerable weakness in external rotation may benefit by performing multi-angle supine external rotation isometrics (Figure 8.6).

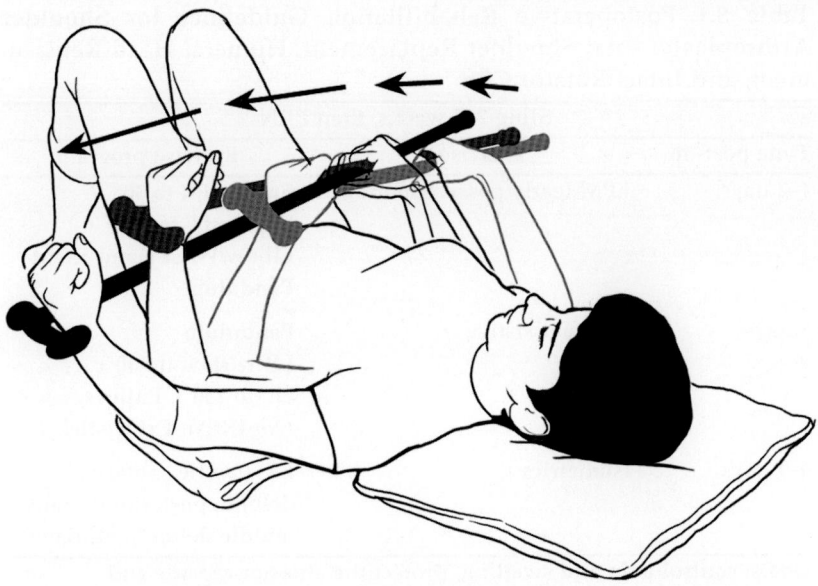

Figure 8.6. Isometric multi-angle external rotation. Lie on your back with a pillow or folded towel under your elbow, hold the cane in your good hand, and hook the other end over the wrist of the involved extremity. Push outward with the wrist of the involved extremity as you use your good hand to hold the cane steady so it doesn't move at all. Hold for the count of 5–10, then relax. Move your wrist away from your body approximately 5–10 degrees and resist in that position holding for the count of 5–10. Repeat this progression until you have reached the end range of motion.

Active Exercise (Early strengthening): Active exercise is considered early strengthening. Isometrics can be eliminated as the patient proceeds in the active program. Active exercise for total shoulder and humeral head replacement with an intact rotator cuff is usually initiated at 10 days to 2 weeks, starting in the supine position and progressing to standing (see Table 8.1). Pain-free functional activity below the horizontal is encouraged during the day. Patients are instructed not to lift any weighted objects. Supine exercise is the first step in progressive strengthening of the rotator cuff and deltoid. It is an effective position to begin gradual strengthening of the sometimes weak muscles that result from long standing pathology and severe traumatic injury. In the supine position the effect of gravity on the weight of the extremity, approximately 5% of body weight [44], is reduced. When approaching 60 to 120 degrees of forward elevation, the arc of maximal subacromial contact [45], a decrease in the amount of compressive force is realized. Exercise in the supine position decreases the effects of gravity on the weight of the extremity, therefore reducing the intratendinous sheer and the extratendinous compressive forces from the coracoacromial arch on the interposing soft tissues and rotator cuff [46]. The rotator cuff must generate a sufficient force to maintain a fulcrum while lifting the weight of the extremity. If the force couple of the rotator cuff and deltoid is lost in elevation, superior translation of the humeral head

Table 8.1. Postoperative Rehabilitation Guidelines for Shoulder Arthroplasty: Total Shoulder Replacement, Humeral Head Replacement, and Intact Rotator Cuff

Sling 2–3 weeks, then PRN		
Time post-op	Exercise	Exercise program
1–2 days	EPM (early passive motion)	Supine ER to 30° Supine FF to 130° Elbow/Wrist/Hand ROM Pendulum
3 days	Active assistive	Pendulum ER w/stick (to 30°) FF (to 130°), Pulleys, *No IR*No Ext w/stick
6–9 days	Isometrics	ER, (*No* IR), anterior deltoid, posterior deltoid, middle deltoid, multiangle

Goals: control pain and swelling, protect the anterior capsule and subscapularis tendon repair, prevent adhesion formation, increase ROM (scapular plane), educate (importance of medication, ice/heat application, compliance to the program, frequent gentle exercise, rest, positioning for comfort at home, family/friend instruction), establish a well understood home program, with a gradual introduction of exercises.

Time post-op	Exercise	Exercise program
10 days	Active	Supine FF w/stick Supine FF w/stick + weight (1–2 lbs.) Supine FF, ER side lying, Eccentric Pulleys, Standing press w/stick, Eccentric standing press w/stick, Prone ext./abd to midline
6 weeks	Advanced stretching, Resistive (scapular)	Follow exercise figures Follow exercise figures

Goals: control pain and swelling, increase active ROM, increase strength, development of neuromuscular control of the shoulder complex, improve proprioception, normalize response to dynamic challenges.

* {Ext. (Extension) and IR (Internal rotation) not performed until 6 weeks postop}. FF = forward flexion, ER = external rotation, Abd. = abduction, w = with, TSR = total shoulder replacement, HHR = humeral head replacement.

accompanied by a shoulder shrug will be observed. The supine position reduces the normal strength requirement for forward elevation in the plane of the scapula. Gradual loading and conditioning in this position allow for the rotator cuff to strengthen without compromise of joint mechanics.

Arthroplasty with medium rotator cuff repair allows for initiation of active exercise at 3 to 4 weeks (Table 8.2) while large to massive tears require a longer protection period. Active exercises begin at approximately 8 weeks (Table 8.3). With proximal humeral fractures, active exercise is usually started at 6 weeks (Table 8.4).

Table 8.2. Postoperative Rehabilitation Guidelines for Shoulder Arthroplasty: Proximal Humeral Fracture

Time post fx	Exercise	Exercise program
3–5 days	EPM (early passive motion)	Supine ER to 30° Supine FF to 130° Elbow/Wrist/Hand ROM
7–10 days	Active assistive	Pendulum
		ER w/Stick FF, *No* IR, *No* Ext w/stick
3 weeks	Active assistive Isometrics (submaximal)	(*No* IR), ER, anterior deltoid, posterior deltoid, middle deltoid, Multiangle

Goals: control pain and swelling, protect fracture site and tuberosity fixation/repair, prevent adhesion formation, increase ROM (scapular plane), educate (importance of medication, ice/heat application, compliance to the program, frequent gentle exercise, rest, positioning for comfort at home, family/friend instruction), establish a well understood home program, with a gradual introduction of exercises.

Time post fx	Exercise	Exercise program
4–6 weeks	Active	Pulley Supine FF w/stick Supine FF w/stick + wt. (1–2 lbs) Supine FF Eccentric pulleys, Active ER side lying, Eccentric Pulleys, Standing press w/stick, Eccentric standing press w/stick, Active FF, Prone ext./abd
12 weeks	Advanced stretching Resistive exercises	Follow exercise figures Progress as tolerated

Goals: control pain and swelling, increase active ROM, increase strength, development of neuromuscular control of the shoulder complex, improve proprioception, normalize response to dynamic challenges.

* {Ext. (Extension) and IR (Internal rotation) not performed until 6 weeks postop}. FF = forward flexion, ER = external rotation, Abd. = abduction, w = with, HHR = humeral head replacement.

Table 8.3. Postoperative Rehabilitation Guidelines for Shoulder Arthroplasty: Large or Massive Rotator Cuff Repair

TSR, HHR w/Cuff Involvement Large Rotator Cuff Repair 3–5 cm./Massive Repair >5 cm. Sling 6–8 weeks		
Time post-op	Exercise	Exercise program
1–2 days	EPM (early passive motion)	Supine ER to 30° Supine FF to 130° Elbow/Wrist/Hand ROM Pendulum
6–8 weeks	Active assistive	Pendulum ER w/stick (to 30°) FF (to 130°), Pulleys, *No IR*No Ext w/stick
6–8 weeks	Isometrics	ER, (No IR), anterior deltoid, posterior deltoid, middle deltoid, multiangle

Goals: control pain and swelling, protect the anterior capsule and subscapularis tendon repair, prevent adhesion formation, increase ROM (scapular plane), educate (importance of medication, ice/heat application, compliance to the program, frequent gentle exercise, rest, positioning for comfort at home, family/friend instruction), establish a well understood home program, with a gradual introduction of exercises.

Time post-op	Exercise	Exercise program
8 weeks	Active	Supine FF w/stick Supine FF w/stick + weight (1–2 lbs.) Supine FE, ER side lying, Eccentric Pulleys, Standing press w/stick, Eccentric standing press w/stick, Prone ext/abd
12 weeks	Advanced stretching Resistive (scapular),	Follow exercise figures Progress as tolerated

Goals: control pain and swelling, increase active ROM, increase strength, development of neuromuscular control of the shoulder complex, improve proprioception, normalize response to dynamic challenges.

* {Ext. (Extension)/IR (Internal rotation) not performed until 10–12 weeks postop}. FF = forward flexion, ER = external rotation, Abd. = abduction, w = with, TSR = total shoulder replacement, HHR = humeral head replacement.

Forward elevation with a stick in the supine position initiates active contraction and strengthening of the rotator cuff and deltoid (Figure 8.7). The stick should be held at shoulders' width. The use of the other extremity facilitates easier controlled motion. In this position, the patient is less fearful of lifting the arm for the first time, since the other extremity can supply support and power if pain or weakness is encountered. As the patient proceeds beyond 90 degrees, the effect of gravity

Table 8.4. Postoperative Rehabilitation Guidelines for Shoulder Arthroplasty: Medium Rotator Cuff Repair

	TSR, HHR w/Cuff Involvement Medium Repair Approx. 2–3 cm. Sling 2–3 weeks, then PRN	
Time post-op	Exercise	Exercise program
1–2 days	EPM (early passive motion)	Supine ER to 30° Supine FF to 130° Elbow/Wrist/Hand ROM Pendulum
3 days	Active assistive	Pendulum ER w/stick (to 30°) FF (to 130°), Pulleys, *No IR*No Ext w/stick
2–3 weeks	Isometrics	ER, (No IR), anterior deltoid, posterior deltoid, middle deltoid, multiangle

Goals: control pain and swelling, protect the anterior capsule and subscapularis tendon repair, prevent adhesion formation, increase ROM (scapular plane), educate (importance of medication, ice/heat application, compliance to the program, frequent gentle exercise, rest, positioning for comfort at home, family/friend instruction), establish a well understood home program, with a gradual introduction of exercises.

Time post-op	Exercise	Exercise program
3–4 weeks	Active	Supine FF w/stick Supine FF w/stick + weight (1–2 lbs.) Supine FF, ER side lying, Eccentric Pulleys, Standing press w/stick, Eccentric standing press w/stick, Prone ext/abd
6 weeks	Advanced stretching, Resistive (scapular)	Follow exercise figures Progress as tolerated

Goals: control pain and swelling, increase active ROM, increase strength, development of neuromuscular control of the shoulder complex, improve proprioception, normalize response to dynamic challenges.

* {Ext. (Extension) and IR (Internal rotation) not performed until 6 weeks postop}. FF = forward flexion, ER = external rotation, Abd. = abduction, w = with, TSR = total shoulder replacement, HHR = humeral head replacement.

helps with stretching toward flexion. As they return toward the starting position an eccentric component is initiated. As the ease of the exercise improves, a 1 lb to 2 lb. weight is added to the stick, which increases the amount of work performed. The patient is then progressed to active forward elevation supine and external rotation side-lying. This is the first time the patient moves their upper extremity without support. A rolled towel or a small pillow under the arm will maintain position in

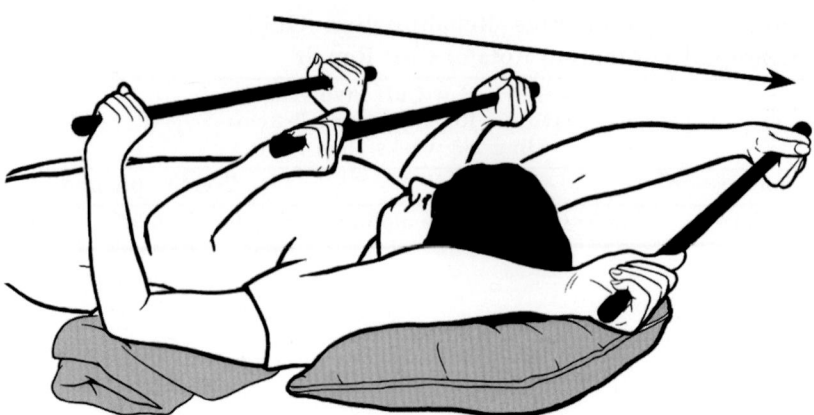

Figure 8.7. Supine forward elevation with a stick. Lie on your back with your elbow supported with a small pillow or a rolled towel. Hold the stick at its ends. Raise your elbows off the mat and reach over your head in a single, slow, smooth motion, straightening your elbow so that you can reach high over your head. The stick should pass close by your face. Then lower your arms along the same path to the starting position.

the scapular plane. These concentric, eccentric exercises help the patient gain neuromuscular control of the proximal muscles and upper extremity.

Constant reassessment of the exercise progression by the therapist must be an ongoing process. Patients with adequate strength may move quickly through this progression. Others with prior weakness and soft tissue pathology may have difficulty at first and be more challenged by these exercises.

Isolation of the posterior cuff and periscapular muscles is accomplished with prone abduction palm down position, and then to the more challenging position of prone abduction with the thumb pointing up. Limiting the range of motion well below the horizontal ensures safety of the anterior structures with this exercise. These exercises can be used in the resistive exercise program with addition of a 1 lb to 2 lb. weight at a later time. Periscapular muscle reeducation is further initiated with prone extension to midline with the arm bent, then with the arm extended. In individuals who have difficulty assuming a prone position, such as the elderly or severely arthritic and kyphotic patient, the difficulty far outweighs the benefit. As the patient demonstrates progress in dynamic control, comfort, and confidence, they are advanced to an erect exercise position. The osteoarthritic patient may progress easily through this part of the program, while the rheumatoid patient with a rotator cuff tear and underlying weakness may move through more slowly. It is dependent on the therapist to ensure the proper performance of the exercise, while at the same time, avoiding pain and overloading, which may cause unnecessary discomfort and delay of the rehabilitation.

Eccentric pulleys allow controlled eccentric loading of the deltoid and rotator cuff with the added protection of the opposite extremity (Figure 8.8). The pulley is positioned and aligned with the shoulder to

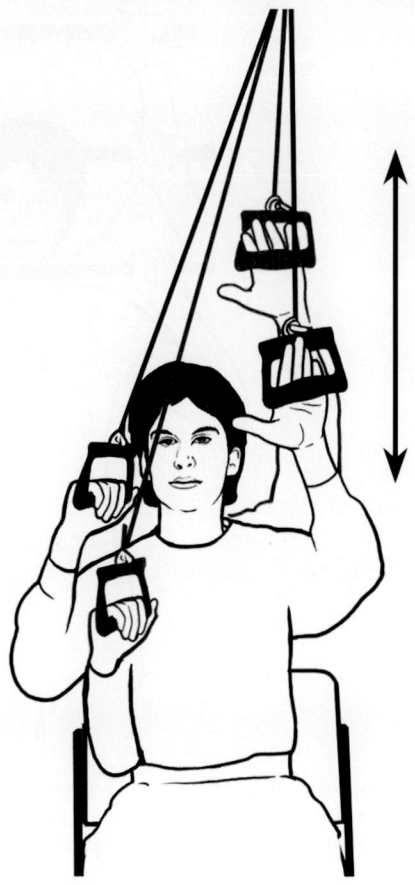

Figure 8.8. Eccentric pulleys. Grasp the handles of the pulleys, and use your good arm to stretch the affected arm as high as it can go. Then, let the affected arm lower slowly down on its own power to the starting position.

maintain the plane of the scapula during elevation. The patient performs the exercise in the functional position with a slightly bent elbow. As the patient slowly lowers the arm and approaches the critical range of 120 degrees to 60 degrees, the therapist must watch the mechanics of the active eccentric exercise. If an anterior/superior translation of the humeral head is observed, accompanied by a shrug sign, the exercise may be overloading the rotator cuff's ability to control, depress, and centralize the humeral head as well as counter the deltoid force while lowering the arm. In this case, the exercise is modified, and the opposite extremity is recruited to take some of the weight of the arm. If anterior/superior translation of the humeral head is accompanied by pain, the exercise should be stopped. It is then prudent to reduce the load on the soft tissues and continue with supine exercise for a longer time until the soft tissues gain sufficient strength to tolerate the more demanding activity.

Following the supine exercises, concentric-eccentric standing press (Figure 8.9) is initiated. The same rule applies; to avoid the shrug sign during these exercises. As strength and control improve, the patient progresses to a more demanding eccentrically specific standing press. The patient is instructed to lift his or her hand off the stick and follow it to the resting position at chest level. Again, good mechanics should

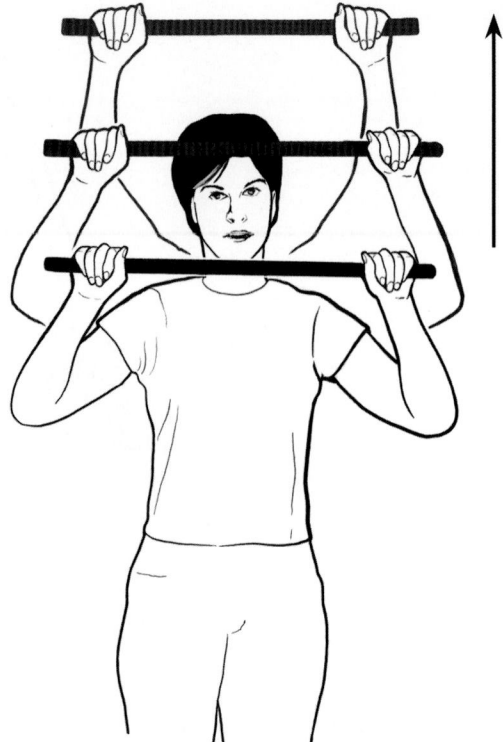

Figure 8.9. Standing press with stick. Stand up with your arm bent at the elbows, grasp the stick at it s ends, and hold it level with our chin. Slowly raise the stick over your head and then lower it to the starting position.

be observed, and pain should not be present with the exercise. All exercises are performed in a functional manner with a flexed elbow. As the performance of exercise becomes easier, it is apparent that the patient has gained sufficient strength to progress to more challenging exercise.

Advanced Stretching Exercise: Advanced stretching is initiated at the 6th postoperative week with an intact rotator cuff as well as with a medium cuff repair. With large/massive rotator cuff repairs and humeral fractures, advanced stretching is deferred until 12 weeks postoperatively. Advanced stretching is initiated at approximately the same time as resistive exercise. The stretching exercise can become more aggressive and forceful at this point in the program. In cases of excessive stiffness, more emphasis is placed on attaining normal range of motion instead of strengthening. However, strengthening does continue and becomes the focus of exercise when range of motion goals are realized. Maximal end-range planar motion and combined motion stretching for functional requirements above and below the horizontal are the goals of this portion of the program. The one arm wall stretch (Figure 8.10) is initiated with the patient holding the wrist of the affected extremity and sliding it up on a smooth surface. Using the finger-walk up the wall is not advocated for this exercise. As the patient begins to reach up, the wrist is released and the patient leans into the wall, while at the same time stretching up toward the ceiling. The goal of this exer-

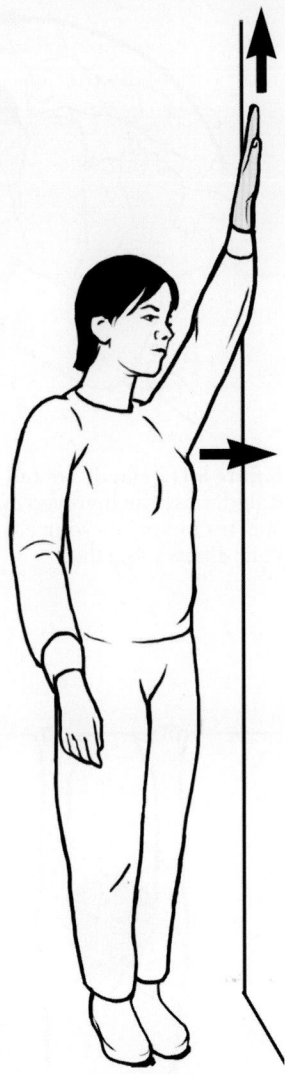

Figure 8.10. Wall stretch, one arm. Place the involved hand on the flat surface of a door; as you reach and stretch to the top of the door attempt to press your arm pit on to the door. Keep your elbow straight.

cise is to have contact of the axilla and arm with the wall. An added benefit to this exercise is the initiation of periscapular upward rotation in the erect position. As the patient progresses to 140 degrees of forward elevation comfortably, combined flexion, external rotation, and abduction stretch can be initiated (Figure 8.11). This position is usually more challenging for the patient. This stretch focuses on the anterior and inferior structures of the shoulder as the patient moves above the horizontal. The requirement of combined flexion abduction and forward elevation are addressed to maximize proper mechanics and function overhead. Patients can be very stiff in this position in spite of good planar motion. A slow gentle progression of intensity of stretching is encouraged since patients can become quite sore with this exercise.

The over-the-door hang (Figure 8.12) is more aggressive and applies more force to the overhead stretch. Patients are reminded that this is

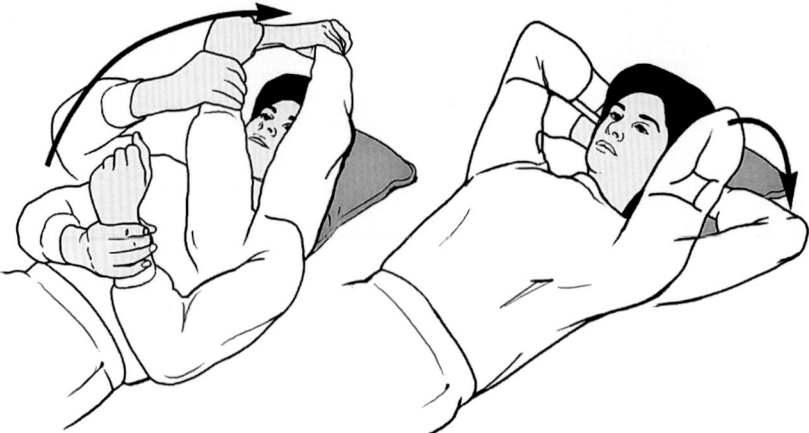

Figure 8.11. Hands behind head with elbows abducted. In one motion as illustrated, raise the involved extremity to the back of your head. Clasp your hands and try to spread your elbows our to the side and touch the mat. Then bring your elbows together.

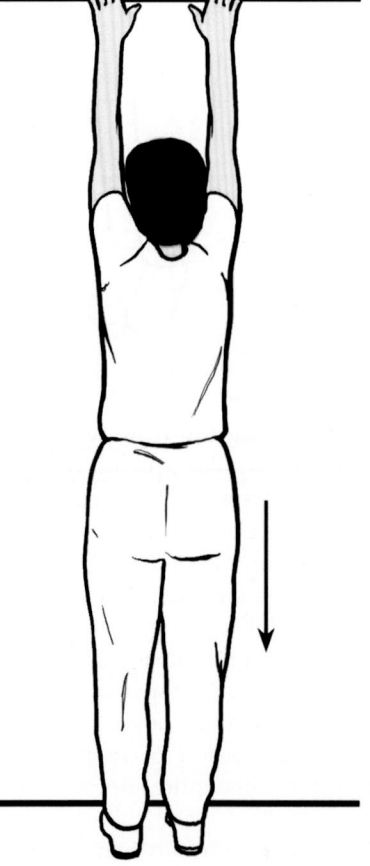

Figure 8.12. Over door hang. Slide both hands to the top of the door and grasp with your finger tips. Relax your arms and shoulders. Bend your knees, gently applying a stretch to your shoulders. Increase intensity as tolerable. Hold to the count of 5–10, and then repeat.

Figure 8.13. Standing 90/90 stretch. Arms out to the side with our elbows bent at 90 degrees. Lean forward into the corner. Hold to the count of 5–10, then repeat.

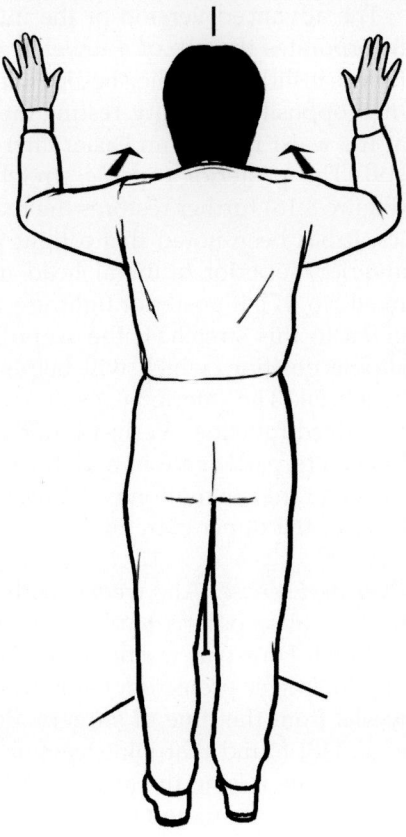

not a *pull-up* but a *hang-down* exercise. Shorter patients can use a stool, or a portable chin-up bar is sometimes recommended. The patient is instructed to reach to the top of the door and only tighten the fingertips, relaxing the rest of the extremity. They then can apply stretch by gently bending their knees and allowing the weight of their body to increase the force applied to the soft tissues of the shoulder joint. The stretch should be gradual and not excessive.

The standing 90/90 stretch (Figure 8.13) continues to address the anterior and inferior soft tissue of the shoulder. When patients are asked to assume this position, many present with an adducted internally rotated position when compared with the opposite side. The patient is directed to approach the corner of a room and position his arms as illustrated. He is then instructed to gently lean into the corner of the wall. Patients should not lead with their hips when leaning but with their upper body to avoid substitution and hyperextension of the lower back. With younger patients who have had shoulder arthroplasty, supine external rotation at 90 degrees of abduction and 90 degrees of elbow flexion may be additionally effective in regaining motion in this position. It is important that a towel be placed under the upper arm, avoiding excessive abduction, which will over stretching the anterior/inferior structures and lead to possible apprehension.

The advanced version of the internal rotation stretch (Figure 8.14) incorporates the use of a towel or a silk scarf/tie, which reduces friction as it slides over the shoulder. In patients who have difficulty using their opposite extremity, resting the hand on a countertop and bending at the waist may be an easier alternative to this exercise (Figure 8.15) [19]. The posterior capsule stretch or cross body adduction stretch (Figure 8.16) further restores the requirement for normal joint mechanics. It has been noted that a tight posterior capsule can contribute to anterior/superior humeral head migration contributing to impingement [46, 47]. If posterior tightness is present, close attention should be given to this stretch. If the scapula is very mobile, stretching in the supine position, which will help stabilize the scapula, may be more beneficial. The inferior capsule stretch further restores flexibility for improved function overhead. In the younger, more active patient who intends to participate in athletic activities, a balance of flexibility and full end range of motion is important to safely accomplish the required tasks of the upper extremity.

Resistive Exercise: At 6 weeks, with intact soft tissues and a sufficiently healed subscapularis tendon repair, the resistive exercise program is initiated. Four-part fractures and large to massive rotator cuff repairs require longer protection before resistive exercise is begun, usually 12 weeks from the time of surgery. Poppen and Walker [44] and Inman et al. [48] found that joint reaction force at the normal glenohumeral joint, while raising the arm in abduction, approximates body weight. A considerable amount of force occurs at the glenohumeral joint during

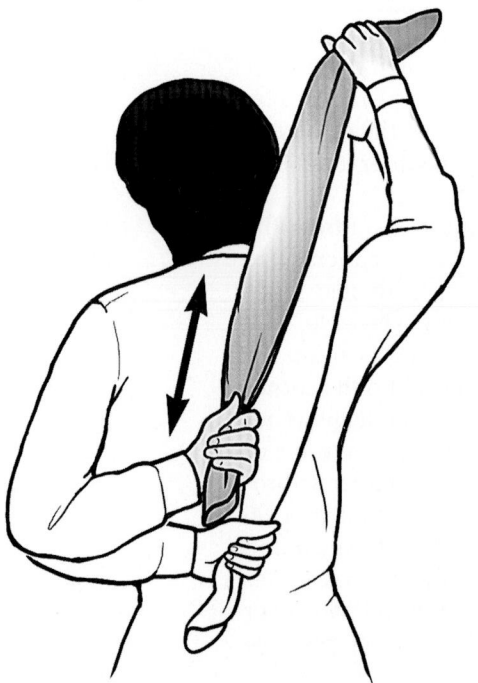

Figure 8.14. Internal rotation using a towel. Standing, grasp a towel or an old silk tie. Use your uninvolved arm to pull the involved arm up your back. Hold to the count of 5–10, then repeat.

Figure 8.15. Internal rotation stretch using a counter top. With your back to the counter, place your hand on the counter top. Bend at the knees slowly until you feel a stretch. Hold to the count of 5–10, then repeat.

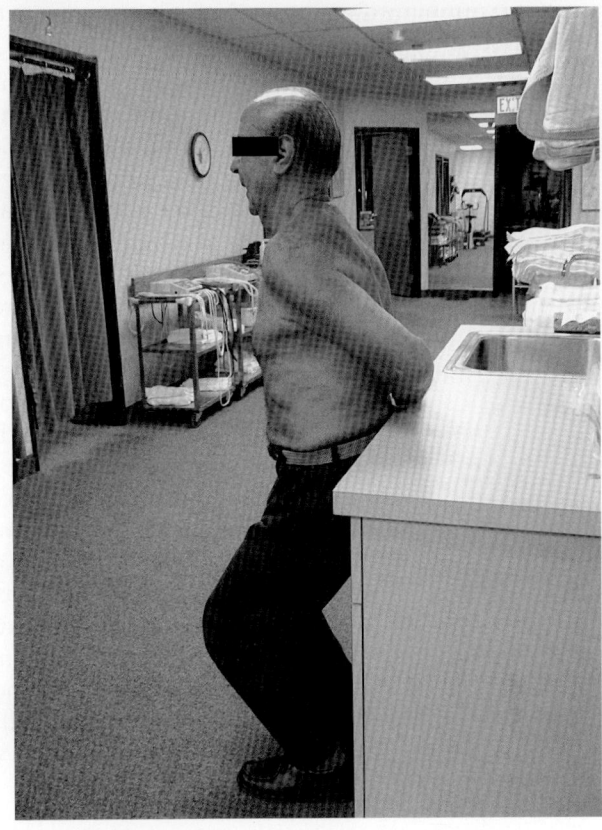

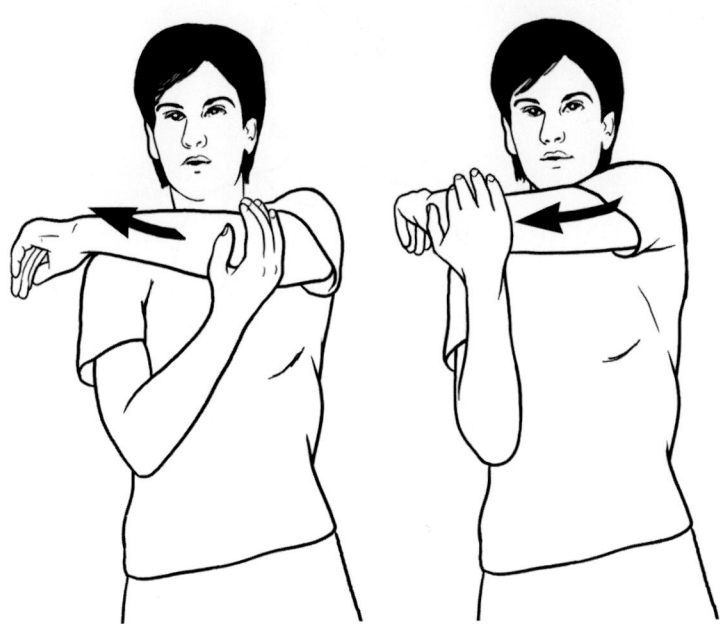

Figure 8.16. Posterior capsule stretch. Raise involved arm to horizontal position. With the other hand, push your elbow toward the opposite shoulder. Hold to the count of 5–10, then repeat.

elevation and should be considered during resistive exercise. Attention must be paid to the arthrokinematics while the resistance is applied. The patient should not experience pain with the strengthening exercises. A progressive system of increasing resistance using elastic tubing or bands is introduced. As patients become accustomed to the resistive exercise, light weights, starting from 1 lb to 5 lbs, are introduced. As the intensity of the exercise increases, the frequency of the resistive exercise may be reduced from once a day to every other day as progression through the program continues.

Rotator cuff function and strengthening is one of the most important aspects of the program. Off-center loading of the glenoid and shear has been associated with superior migration of the humeral head, which can be due to a deficient rotator cuff as well as an overloaded or weak rotator cuff [49]. Riding of the humeral head on the superior/posterior glenoid can be one of the factors contributing to a rocking horse effect and the possibility of glenoid component loosening [50–53]. Overloading the rotator cuff can encourage this phenomenon.

Careful consideration must be given to appropriate resistance during strengthening with focus on proper mechanics, humeral head depression, and centralization. External rotation with resistive tubing strengthens the posterior cuff muscles (Figure 8.17). Positioning with a towel between the arm and the trunk keeps the shoulder in the plane of the scapula, avoiding substitution and facilitating effective strengthening. Patients with weakness who have difficulty handling light resis-

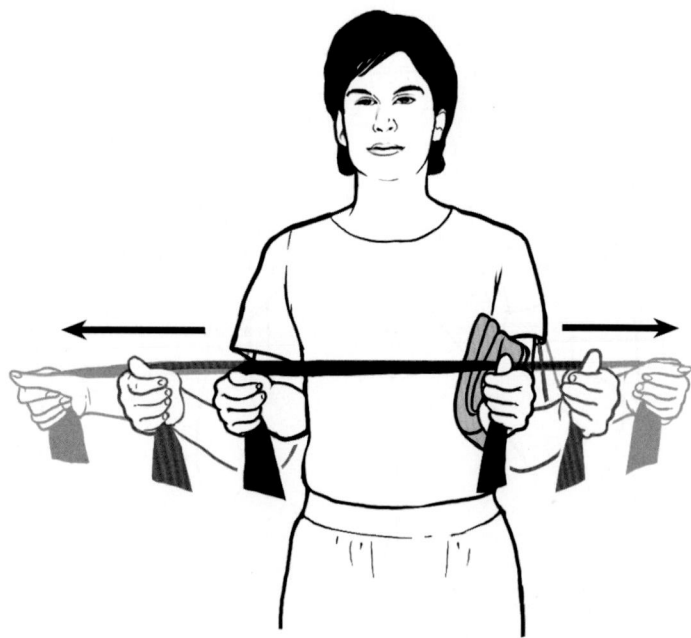

Figure 8.17. Resisted external rotation. While standing, hold the elastic tubing in front of you with both hands. Place a folded towel between your waist and upper arm for proper position. Keeping your elbow pressed to the towel. Pull the elastic tubing outward with your hands. Then slowly return to the starting position, and then repeat.

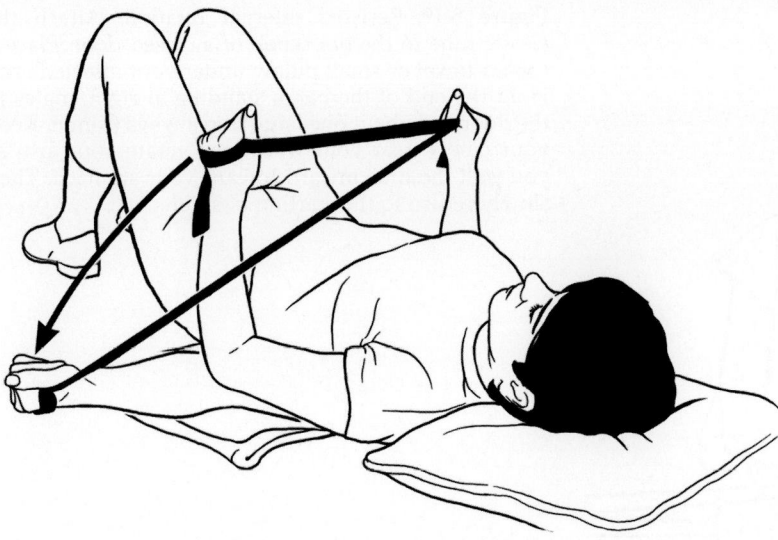

Figure 8.18. Resisted supine external rotation. Lie supine (on the table) with a folded towel or small pillow under the affected arm for proper position. Hold the elastic band in both hands, and pull outward with your affected arm, keeping your elbow bent at 90 degrees. Slowly return to the staring position.

tance tend to rotate more of their trunk and shoulder girdle rather than rotating their forearm. In these cases, supine external rotation helps avoid substitution, and proper resistive band strength can be assessed and appropriate resistance applied (Figure 8.18).

Internal rotation may be very weak due to the direct effects of surgery and contracture release. This exercise should be performed with a towel placed between the upper arm and the trunk (Figure 8.19). A controlled inward rotation to the belly press position followed by a controlled eccentric rotation to the starting position ensures proper strengthening. Subscapularis integrity and strength is pivotal for shoulder stability and function [54, 55]. Internal rotation strength may be the slowest to improve after surgery since it is the only muscle released for access to the glenohumeral joint during surgery. Required lengthening due to contracture to reestablish external rotation may also contribute to a lengthened time of strength gain.

Resistive abduction, a complex exercise (Figure 8.20) focuses primarily on strengthening the middle deltoid and supraspinatus with the abduction motion. Additionally, maintaining the forearm and hand at a constant position through the exercise also loads the infraspinatus and teres minor muscles. Weakness of either muscle group results in excessive scapular upward rotation and drifting of the hand and forearm inward. Care should be taken to appropriately load this combined activity.

Posterior deltoid strengthening (Figure 8.21) is accomplished by attaching an elastic tube to a door handle and pulling toward extension. This exercise is usually the most comfortable. Anterior deltoid strengthening is performed by attaching an elastic band to a door knob and performing an upward punching motion (Figure 8.22). Observing

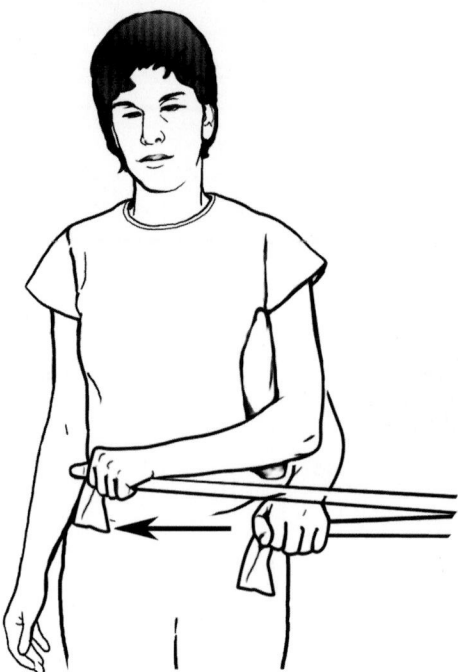

Figure 8.19. Resisted internal rotation. Attach the elastic tube to the doorknob of a closed door. Place a folded towel or small pillow under your affected arm. Hold the end of the band, standing at right angles to the door and about one large step always from it. Keep your elbow near your waist, and rotate your arm as you pull the tube inward toward your stomach. Then slowly return to the starting position.

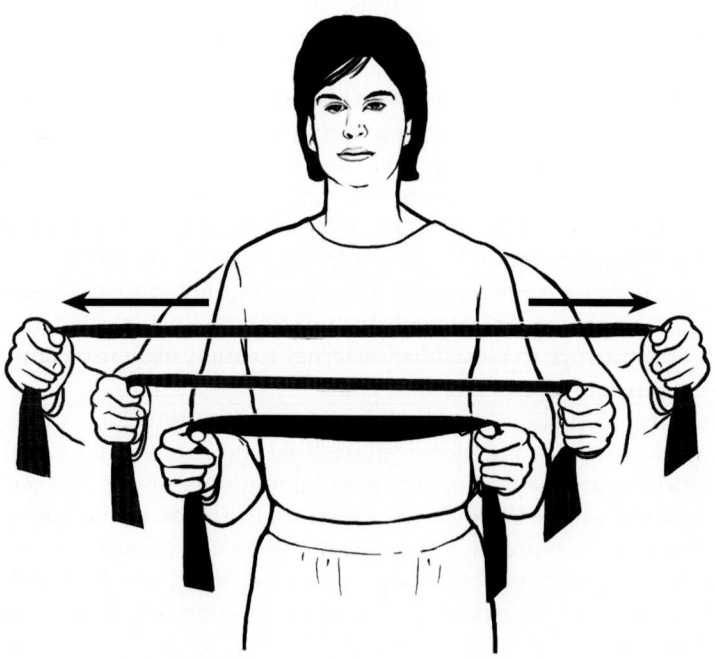

Figure 8.20. Resisted abduction. While standing, hold the Thera-Band in front of your with both hands. Keep your elbows at a 90-degree angle, but do not keep them at your waist. Instead, raise your elbows and hands to the side as you stretch the band outward and upward.

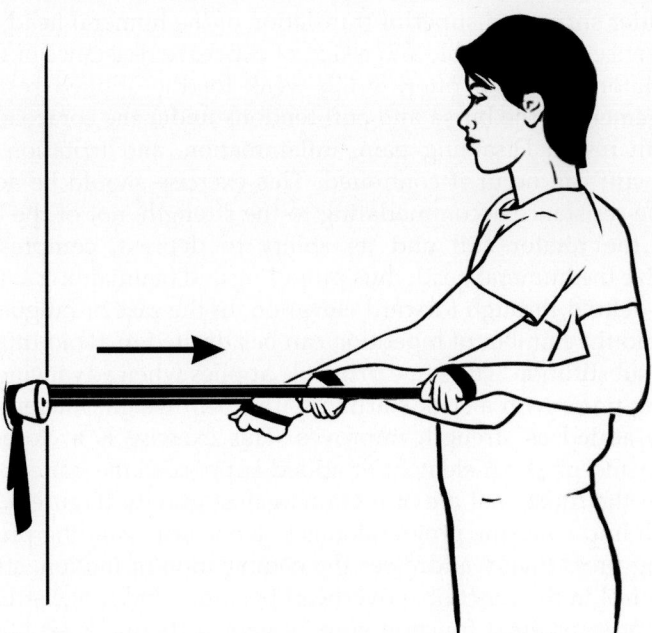

Figure 8.21. Resisted extension. Attach the elastic tubing to the doorknob of a closed door. Face the door, about one step away from it. Hold the end of the elastic band and pull straight backward until your hand is even with your waist. Then return to the starting position.

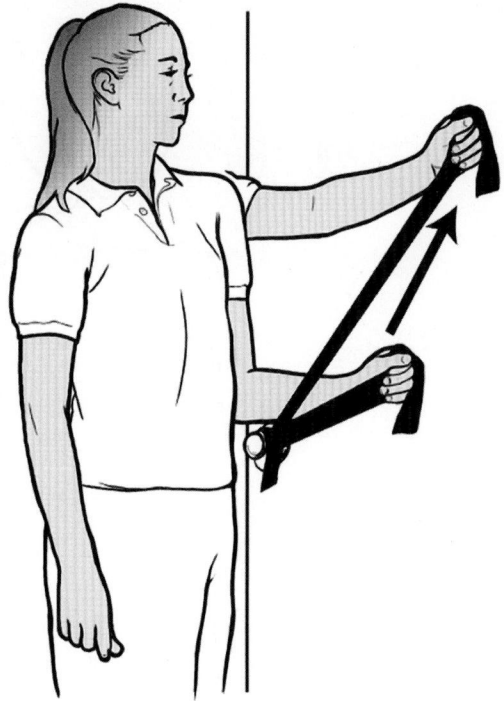

Figure 8.22. Resisted forward flexion. Attach the elastic tube to the doorknob of a closed door. Hold the end of the elastic tube, standing at right angles to the door, but this time, stand near the door. Start with your elbow at your waist. Perform an upper cut by raising your hand above your head. Then return to the starting position.

a shoulder shrug and superior translation of the humeral head during this exercise is undesirable and a sign of excessive resistance or fatigue. The rotator cuff most often is too weak for the applied resistance. Impingement of the bursa and cuff tendons under the coracoacromial arch can result. Disabling pain, inflammation, and irritation of the rotator cuff can occur if continued. This exercise should be adjusted with the resistance accommodating to the strength, not of the deltoid but of the rotator cuff and its ability to depress, compress, and centralize the humeral head, thus providing and maintaining a fulcrum for the deltoid through forward elevation. In the case of fatigue, resistance and the number of repetition can be adjusted to avoid this undesirable substitution. The same principle applies when advancing to the standing press with a stick starting with a 1-lb weight. Increments of 1 lb are added as strength improves. This exercise is a closed loop exercise and gives an element of added support as the patient moves through the functional arc of motion against gravity (Figure 8.23). As strength improves, the progression is to a one arm standing press The standing press finally addresses the combination of motion, strength, and control in the functional overhead position. End range strength is necessary if maximal function is to be gained (Figure 8.24) [27]. This can take time since end range strength can sometimes lag in the recov-

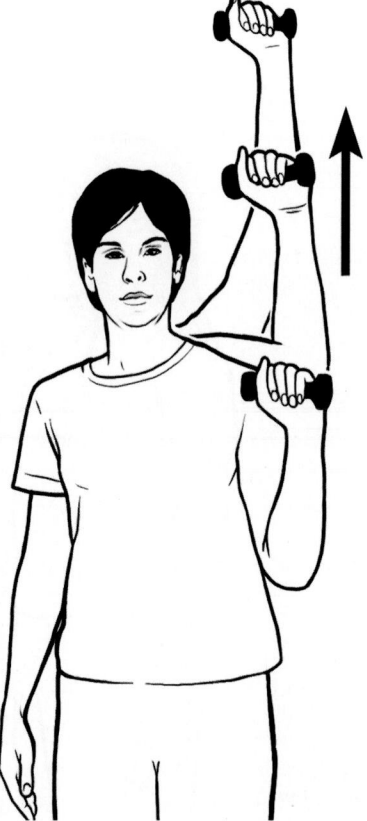

Figure 8.23. Standing press with weight. Hold a weight (1–5 lbs) at shoulder level. Press upward until your arm is straight, and then return to the starting position.

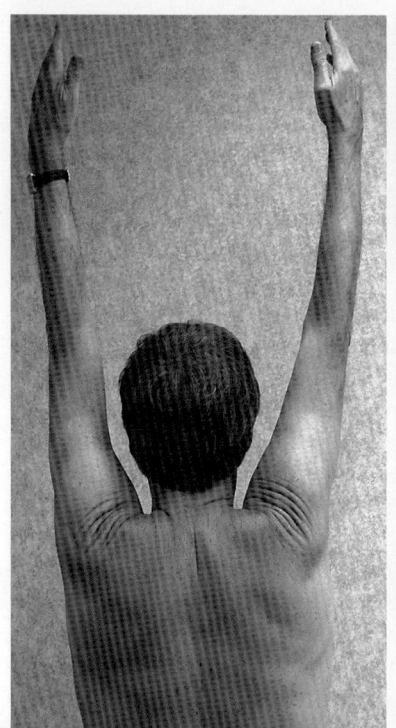
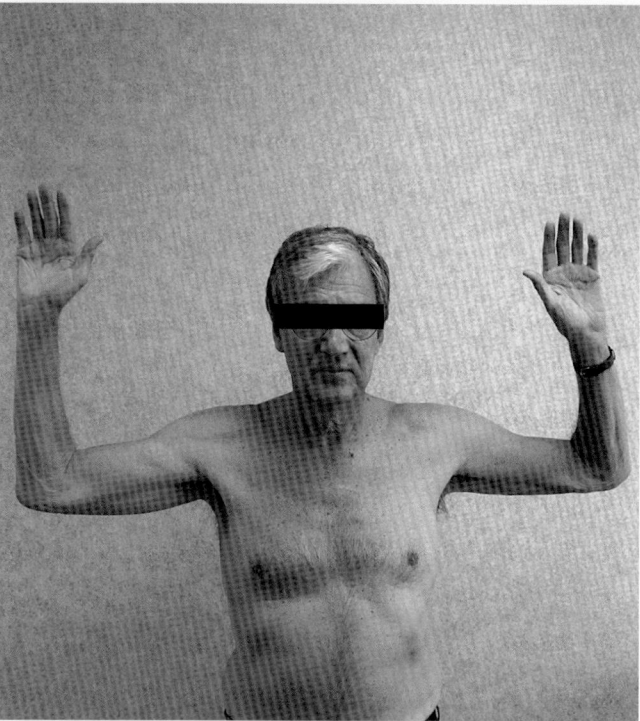

A

B

Figure 8.24. (**A**) Notice the *dimpling* and equal contours of both shoulders, which demonstrates good glenohumeral translation. (**B**) Note the accomplished goal of 90 degrees of external rotation in abduction and no Hornblower's Sign.

ery process. If the resistive exercise causes pain, the amount of weight or the strength of the elastic band should be reduced.

Periscapular muscle strength is usually adequate for proper mechanics following arthroplasty. The upward rotation and setting of the scapular, to maintain the humeral head centered on the glenoid, is necessary if stability in overhead function is to be achieved. This requires good strength of the trapezius, rhomboids, levator scapula, and serratus anterior muscles. Abnormal scapular patterns before surgery appear to be a secondary phenomenon due to the destruction of the glenohumeral joint, lack of motion, and weakness of the rotator cuff. The continued use of the extremity before arthroplasty tends to shift motion to the scapular for required function. These abnormal patterns acquired, due to altered mechanics at the glenohumeral joint, tend to normalize through the progressive range of motion, stretching, and strengthening program as glenohumeral mobility and cuff strength returns after arthroplasty. During the exercise progression dynamic proximal stability and proper setting of the scapular is initiated. As activity overhead becomes more prevalent with improved range of motion and strength, completion of the program is directed to scapular strengthening. The supine position helps isolate scapula motion (Figure 8.25). Increments of 1 lb. are added to a maximum of 5 lbs. as strength improves. Progression to a closed chain wall push up plus, and then to a more demanding modified closed chain quadruped push up plus exercise are selectively applied to the individual patient. For patients with proximal weakness or patients who are going to participate in athletic activity, isolated scapular strengthening is advocated.

The Weak Shoulder: The neuromuscular and biomechanical components of active exercise during rehabilitation can be challenged by the following: shoulder arthroplasty associated with severe weakness after large and massive cuff tear, long-standing degenerative changes, instability, and fracture due to severe trauma involving neurovascular injury. A modified program of exercise is applied if the patient presents with inability to raise the arm over head (Figure 8.26). The potential for good function is usually present, but unless the appropriate exercise is applied, the potential may never be realized. Rehabilitation of the profoundly weak shoulder is a challenge to all clinicians.

With fracture and rotator cuff tear, a variety of mechanical, muscular, and neural deficits can be present. Range of motion and available strength must be carefully assessed so the exercise program can be tai-

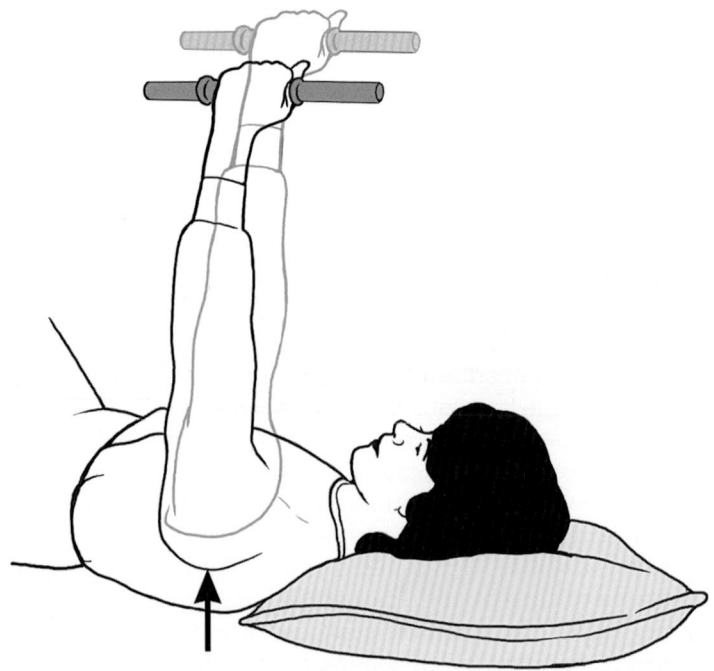

Figure 8.25. Scapular protraction with weight. Lie on your back and hold a weight (1–5 lbs) straight up in the air with your affected arm. Keeping your elbow locked, raise your shoulder off the table, and reach toward the ceiling. Slowly return to the starting position.

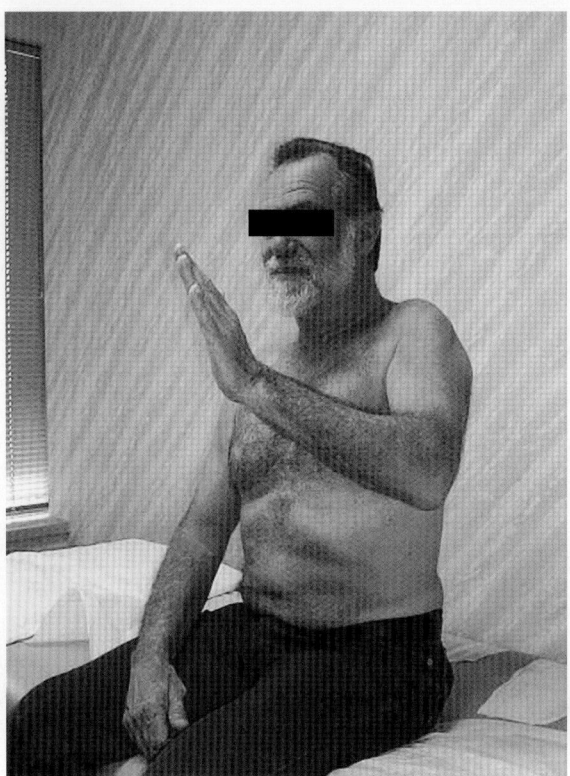

Figure 8.26. This patient has difficulty elevating his upper extremity and displays a shrug sign.

lored to the individual patient. Overloading muscle groups by instructing the weak shoulder patient in a standard exercise progression may not be an effective way to restore strength, muscular balance, and function. The weak shoulder program focuses on supine exercise with gravity eliminated, thus motion is accomplished with reduced weight of the upper extremity A gradual progression from supine to an erect position introduces the increasing effect of gravity on the extremity. The progression also allows for comfortable neuromuscular reeducation and good mechanics avoiding anterior superior translation of the humeral head while appropriate resistance less than the weight of the extremity is experienced (Figure 8.27). Active exercise with a stick is initiated. The table back is then elevated to 30 degrees, which increases the weight of the extremity due to gravity as it moves into the critical range of 60 to 120 degrees of forward elevation. The rotator cuff therefore has less weight applied to it as it develops a fulcrum for the deltoid to raise the arm through the arc of motion. If the patient demonstrates a shoulder shrug through the arc of motion, strengthening continues in the supine position with progressive forms of resistance, that is, weight, elastic band, or manual resistance by the therapist [31]. As the patient demonstrates improvement in strength, they are then progressed to the next elevation. The progression proceeds to 60 degrees of elevation and then to an erect position.

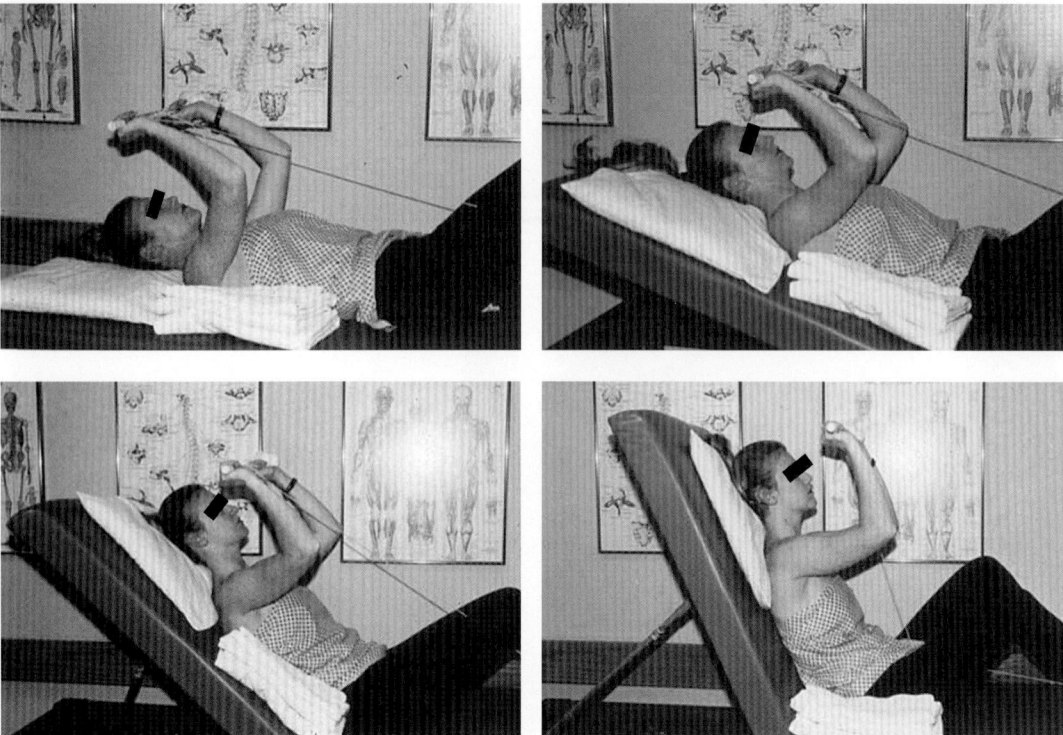

Figure 8.27. A progression from supine to 30 degrees to approximately 60 degrees and finally 90 degrees of trunk elevation increases the weight of the extremity with regard to gravity and the resistance the weight of the upper extremity exerts on the rotator cuff and deltoid.

Forward elevation with the beach ball is effective in developing co-contraction around the shoulder as elevation is performed (Figure 8.28). The patient is instructed to press in on the ball as they raise both extremities through a full range of motion. Co-contraction of the internal rotators facilitates joint compression. This concavity compression effect centralizes the humeral head and assists in establishing a fulcrum for elevation, which enhances good mechanics for strengthening and muscle reeducation through the functional range [56].

Weakness of external rotation during forward elevation is approached in the same manner. The program can be started with supine multi-angle isometrics (see Figure 8.6). The patient is able to contract and relax at multiple positions of external rotation, working into the weakest points. The patient is then given a thin elastic tube and is instructed to perform external rotation at multiple levels as he elevates both extremities (Figure 8.29). Manual resistance can be applied as the patient performs forward elevation in the side-lying position (Figure 8.30) and at multiple levels supine. Progress can be slow with this program. Commitment by all involved results in the best possible outcome.

Cuff Tear Arthropathy – Limited Goals program: Pain-free function below the horizontal with good stability, are the intended goals of surgery and

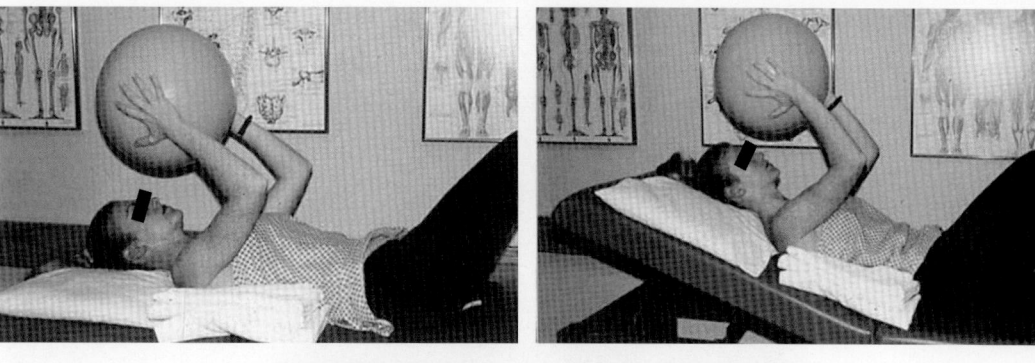

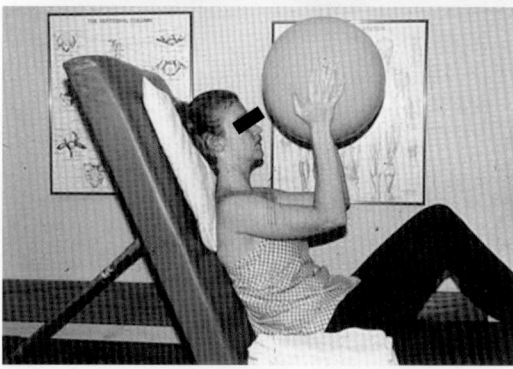

Figure 8.28. The patient is instructed to compress and forward elevate simultaneously, which requires activation and co-contraction of the internal rotators rotator cuff and deltoid. The supine position decreases the effect of gravity on the weight of the extremity as critical ranges are approached.

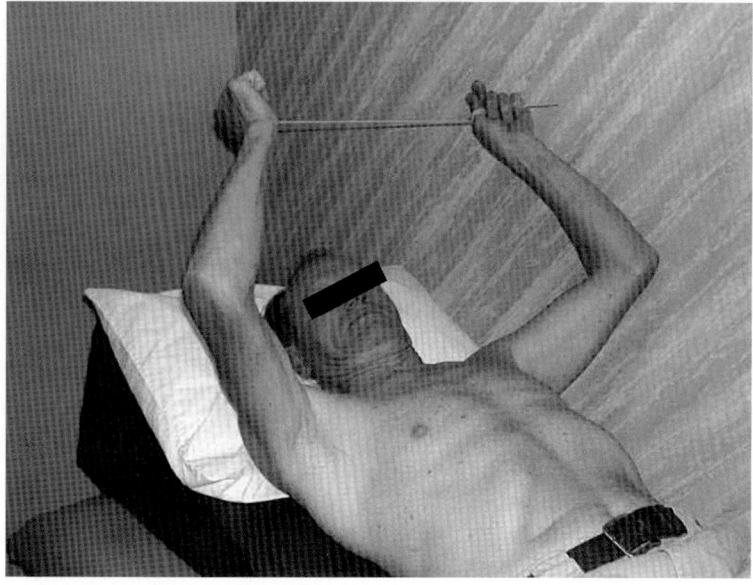

Figure 8.29. Manuel exercise can be applied, which allows the therapist to control the amount of resistance and direct the force at the varying points in the range. Hand placement facilitates combined forward elevation and external rotation through a functional motion. This activity also facilitates neuromuscular re-education and allows for controlled smooth excursion through the range.

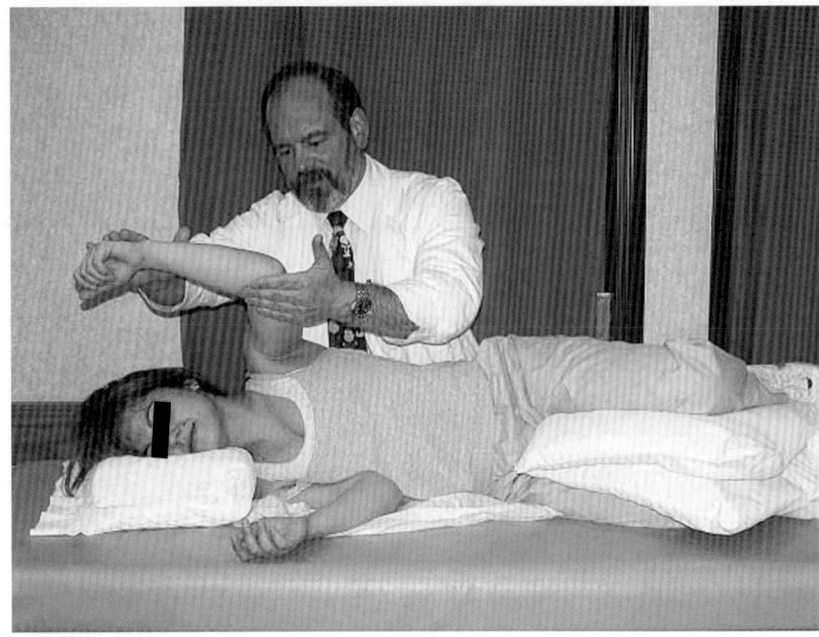

Figure 8.30. Manual exercise give the therapist vital information about the strength and coordination of the upper quarter and should be part of shoulder rehabilitation program.

postoperative rehabilitation [8, 12]. Attempts are made to repair as much soft tissue as possible to ensure stability of the humeral head. The exercise program consists of pendulum exercise, early passive motion exercise to 30 degrees of external rotation, and supine forward elevation to 130 degrees for 8 to 12 weeks as determined by the surgeon (Table 8.5). Active assistive exercise and isometrics are started below the horizontal at 12 weeks. When the patient demonstrates good control, active exercise to tolerance is initiated. A gradual gentle progression to resistive exercise can be initiated as comfort and function permits.

Athletic Activity: Little information exists in the literature concerning athletic activity following unconstrained shoulder arthroplasty [12, 57]. The primary indication for shoulder replacement continues to be for the relief of pain. The demand for normal function thus improving the quality of life, has also become equally important. With third-generation prosthetic design and improved outcomes, the expectations of athletic patients who have arthroplasty is to return to more demanding activities. Of concern are component loosening, stability, and wear. A number of authors advocate an uncemented humeral component in the young active patients who have a well-conformed healthy glenoid [33]. Jensen and Rockwood [57] retrospectively evaluated 24 patients who had shoulder arthroplasty and played recreational golf. Of the 24 patients, 23 were able to return to the sport. Twenty patients had TSA, one had bilateral shoulder arthroplasty, and 6 had humeral head

Table 8.5. Postoperative Rehabilitation Guidelines for Shoulder Arthroplasty: Cuff Tear Arthropathy

TSR, HHR w/Cuff Involvement *Limited Goals* Cuff Tear Arthropathy, Instability, Poor Deltoid Sling 8–12 weeks		
Time post-op	Exercise	Exercise program
8–12 week	EPM (early passive motion)	Supine ER to 30° Supine FF to 130° Elbow/Wrist/Hand ROM Pendulum
12 weeks	Active assistive	Pendulum ER w/stick FF, Pulleys, Ext w/stick IR
12 weeks	Isometrics	ER, IR, anterior deltoid, posterior deltoid, middle deltoid, multiangle

Goals: control pain and swelling, protect the anterior capsule and subscapularis tendon repair, prevent adhesion formation, increase ROM (scapular plane), educate (importance of medication, ice/heat application, compliance to the program, frequent gentle exercise, rest, positioning for comfort at home, family/friend instruction), establish a well understood home program, with a gradual introduction of exercises.

Time post-op	Exercise	Exercise program
As tolerated	Active (below horizontal)	
		Supine FF w/stick Supine FF w/stick + weight (1–2 lbs.) Supine FE, ER side lying, Eccentric Pulleys, Standing press w/stick Eccentric standing press w/stick, Prone ext/abd
	Advanced stretching	Follow exercise figures
	Resistive	Progress as tolerated

Goals: control pain and swelling, increase active ROM, increase strength in a stable range below the horizontal.

FF = forward flexion, ER = external rotation, IR = internal rotation, Ext. = extension, Abd. = abduction, w = with, TSR = total shoulder replacement, HHR = humeral head replacement.

replacement. The average time from surgery to playing a full round of golf was 4.5 months. Eighteen patients had a change in their preoperative handicap with an improvement of 5 strokes. Their was no significant difference in radiolucent lines in the people with arthroplasty who did not play golf from those with arthroplasty who did play golf. Rehabilitation consisted of a two-phase physician-directed home program. Phase 1 consisted of passive stretching, to achieve full range of motion. When full range of motion was achieved, the patient proceeded to phase 2, which consisted of deltoid, rotator cuff, and scapular rotator strengthening exercise. Active motion such as putting and chip shots were allowed after healing of the subscapularis muscle. A questionnaire was submitted to the ASES with 44 of the 50 members responding. Ninety-one percent encouraged return to golf. The recommended time to return to golf was 4.3 months. Half of the surgeons gave special instructions to their patients with respect to a gradual progression into the sport. Progression through putting, chip shot, and eventually to longer irons at a later time was recommended. Avoiding divots by teeing up even on the fairway was encouraged. Delay in using a driver was advocated until a later time. Slightly less than 75 percent of the surgeons believed that carrying a golf bag while playing golf was not a problem. Healy, Iorio, Lemos [58] surveyed 35 members of the American Shoulder and Elbow Society regarding their patients who had arthroplasty and participation in sports and athletic activities. The recommended or allowed activity largely consisted of lower extremity intense activity with upper extremity requirements at a moderate velocity below the horizontal. Above the horizontal activity included swimming, doubles tennis (did not specify dominant side), and dancing–ball room, square, and jazz. Golf, ice skating, shooting, and downhill skiing were allowed with prior experience. Activities not recommended included elements of high velocity, high load, above and below the horizontal, and contact sports, such as football, gymnastics, hockey, and rock climbing. Neer [12] found in a series of 408 patients, average age of 39, who had undergone arthroplasty for arthritis of recurrent dislocations with an a minimum 2-year follow-up, had excellent result in 232, satisfactory results in 54, and unsatisfactory results in 49. The remainder were in a limited goals program with 1 unsatisfactory result. Many in the series were athletic individuals. Neer recommended golf, tennis, and noncontact sports. He discouraged lifting heavy weights overhead, limiting the amount to 50 lbs. He also felt that sports involving hard falls, such as downhill skiing, should be avoided.

Although it is an individual decision, the surgeon and patient should discuss the gains and possible detriment of the activity. Educating the patient maximizes his/her expectations and, it is hoped, minimizes potential complications in the future.

Acknowledgment
Thanks to Nancy Heim, Medical Illustrator, Center for Biomedical Communications, Columbia University, New York, for Figures 8.3 through 8.14, 8.16 through 8.23, and 8.25.

References

1. Fehringer EV, Kopjar B, Boorman RS, Churchill RS, Smith KL, Matsen FA III. Characterizing the functional improvement after TSA for osteoarthritis. J Bone Joint Surg Am 2002;84-A:8,1349–1353.
2. Bigliani LU, Kelkar R, Flatow EL, Pollock RG, Mow V. Glenohumeral stability: biomechanical properties of passive and active stabilizers. Clin Orthop 1996;330:13–30.
3. Arntz CT, Jackins S, Matsen FA III. Prosthetic replacement of the shoulder for the treatment of defects in the rotator cuff and the surface of the Glenohumeral Joint. J Bone Joint Surg 1993;75-A:4,485–491.
4. Cofield RH, Iannotti JP, Matsen FA III, Rockwood CA Jr. Shoulder Arthoplasty: Current Techniques. AAOS Instructional Course Lecture No. 148. March 1998.
5. Robinson MC, Page RS, Hill R, Sanders DL, Court-Brown CM, Wakefield AE. Primary hemiarthroplasty for treatment of proximal humeral fractures. J Bone Joint Surg Am 2003;85-A:7,1215–1223.
6. Demirhan M, Kilicoglu O, Altinel L, Eralp L, Akalin Y. Prognostic factors in prosthetic replacement for acute proximal humerus fractures. J Orthop Trauma 2003;17:181–188.
7. Crosby LA. Total Shoulder Arthroplasty: Monograph Services. AAOS Instructional Lecture Course, 2000.
8. Rockwood CA, Matsen FA II. The Shoulder. Philadelphia: WB Saunders, 1990;678–749.
9. Bigliani LU. Complications of Shoulder Surgery. Philadelphia: Williams and Wilkens 1993.
10. Hartsock LA, Estes WJ, Craig MA, Friedman RJ. Shoulder hemiarthroplasty for proximal humeral fractures. Ortho Clinic North Am 1998;29: 467–475.
11. Compito CA, Self EB, Bigliani LU. Arthroplasty and acute shoulder trauma. Clin Orthop 1994;307:27–36.
12. Neer CS II. Shoulder Reconstruction. Philadelphia: WB Saunders, 1990; 143–271.
13. Moeckel BH, Altchek DW, Warren RF, Wickiewicz TL, Dines DM. Instability of the shoulder after arthroplasty. J Bone Joint Surg 1993;75-A:4,492–497.
14. Post M, Bigliani LU, Flatow EL, Pollack RG. The Shoulder Operative Techniques. Philadelphia: Williams and Wilkins, 1998;43–71.
15. Norris TR, Hatzidakis AM. Prosthetic replacement for proximal humeral fractures: indications and results. AAOS Instructional Lecture Course. February 2003.
16. Ramsey ML, Warner JJP, Williams GR Jr, Iannotti JP. Proximal humeral fractures I: Alternatives to Arthroplasty. AAOS Instructional Lecture Course, February 5, 2003.
17. Basti JB, Dionysian E, Sherman PN, Bigliani LU. Management of Proximal Humeral Fractures. J Hand Therapy 1994;April–June.
18. Bigliani LU, McCluskey GM, Fisher RA. Failed Prosthetic Replacement in Displaced Humeral Fractures. Ortho Trans 1991;15:747–748.
19. Goldman RT, Koval KJ, Cuomo F, Gallagher MA, Zucherman JD. Functional outcome after humeral head replacement for acute three- and four-part proximal humeral fractures. J Shoulder Elbow Surg 1995; 4:81–86.
20. Mighell MA, Kolm GP, Collinge CA, Frankle MA. Outcomes of hemiarthroplasty for fractures of the proximal humerus. J Shoulder Elbow Surg 2003;12:6.

21. Boileau P, Trogani C, Walsh G, Sumant KG, Romeo A, Sinnerton R. Shoulder arthroplasty for treatment of the sequela of fractures of the proximal humerus. J Shoulder Elbow Surg 2001;10:4.

22. Prekash U, McGurty DW, Dent JA. Hemiarthroplasty for severe fractures of the proximal humerus. J Shoulder Elbow Surg 2002;11:428–430.

23. Norris RT. Fractures of proximal humerus and dislocation of the shoulder. In Skeletal Trauma, vol. 2, BD Brown, Jupiter JB, Levine AM, Trafton PG, Editors. Philadelphia, WB Saunders, 1992;1201–1290.

24. Shapiro J, Zuckerman J. Glenohumeral arthroplasty: indications and preoperative considerations. AAOS Instructional Course Lecture, 2002.

25. Iannotti JP, Norris TR. Influence of preoperative factors on outcome of shoulder arthroplasty for glenohumeral osteoarthritis. J Bone Joint Surg Am 2003,85-A:2,251–258.

26. Bradley ET, Aziz B, Jean-Francois K, Boileau P, Chantel N, Walch G. The influence of rotator cuff disease on the results of shoulder arthroplasty for primary osteoarthritis: results of a multi-center study. J Bone Joint Surg 2002;84-A(12):2240–2248.

27. Bigliani LU, Brems JJ, Burkhead WZ, Flatow EL, Zuckerman JD. Shoulder arthroplasty: current techniques. AAOS Instructional Course Lecture., February 7, 2003.

28. Cofield RH. Total shoulder arthroplasty with the Neer prosthesis. J bone Joint Surg 1984;66-A:899–906

29. Hasan SS, Romeo AA. Nontraumatic osteonecrosis of the humeral head. J Shoulder Elbow Surg 2002;11:281–298.

30. Hattrup SJ. Indications, techniques and results of shoulder arthroplasty in osteonecrosis. Total Shoulder Arthroplasty 1998;29:445–451.

31. Marx RG, McCarty EC, Montemurno TD, Altchek DW, Craig EV, Warren RF. Development of arthrosis following dislocation of the shoulder: a case-control study. J Shoulder Elbow Surg 2002;11:1–5.

32. Zuckerman JD, Matsen FA II. Complications about the glenohumeral joint related to the use of screws and staples. J Bone Joint Surg Am 1984; 66:175–180.

33. Brems JJ. Arthritis of dislocation. Orthop Clin North Am 1998;29:3.

34. Matsen FA II, FU FH, Hawkins RJ. The shoulder abalance of mobility and stability. AAOS, 1992;279–304.

35. Van der Zwaag HM, Brand R, Obermann WR, Rozing PM. Glenohumeral osteoarthrosis after Putti-Platt repair. J Shoulder Elbow Surg 1999;8: 252–258.

36. Bigliani LU, Weinstein DM, Glasgow MT, Pollock RG, Flatow EL. Glenohumeral arthroplasty for arthritis after instability surgery. J Shoulder Elbow Surg 1995;4:87–94.

37. Neer CS II, McCann PD, Macfarlane EA, Padilla N. Early passive motion following shoulder arthroplasty and rotator cuff repair: a prospective study. Orthop Trans 1987;11:231.

38. Hughes M, Neer CS II. Glenohumeral joint replacement and postoperative rehabilitation. Physical Therapy 1995;55(Aug):8.

39. Brems JJ. Rehabilitation following total shoulder arthroplasty. Clin Orthop 1994;307:70–85.

40. Brown DD, Friedman RJ. Postoperative rehabilitation following total shoulder arthroplasty. Total Shoulder Arthroplasty 1998;29:535–547.

41. Boardman ND II, Cofield RH, Bengston KA, Little R, Jones MC, Rowland CM. Rehabilitation after total shoulder arthroplasty. J Arthroplasty 2001; 16:483–486.

42. DiGiovani J, Marra G, Park JY, Bigliani LU. Hemi-arthroplasty for gleno-humeral arthritis with massive cuff tears. Orthop Clin North Am 1998; 29:477–488.

43. McCann PD, Wootten MS, Kadaba MP, Bigliani LU. A kinematic and electromyographic study of shoulder rehabilitation exercises. Clin Orthop Related Res 1993;288:179–188.

44. Poppen NK, Walker PS. Forces at the glenohumeral joint in abduction. Clin Orthop 1978;135:165–170.

45. Soslowsky LJ, Flatow EL, Pawluk RJ, Ark CM, Boulris CM, Helper MD, et al. Subacromial contact (impingement) on the rotator cuff in the shoulder: 38th Annual Meeting, Orthopaedic Research Society, 1992. February 17–20 Washington, DC.

46. Bigliani LU, Levine WN. Subacromial impingement syndrome. J Bone Joint Surg 1997;79:1854–1868.

47. Harryman DT, Sidles JA, Harris SL, Matsen FA II. Laxity of the normal glenohumeral joint: a quantitative in vivo assessment. J Shoulder Elbow Surg 1992,1:66–76.

48. Inman VT, Saunders JB, Abbott LC. Observations on function of the shoulder joint. J Bone Joint Surg 1944;26:1

49. Severt R, Thomas BJ, Tsenter MJ, Amstutz HC, Kabo JM. The influence of conformity and constraint on translational forces and frictional torque in total shoulder arthroplasty. Clin Orthop Related Res 1993;293:151–158.

50. Flatow EL. Prosthetic design considerations in total shoulder arthroplasty. Sem Arthroplasty 1995;6:233–244.

51. Anglin C, Wyss UP, Pichora DR. Mechanical testing of shoulder prostheses and recommendations for glenoid design. J Shoulder Elbow Surg 2000; 9:323–331.

52. Stone KD, Grabowski JJ, Cofield RH, Morrey BF, An KN. Stress analysis of glenoid components in total shoulder arthroplasty. J Shoulder Elbow Surg 1999;8:151–158.

53. Severt R, Thomas BJ, Tsenter MJ, Amstutz HC, Kabo JM. The Influence of conformity and constraint on translational forces and frictional torque in total shoulder arthroplasty. Clin Orthop 1993;292:151–158.

54. Miller SL, Hazrati Y, Klepps S, Chiang A, Flatow EL. Loss of subscapularis function after total shoulder replacement: A seldom recognized problem. J Shoulder Elbow Surg 2003,1:29–34.

55. Cuomo F, Cheiroun A. Avoiding pitfalls and complications in total shoulder arthroplasty. Ortho Clin North Am 1998;29:3.

56. Lippitt SB, Vanderhoof JE, Harris SL, Sidles JA, Harryman DT, Matsen FA III. Glenohumeral stability from concavity-compression: a quantitative analysis. J Shoulder Elbow Surg 1993;2:27–33.

57. Jensen KL, Rockwood CA. Shoulder arthroplasty in recreational golfers. J Shoulder Elbow Surg 1998;7:362–367.

58. Healy WL, Iorio R, Lemos M. Athletic activity after joint replacement. Am J Sports Med 2001;29:377–388.

Index

A

Abduction exercise, outpatient rehabilitation program with, 193, 194

Acromioclavicular arthritis, glenohumeral inflammatory arthritis with, 80

Acromiohumeral articulation, rotator cuff deficiency with, 149

Acromio-humeral interval (AHI), physical examination with, 9, 10

Active assistive exercise, outpatient rehabilitation program with, 177–178, 180, 181, 182, 183, 203

Active exercise, outpatient rehabilitation program with, 179–186, 203

Active supine external rotation exercise, postoperative rehabilitation program with, 175, 176, 180, 181, 182, 183, 203

Advanced stretching exercise
combined flexion/external rotation/abduction stretch in, 187, 188
combined motion stretching in, 186
end-range planar motion in, 186
internal rotation stretch in, 190, 191

one arm wall stretch in, 186–187

outpatient rehabilitation program with, 180, 181, 182, 183, 186–190, 203

over-the-door hang in, 187–189

posterior capsule stretch in, 190, 191

rehabilitation principles with, 172, 173

standing 90/90 stretch in, 189

AHI. *See* Acromio-humeral interval

Allograft, proximal humeral bone deficiency with, 129, 131

Allograft-prosthetic composites, 129, 131

Anesthesia
postoperative rehabilitation program with, 173
rotator cuff deficiency with, 155–156
scalene regional block as, 155
shoulder arthroplasty, 12

Anterior deltoid attachment, revision shoulder arthroplasty with, 124, 125

Anterior deltoid strengthening, outpatient rehabilitation program with, 193, 195

Anterior superior instability, rotator cuff deficiency surgery with, 164

Anterosuperior instability, TSA followed by, 139, 140

Arthritis. *See also* Glenohumeral inflammatory arthritis
capsulorraphy, 2
CTA as, 2
cuff tear arthropathy with, 149
juvenile chronic, 63
osteoarthritis, 1, 5, 6
rehabilitation for, 167–170, 184, 204
rheumatoid, 1–2, 5, 7, 63, 168, 169
rotator cuff deficiency with, 149, 150, 151, 162, 164
seronegative spondyloarthropathies as, 63
TSA with, 1–2

Articular impression fractures, 92

Articular surface fractures, 92

Athletic activity, outpatient rehabilitation program with, 202–204

Autograft, proximal humeral bone deficiency with, 129, 131

Avascular necrosis
preoperative evaluation with, 2
rehabilitation for, 169